KEY TOPICS IN

GENERAL SURGERY

SECOND EDITION

The KEY TOPICS Series

Advisors:

T.M. Craft *Department of Anaesthesia and Intensive Care, Royal United Hospital, Bath, UK*
C.S. Garrard *Intensive Therapy Unit, John Radcliffe Hospital, Oxford, UK*
P.M. Upton *Department of Anaesthesia, Royal Cornwall Hospital, Treliske, Truro, UK*

Accident and Emergency Medicine, Second Edition
Anaesthesia – Clinical Aspects, Third Edition
Cardiovascular Medicine
Chronic Pain, Second Edition
Critical Care
Evidence-Based Medicine
Gastroenterology
General Surgery, Second Edition
Neonatology
Neurology
Obstetrics and Gynaecology, Second Edition
Oncology
Ophthalmology, Second Edition
Oral and Maxillofacial Surgery
Orthopaedic Surgery
Orthopaedic Trauma Surgery
Otolaryngology, Second Edition
Paediatrics, Second Edition
Psychiatry
Renal Medicine
Respiratory Medicine
Thoracic Surgery
Trauma

Forthcoming titles include:

Acute Poisoning
Cardiac Surgery
Urology

KEY TOPICS IN
GENERAL SURGERY

SECOND EDITION

C.R. Lattimer
FRCS
Queen Elizabeth the Queen Mother Hospital,
Margate, UK

N.M. Wilson
BSc, MS, FRCS
Royal Hampshire County Hospital,
Winchester, UK

N.R.F. Lagattolla
FRCS
Dorset County Hospital,
Dorchester, UK

BIOS

© BIOS Scientific Publishers Limited, 2002

First published 1996 (ISBN 1 872748 02 3)
Second edition 2002 (ISBN 1 85996 164 9)

A CIP catalogue record for this book is available from the British Library.

ISBN 1 85996 164 9

BIOS Scientific Publishers Ltd
9 Newtec Place, Magdalen Road, Oxford OX4 1RE, UK
Tel. +44 (0)1865 726286. Fax +44 (0)1865 246823
World Wide Web home page: http://www.bios.co.uk/

Important Note from the Publisher
The information contained within this book was obtained by BIOS Scientific Publishers Ltd from sources believed by us to be reliable. However, while every effort has been made to ensure its accuracy, no responsibility for loss or injury whatsoever occasioned to any person acting or refraining from action as a result of information contained herein can be accepted by the authors or publishers.

The reader should remember that medicine is a constantly evolving science and while the authors and publishers have ensured that all dosages, applications and practices are based on current indications, there may be specific practices which differ between communities. You should always follow the guidelines laid down by the manufacturers of specific products and the relevant authorities in the country in which you are practising.

Production Editor: Nadine Séveno
Typeset by Jayvee Computer Services, Trivandrum, India
Printed by The Cromwell Press, Trowbridge, UK

CONTENTS

[a] Contributed by O. Faiz, Queen Elizabeth the Queen Mother Hospital, Margate, UK.
[b] Contributed by S.A.L. Gibbs, Queen Elizabeth the Queen Mother Hospital, Margate, UK.
[c] Contributed by N. Gureja, Queen Elizabeth the Queen Mother Hospital, Margate, UK.
[d] Contributed by D. Marzouk, Queen Elizabeth the Queen Mother Hospital, Margate, UK.
[e] Contributed by C. Perera, Queen Elizabeth the Queen Mother Hospital, Margate, UK.
[f] Contributed by A. Simoes, Queen Elizabeth the Queen Mother Hospital, Margate, UK.
[g] Contributed by P. Sinha, William Harvey Hospital, Ashford, UK.

ABBREVIATIONS

5-ASA	5-aminosalicylic acid
AAA	abdominal aortic aneurysm
ABPI	ankle brachial pressure index
ACD	acid-citrate-dextrose
ACPO	acute colonic pseudo-destruction
ACTH	adrenocorticotrophic hormone
ADH	antidiuretic hormone
A/E	Accident and Emergency
AFP	α-fetoprotein
AIDS	acquired immunodeficiency syndrome
APC	adenomatous polyposis coli
APTT	activated partial thromboplastin time
ARDS	adult respiratory distress syndrome
ASA	American Society for Anesthesiology
AST	aspartate transaminase
ATLS	Advanced Trauma Life Support
ATP	adenosine triphosphate
AV	arteriovenous
AXR	abdominal X-ray
β-HCG	β-human chorionic gonadotrophin
BCC	basal cell carcinoma
BPH	benign prostatic hyperplasia
CAPD	continuous ambulatory peritoneal dialysis
CAVHD	continuous arteriovenous haemodialysis
CAVHF	continuous arteriovenous haemofiltration
CDC	Centers for Disease Control
CEA	carcinoembryonic antigen
CEPOD	Confidential Enquiry into Perioperative Deaths
CHI	Commission for Health Improvement
CIS	carcinoma-in-situ
CNS	central nervous system
CPAP	continuous positive airways pressure
CPP	cerebral perfusion pressure
CSF	cerebrospinal fluid
CT	computensed tomography
CVA	cerebrovascular accident
CVP	central venous pressure
CXR	chest X-ray
DCIS	ductal carcinoma-in-situ
DDC	dideoxycytidine
DDI	dideoxyinosine
DIC	disseminated intravascular coagulation
DRE	digital rectal examination

DSA	digital subtraction angiography
DU	duodenal ulcer
DVT	deep vein thrombosis
EAS	external anal sphincter
EATL	enteropathy associated T-cell lymphoma
ECF	extracellular fluid
ECG	electrocardiograph
ECMO	extracorporeal membrane oxygenation
EEG	electroencephalography
EGF	epithelial growth factor
ELAP	endoscopic laser ablation of the prostate
EMG	electromyography
EPTFE	expanded polytetra flouvoethylene
ERCP	endoscopic retrograde cholangiopancreatography
ESR	erythrocyte sedimentation rate
ESWL	extracorporeal shock wave lithotripsy
ETAR	endoscopic transanal resection
EUA	examination under anaesthesia
EVAR	endovascular aneurysm repair
FAP	familial adenomatous polyposis
FBC	full blood count
FFP	fresh frozen plasma
FiO_2	fraction of inspired oxygen
FNAC	fine needle aspiration cytology
FNH	focal nodular hyperplasia
GA	general anaesthetic
GCS	glasgow coma scale
GCT	germ cell tumour
GGT	gamma-glutamyl transpeptidase
GI	gastro-intestinal
GIST	GI stromal tissue
GMC	general medical council
GM-CSF	granulocyte–macrophage colony-stimulating factor
GOJ	gastro-oesophageal junction
GORD	gastro-oesophageal reflux disease
GTN	glyceryl trinitrate
GU	gastric ulcer
HCC	hepatocellular carcinoma
HCG	human chorionic gonadotrophin
HCI	hydrochloric acid
HIAA	hydroxyindoleacetic acid
HIFU	high-intensity focused ultrasound
HIV	human immunodeficiency virus
HLA	human leukocyte antigen
HNPCC	hereditary non-polyposis colonic cancer
HP	*Helicobacter pylori*

HPV	human papilloma virus
HPV	human papillomatosis
IAS	internal anal sphincter
IBD	inflammatory bone disease
IBS	irritable bowel syndrome
ICA	internal carotid artery
ICF	intracellular fluid
ICP	intracranial pressure
ICU	intensive care unit
IIS	injury severity scale
IL-1	interleukin 1
IL-6	interleukin 6
INR	international normalised ratio
IPPV	intermittent positive pressure ventilation
IPSID	immunoproliterative small intestinal disease
I-PSS	international prostate symptom score
ISG	immunoscintigraphy
ISS	injury severity score
IVU	intravenous urogram
LCIS	lobular carcinoma-in-situ
LDH	lactate dehydrogenase
LFT	liver function test
LHRH	luteinizing hormone-releasing hormone
LOS	lower oesophageal sphincter
LUTS	lower urinary tract symptoms
MALT	mucosa-associated lymphoid tissue
MEN	multiple endocrine neoplasia
MFH	malignant fibrous histiocytoma
MIBG	metaiodobenzylguanidine
MIBI	technetium 99m sestamibi
MODS	multiple organ dysfunction syndrome
MOF	multiple organ failure
MRA	magnetic resonance angiography
MRCP	magnetic resonance cholangiopancreatography
MRI	magnetic resonance imaging
MRP	maximum resting anal pressure
MRSA	methicillin resistant *Staphylococcus aureus*
MSF	melanocyte-stimulating factor
MSH	melanocyte stimulating hormone
MSP	maximum squeeze pressure
NAH	nodular adrenal hyperplasia
NGCT	non-germ cell tumour
NHS	National Health Service
NICE	National Institute for Clinical Excellence
NIH	national institute of health
NMDA	N-methyl-D-aspartate receptors

NSAID	non-steroidal anti-inflammatory drug
NSAP	non-specific abdominal pain
OPSI	overwhelming post-splenectomy infection
PAN	polyarteritis nodosa
PCA	patient-controlled analgesia
PDGF	platelet-derived growth factor
PDS	polydioxanone
PE	pulmonary embolism
PEEP	positive end expiratory pressure
PEG	percutaneous endoscopic gastrostomy
PEI	percutaneous ethanol injection
PET	positron emission tomography
PFC	perfluorocarbons
PGL	persistent generalized lymphadenopathy
PIN	prostate intraepithelial neoplasia
PLAP	placental alkaline phosphatase
PaO_2	partial pressure of oxygen
PPI	proton pump inhibitor
PSA	prostate-specific antigen
PTC	percutaneous transhepatic cholangiogram
PTH	parathyroid hormone
PTS	paediatric trauma score
QUASAR	quick and simple and reliable
RCC	renal cell carcinoma
RMH	Royal Marsden Hospital
RPLND	retroperitoneal lymph node dissection
RTS	revised trauma score
SAG-M	saline-adenine-glucose-mannitol
SAP	systemic arterial pressure
SCC	squamous cell carcinoma
SEPS	subfascial endoscopic perforating vein surgery
SIMV	selective intermittent mandatory ventilation
SIRS	systemic inflammatory response syndrome
SLE	systemic lupus erythematosis
SVC	superior vena cava
TAPP	transabdominal preperitoneal
TB	tuberculosis
TBG	thyroid binding globulin
TBSA	total body surface area
TCC	transitional cell carcinoma
TCD	transcranial Doppler
TGF	transforming growth factor
TIPS	transjugular intrahepatic partasystemic anastomosis
TISSA	total body surface area
TNF-α	tumour necrosis factor α
TPN	total parenteral nutrition

TRUS	transrectal ultrasound
TS	trauma scale
TSH	thyroid stimulating hormone
TUMT	transurethral microwave thermotherapy
TUNA	transurethral needle ablation
TURP	transurethral resection of the prostate
U&E	urea and electrolytes
UOS	upper oesophageal sphincter
UTI	urinary tract infection
VDRL	venereal disease reference laboratory
VIP	vasoactive intestinal polypeptide
VMA	vanillylmandelic acid
WBC	white blood cell
WCC	white cell count
WHO	World Health Organisation

PREFACE TO SECOND EDITION

The second edition of *Key Topics in General Surgery* has been updated to reflect changes in surgical practice that have occurred since the first edition was published in 1996. The format remains largely unchanged but several old topics have been discarded in favour of new, more relevant chapters. The old Fellowship examination has now been abandoned, and we feel that the book is well suited to trainees preparing for the MRCS.

In keeping with the growth of evidence-based practice, we have attempted to indicate the strength of evidence supporting much of the material included. Where a *systematic review* of randomized controlled trials (the 'gold standard' of evidence-based medicine) is reported, it is identified with the superscript 'a' in the text. (Some meta-analyses are considered to be equivalent to a systematic review.) Where work from a *randomized controlled trial* (RCT) or meta-analysis is reported, it is identified with the superscript 'b' in the text. Other *peer reviewed* work (reviews, uncontrolled studies or case reports) is identified with the superscript 'c'. Alternatively, the references may be cited at the end of the chapter. Much of surgical practice is not yet or cannot be supported by high level evidence, and this is apparent by the paucity of references in some areas.

We are grateful to the many surgical trainers and colleagues with whom we have worked and whose practice constitutes much that is contained in this book. We thank Jonathan Ray, Lisa Mansell and Nadine Séveno of BIOS for their help and patience in its preparation, and are grateful to friends and families for their forbearance during its gestation.

C.R. Lattimer, N.M. Wilson, N.R.F. Lagattolla

PREFACE TO FIRST EDITION

This book is primarily directed at trainees preparing for the Membership and Fellowship examinations of the various Royal Colleges of Surgeons. We feel that the format will remain pertinent throughout the forthcoming changes to these examinations. The book should be used in conjunction with larger texts, but will be particularly useful in the run-up to an examination when key facts need to be crystallized out from the larger pool of information assimilated from other sources. We hope that medical students preparing for finals will also find this book informative and easy to use. Nursing staff managing surgical patients may find it useful as a basic source of reference.

We have attempted to provide a contemporary review of the key topics in gerneral surgery. Each chapter is limited to several pages of concise information presented in a 'short notes' style. Long lists are generally avoided because they are difficult to remember and superfluous information has been omitted to aid concentration.

We are grateful to the many consultants under whose guidance we have learned and practised much that is contained within this book. We thank Jonathan Ray and Priscilla Goldby of BIOS for their help and patience in its preparation, and are grateful to our friends and families for their encouragement and hard work in checking the manuscript.

C.R. Lattimer, N.M. Wilson, N.R.F. Lagattolla

Names of Medical Substances

In accordance with directive 92/27/EEC, this book adheres to the following guidelines on naming of medicinal substances (rINN, Recommended International Non-proprietary Name; BAN, British Approved Name).

List 1 – Both names to appear

UK Name	rINN
[1]adrenaline	epinephrine
amethocaine	tetracaine
bendrofluazide	bendroflumethiazide
benzhexol	trihexyphenidyl
chlorpheniramine	chlorphenamine
dicyclomine	dicycloverine
dothiepin	dosulepin
eformoterol	formoterol
flurandrenolone	fludroxycortide
frusemide	furosemide
hydroxyurea	hydroxycarbamide
lignocaine	lidocaine
methotrimeprazine	levomepromazine
methylene blue	methylthioninium chloride
mitozantrone	mitoxantrone
mustine	chlormethine
nicoumalone	acenocoumarol
[1]noradrenaline	norepinephrine
oxypentifylline	pentoxifylline
procaine penicillin	procaine benzylpenicillin
salcatonin	calcitonin (salmon)
thymoxamine	moxisylyte
thyroxine sodium	levothyroxine sodium
trimeprazine	alimemazine

List 2 – rINN to appear exclusively

Former BAN	rINN/new BAN
amoxycillin	amoxicillin
amphetamine	amfetamine
amylobarbitone	amobarbital
amylobarbitone sodium	amobarbital sodium
beclomethasone	beclometasone
benorylate	benorilate
busulphan	busulfan
butobarbitone	butobarbital
carticaine	articane
cephalexin	cefalexin
cephamandole nafate	cefamandole nafate
cephazolin	cefazolin
cephradine	cefradine
chloral betaine	cloral betaine
chlorbutol	chlorobutanol
chlormethiazole	clomethiazole
chlorathalidone	chlortalidone
cholecalciferol	colecalciferol
cholestyramine	colestyramine
clomiphene	clomifene
colistin sulphomethate sodium	colistimethate sodium
corticotrophin	corticotropin
cysteamine	mercaptamine
danthron	dantron
desoxymethasone	desoximetasone
dexamphetamine	dexamfetamine
dibromopropamidine	dibrompropamidine
dienoestrol	dienestrol
dimethicone(s)	dimeticone
dimethyl sulphoxide	dimethyl sulfoxide
doxycycline hydrochloride (hemihydrate hemiethanolate)	doxycycline hyclate
ethancrynic acid	etacrynic acid
ethamsylate	etamsylate
ethinyloestradiol	ethinylestradiol
ethynodiol	etynodiol
flumethasone	flumetasone
flupenthixol	flupentixol
gestronol	gestonorone
guaiphenesin	guaifenesin

---

[1] In common with the BP, precedence will continue to be given to the terms adrenaline and noradrenaline.

hexachlorophane	hexachlorophene	quinalbarbitone	secobarbital
hexamine hippurate	methenamine hippurate	riboflavine	riboflavin
		sodium calciumedetate	sodium calcium edetate
hydroxyprogesterone hexanoate	hydroxyprogesterone caproate	sodium cromoglycate	sodium cromoglicate
indomethacin	indometacin	sodium ironedetate	sodium feredetate
lysuride	lisuride	sodium picosulphate	sodium picosulfate
methyl cysteine	mecysteine	sorbitan monostearate	sorbitan stearate
methylphenobarbitone	methylphenobarbital	stilboestrol	diethylstilbestrol
oestradiol	estradiol	sulphacetamide	sulfacetamide
oestriol	estriol	sulphadiazine	sulfadiazine
oestrone	estrone	sulphadimidine	sulfadimidine
oxethazaine	oxetacaine	sulphaguanadine	sulfaguanadine
pentaerythritol tetranitrate	pentaerithrityl tetranitrate	sulphamethoxazole	sulfamethoxazole
		sulphasalazine	sulfasalazine
phenobarbitone	phenobarbital	sulphathiazole	sulfathiazole
pipothiazine	pipotiazine	sulphinpyrazone	sulfinpyrazone
polyhexanide	polihexanide	tetracosactrin	tetracosactide
potassium cloazepate	dipotassium clorazepate	thiabendazole	tiabendazole
		thioguanine	tioguanine
pramoxine	pramocaine	thiopentone	thiopental
prothionamide	protionamide	urofollitrophin	urofollitropin

CONTRIBUTORS

Omar Faiz (BSc, MBBS, FRCS)
Queen Elizabeth the Queen Mother Hospital, Margate, UK

Simon A.L. Gibbs (MA, MBBS, FRCS)
Queen Elizabeth the Queen Mother Hospital, Margate, UK

Nitin Gureja (MB, ChBAO, MRCS)
Queen Elizabeth the Queen Mother Hospital, Margate, UK

Deya Marzouk (MB, ChB, MS, MD, FRCS)
Queen Elizabeth the Queen Mother Hospital, Margate, UK

Chris Perera (MD, FFARCSI, DA)
Queen Elizabeth the Queen Mother Hospital, Margate, UK

Adrian Simoes (MS, FRCS)
Queen Elizabeth the Queen Mother Hospital, Margate, UK

Prakash Sinha (MS, FRCS)
William Harvey Hospital, Ashford, UK

ABDOMINAL TRAUMA

Nick Wilson

The majority of abdominal injuries sustained in mainland Britain follow road traffic accidents. Recognition of the presence of an intra-abdominal injury requiring surgery is far more important than its precise definition. A high index of suspicion is necessary, based on the history, especially the mechanism of injury and associated injuries, as physical signs can be misleading initially.

Mechanism of injury

1. Blunt. Direct blow, compression, shearing and tearing forces.

2. Penetrating. Stab wounds – 30% chance of visceral injury. Projectiles – low and high velocity – 95% chance of visceral injury. Laparotomy mandatory if projectile has breached peritoneum.

Management

A rapid primary assessment and resuscitation should be performed (Trauma management, p. 328). It is vital to recognize co-existing cervical and spinal injuries.

1. History
- Mechanism of injury, associated injuries.
- Site and nature of pain.
- Alcohol.

2. Physical signs
- Pulse, blood pressure, venous pressure and urine output – hypovolaemia.
- Seat belt abrasions, bruising and penetrating wounds.
- Generalized or localized abdominal distension – bleeding.
- Generalized tenderness and shoulder discomfort – free intestinal contents or blood.
- Localized tenderness – damage to a particular organ.
- Bowel sounds – unhelpful initially.
- Rectal examination – sphincter tone, blood in rectum, high riding prostate.
- Peripheral pulses. Auscultate for bruits – arterial compression or AV fistula.
- Regular reassessment – initial signs are often misleading.

3. Special investigations
- FBC, U & E, amylase, cross match blood.
- CXR, plain AXR – of limited value.
- Ultrasound scan. Used increasingly in A/E and trauma centres.
- Peritoneal lavage, CT in children.
- CT scan.
- IVU – non-function indicates severe renal disruption or vascular injury.
- If shock and clinical condition indicate need for laparotomy – do not waste time with lavage or CT.

Specific visceral injuries

Do not remove implements embedded in the abdomen until laparotomy. A long midline incision gives good access for most injuries. After opening the abdomen, control bleeding with sucker, clot evacuation and packs in each quadrant. Once blood volume restored, remove packs one by one to determine source of bleeding.

1.   Spleen.   In patients presenting with shock and extensive splenic injury, splenectomy should be performed immediately. In stable patients (particularly children) with less extensive splenic damage, splenic repair may be attempted but is time consuming and requires an experienced surgeon. Postoperative pneumococcal vaccination and prophylactic antibiotic cover should be given.

2.   Liver.   Blunt, macerating injuries are more hazardous than sharp penetrating injuries. No action is required if bleeding from the wound has stopped. Subcapsular haematomas should be explored and bleeding points controlled. Massive bleeding should be controlled by pressure, Pringle's manoeuvre and packs. Devitalized liver tissue should be removed. Heavy bleeding from the hepatic veins may require caval bypass to gain control. Gall bladder and bile duct injuries should be sought. The common bile duct can be repaired over a T-tube, but a damaged common hepatic duct requires drainage into a Roux loop.

3.   Duodenum and pancreas.   These injuries are easily missed. A midline haematoma in the lesser sac must be explored and Kocher's manoeuvre performed. Small duodenal lacerations may be repaired, but larger injuries are best treated by gastroenterostomy, closure of the pylorus and drainage. Distal pancreatectomy should be performed for transection of the pancreatic neck.

4.   Stomach.   Most stomach injuries can treated by wound excision and suture. For severe distal injuries, Polya gastrectomy may be necessary. Injuries to the cardia and the posterior wall are easily missed.

5.   Intestines.   Sharp penetrating injuries of both small and large bowel can usually be excised and primary suture or anastomosis performed. Left colon projectile injuries may require excision, anastomosis and defunctioning or Hartmann's operation. Blunt injuries produce bowel lacerations, transections (which can usually be excised and anastomosed) and mesenteric haematomas (which must be explored to control bleeding points). Tears at the ileocaecal junction, the splenic flexure and rectosigmoid junction are easily overlooked.

6.   Kidneys and ureter.   Haematuria and loin swelling indicate renal injury and IVU will show parenchymal damage and confirm the presence of a normal contralateral kidney. Angiography may be required if a vascular injury is likely. Lateral haematomas overlying the kidneys found at laparotomy need not be explored providing they are not expanding and there is no hypotension. Partial nephrectomy and/or repair of renal vessels should be performed from the front and the renal pedicle controlled before opening the haematoma. Ureteric injuries are rare and often missed. Re-anastomosis with stenting and drainage should be performed for upper injuries and reimplantation for lower injuries. Nephrostomy and late reconstruction may be necessary in extensive injuries.

7.   Bladder and urethra.   Blunt or penetrating injury may rupture a full bladder. Operative repair with catheter drainage is necessary. Blood at the urethral meatus implies urethral injury requiring suprapubic catheterization and subsequent urethral repair.

8.   Major blood vessels.   A midline haematoma should be explored and any underlying aortic, iliac or caval injury sutured, patched or excised and grafted as appropriate. Contained pelvic haematomas are not explored for fear of uncontrollable venous haemorrhage. Pelvic stabilization with an external fixator is usually required.

Complications

1.   General

- Pulmonary dysfunction – atelectasis, infection, ARDS.
- DVT, PE. Appropriate thromboembolic precautions should be taken.
- Shock.
- Ileus.
- Duodenal stress ulceration. Prophylactic measures reduce incidence.
- Peritonitis.
- Intra-abdominal abscess.
- Fistula.
- Nutritional problems.

2.   Local

- Wound – infection, dehiscence, necrotizing fasciitis.
- Liver and biliary tree – continued bleeding, bile leak.
- Spleen – subphrenic abscess, thrombocytosis, OPSI.
- Pancreas – cysts, pseudocysts, abscess.
- Bladder and kidneys – Urine leak.

Further reading

Rowlands BJ, Barros D'Sa AAB. Principles in the Management of Major Trauma. In Burnand KG, Young AE (eds) *The New Aird's Companion in Surgical Studies (2nd Edn)*. London: Churchill Livingstone, 1998; 127–151.

Related topics of interest

Chest trauma (p. 81); Head injury (p. 158); Trauma management (p. 328).

ACUTE APPENDICITIS

Nick Lagattolla

Acute appendicitis is the most common surgical emergency in developed countries. Its incidence has fallen over the last three decades. About one in six of the population undergo appendicectomy. It is rare before the age of 2 years, reaches maximal incidence in childhood and declines thereafter with increasing age.

Pathogenesis

Appendiceal inflammation arises from luminal obstruction, usually secondary to obliteration of the lumen by a faecolith or possibly from lymphoid hyperplasia in response to an infection. Importantly, obstructive appendicitis can also be caused by tumours of the appendix or caecal pole. The extent of inflammation varies greatly from a mild self-limiting inflammation with resolution, through the spectrum of suppurative appendicitis, to frank gangrene. Faecoliths are found in 30–40% of appendicectomies and in these gangrene is twice as common (75–80%).

Disease course

Progression to peritonitis or perforation may occur if an inflamed appendix is not removed, but this is not inevitable. Perforation occurs in 25% of patients with a history of pain of less than 24 hours and in 35% with a history exceeding 48 hours. Perforation may occur particularly rapidly in children. Perforation, gangrene, or the presence of generalized peritonitis all carry a higher incidence of complications, even when operated.

Clinical features

Typically a patient presents with gradual onset of colicky, central abdominal pain with anorexia and vomiting. Within several hours this visceral mid-gut pain localizes to the right iliac fossa as transmural inflammation causes parietal peritoneal irritation. Only 50% of patients give such a classical history. In 30% the history exceeds 24 hours and the pain starts in the right iliac fossa. The systemic response of tachycardia, fever and dehydration is variable. The abdominal examination is pivotal in the diagnosis. The point of maximal tenderness may not be in the right iliac fossa, reflecting the true position of the inflamed part of the appendix. With a high retrocaecal appendix pain and tenderness may be felt in the loin, while in a pelvic appendix tenderness may only be apparent on rectal examination. Diffuse peritonism occurs most commonly in the very young and elderly, and can be indistinguishable from other causes of peritonitis. A tender right iliac fossa mass suggests the formation of an inflammatory mass or abcess around the appendix.

Differential diagnosis

Diagnosis is particularly difficult in young children, young or pregnant women and in the elderly. Among young men the negative appendicectomy rate is relatively low (5–20%). The figure rises to in excess of 30% in young women and children. The difficulty of diagnosing appendicitis in the elderly is reflected by the high incidence of perforation (>50%), rather than by a high negative appendicectomy rate. There are numerous conditions which have been mistaken for acute appendicitis. In children the most common differential diagnosis is mesenteric adenitis (viral upper respiratory tract infection and high fever), while in young women it is important to distinguish appendicitis from pelvic inflammatory disease or a urinary tract infection. Pain of immediate onset without prior warning is rarely due to appendicitis. The more common differential diagnoses are listed below.

- Mesenteric adenitis.
- Lower urinary tract infection
- Pyelonephritis.
- Salpingitis.
- Ectopic pregnancy.
- Ruptured ovarian follicle (Mittelschmerz syndrome).
- Torsion or ruptured ovarian cyst.
- Acute cholecystitis.
- Terminal ileitis.
- Inflammatory or perforated caecal carcinoma.

Aids in diagnosis

A high rate of negative appendicectomy is undesirable. Removal of a normal appendix is associated with all the usual postoperative complications. Additionally, patients can suffer late complications such as adhesive intestinal obstruction. Considerable efforts are being made to improve diagnostic accuracy and prevent unnecessary appendicectomies using the following:

1. **White cell count.** High sensitivity for appendicitis, as only 4% of patients with appendicitis have normal counts, but of low specificity as it is raised in many other conditions.

2. **Urine analysis.** Useful in excluding significant urinary tract infection, particularly in children and young women. A positive pregnancy may indicate an ectopic pregnancy.

3. **Barium enema.** Accurate in the diagnosis of appendicitis, revealed by non-filling of the appendiceal lumen, but failure to reach the appendix can result in false positives, and generally an unnecessary and time-consuming investigation.

4. **Ultrasound.** Visualization of the appendix by ultrasonography may be diagnostic for acute appendicitis. The sensitivity of the technique is reduced in early appendicitis and in retrocaecal appendix. Ultrasound can accurately diagnose other conditions mimicking appendicitis, and not requiring surgery, like mesenteric adenitis, renal abnormalities and ovarian disorders, as well as diagnosing disorders where surgical intervention is indicated, such as ectopic pregnancy.

5. **CT scan.** This has been advocated as the ultimate in achieving high sensitivity and specificity in acute appendicitis, as very few cases are missed, and other pathologies are also confidently diagnosed. However, the cost may be prohibitive.

6. **Laparoscopy.** Appendicitis can be excluded if a normal appendix is seen or another cause of intra-abdominal pathology revealed, particularly gynaecological disorders. It is an invasive procedure requiring general anaesthesia with specific complications.

7. **Catheter peritoneal aspiration.** This technique does not distinguish between appendicitis, salpingitis and mesenteric adenitis as all can cause an abnormal number of leucocytes on a smear, however, negative cytology will exclude all three conditions. Complications may arise from inadvertent visceral puncture.

8. **Active observation.** This is safe in patients with an equivocal clinical picture. Repeated examinations are performed and appendicectomy undertaken if definitive signs develop.

9. **Computer-aided diagnosis.** In conjunction with structured patient interview, this technique is highly accurate in diagnosing acute appendicitis and reduces the negative exploration rate.

Management

Appendicectomy and local peritoneal and/or pelvic lavage is the treatment for acute appendicitis, performed as soon as the patient's condition permits. Normally this is by open operation, although there is evidence for diagnostic laparoscopy and laparoscopic removal. There are a number of specific situations that can arise:

1. **Preoperative palpable mass.** A mass may not be palpable while a patient is awake and tender, as local guarding frequently conceals an underlying inflammatory mass or abcess. If symptoms are recent, within 3 or 4 days, appendicectomy is the correct management for both inflammatory mass and abcess in experienced hands. This is safe and expeditious. An established appendix mass may be treated conservatively with intravenous antibiotics, repeated clinical evaluation, and deferred appendicectomy. A mass palpable only on the operating table may cause the surgeon to reconsider the intended incision. In the elderly, a caecal carcinoma must be strongly suspected, and a right hemicolectomy should be undertaken if this is felt likely.

2. **Normal appendix.** The terminal ileum should be inspected for a Meckel's diverticulum, mesenteric adenitis or terminal ileitis. The right tube and ovary must be visualized and the left ovary palpated. In terminal ileitis, if the caecal pole is healthy, the appendix should be removed.

3. **Appendiceal tumours.** These are usually carcinoid tumours, and are usually only discovered histologically. Appendicectomy is adequate treatment if the carcinoid is less than 2 cm in diameter. If greater than 2 cm or incompletely excised, right hemicolectomy is necessary. Appendiceal villous adenomas occur, and these may result in a grossly distended, non-inflamed mucocele of the appendix. Primary adenocarcinomas occur but are rare.

Complications

Overall mortality for appendicitis is less than 1% but rises to over 5% in the presence of perforation, especially in the elderly. The most frequent complication is wound sepsis. With appropriate perioperative antibiotic prophylaxis the prevalence, even in cases of perforation, can be reduced to 5%. Inadequate peritoneal toilet can lead to subsequent intra-abdominal or pelvic abscess formation.

Further reading

Reviews

Hoffmann J, Rasmussen OO. Aids in the diagnosis of acute appendicitis. *British Journal of Surgery*, 1989; **76**: 774–779.

Paterson-Brown S, Vipond M. Modern aids to clinical decision-making in the acute abdomen. *British Journal of Surgery*, 1990; **77**: 13–18.

Observational study

Galindo Gallego M *et al.* Evaluation of ultrasonography and clinical diagnostic scoring in suspected appendicitis. *British Journal of Surgery*, 1998; **85**: 37–40.

Korner H *et al.* Structured data collection improves the diagnosis of acute appendicitis *British Journal of Surgery*, 1998; **85**: 341–344.

Metanalysis

McCall JL *et al.* Systematic review of randomized controlled trials comparing laparoscopic with open appendicectomy. *British Journal of Surgery*, 1997; **84**: 1045–1050.

Related topic of interest

Non-specific abdominal pain (p. 231).

ACUTE PANCREATITIS

Nick Lagattolla

This is acute inflammation of the pancreas which ranges from very mild and self-limiting, to fulminant and fatal. The incidence appears to have increased over the last 40 years. In the UK the condition is a common cause of acute abdomen requiring hospital admission. The overall mortality has remained unchanged at 10%. In approximately 75% of patients complete recovery occurs after a few days of bed rest and alimentary rest, however in the remainder the attack is severe, with a mortality of 25–30%. There is thus a clear need for the early identification of this group of patients.

Epidemiology

Clinical series under-report the incidence as cases diagnosed at post-mortem are omitted. The incidence varies in relation to alcohol consumption, which is the main cause in the young, and the prevalence of gallstones, which is the predominant cause in the elderly. In many cases, no cause is evident, and these idiopathic cases are often referred to as the third most common cause of acute pancreatitis.

Aetiology

The common predisposing conditions are well known as gallstones and alcohol consuption. In Britain gallstones account for 50–60% of cases. Alcohol accounts for most of the rest, but other causes include:

- Trauma (blunt, penetrating, iatrogenic, post ERCP).
- Obstruction of the pancreatic duct (neoplasm, pancreas divisum).
- Hypercalcaemia.
- Hypertriglyceridaemia.
- Hypothermia.
- Drugs (thiazides, corticosteroids, oestrogens).
- Renal failure.
- Post-operative (cardio-pulmonary bypass).
- Viral infections (mumps, coxsackie).

Pathophysiology

The precise mechanisms by which the above factors can induce acinar rupture with release of activated enzymes within the gland parenchyma with autolysis of the gland are still not well understood. However, a severe systemic inflammatory response occurs, characterized by multiple inflammatory mediators (interleukin-6 and -8, and tumour necrosis factor-α) and activation of the cytokine cascade. Fluid sequestration, hypoalbuminaemia, intraperitoneal fat necrosis, and hypocalcaemia are all characteristic findings. The gland may become haemorrhagic.

Diagnosis

Typically the patient complains of sudden-onset, severe upper abdominal pain radiating into the back. Repeated vomiting is very characteristic. Sitting upright may ease the pain. Abdominal findings range from mild epigastric tenderness to generalized peritonism. Intradermal staining by extravasated blood in the flank (Grey Turner's sign) or at the umbilicus (Cullen's sign) heralds an attack of severe haemorrhagic pancreatitis which carries a high mortality. The diagnosis is usually confirmed by an elevated serum amylase. Urinary amylase can also be estimated rapidly by reagent strips. It is essential to exclude hyperamylasaemia in every acute abdomen. False positive test results (non-pancreatitis hyperamylasaemia) are common, and may be caused by:

- Perforated peptic ulcer.
- Biliary disease particularly gallstone related.
- Afferent loop obstruction following gastrectomy.
- Ruptured aortic aneurysms.
- Mesenteric infarction.
- Ruptured ectopic pregnancy
- Salivary hyperamylasaemia.

The amylase level is often just above the recognized upper limit of normal. False negatives can occur if presentation is very early (within the first 3–4 hours) or late in the episode. In chronic alcohol dependency, previous destruction of the gland parenchyma accounts for very slowly rising levels.

Determination of severity

The degree of hyperamylasaemia does not correlate with the severity of the disease. Early identification of the 25% of patients with a severe, life-threatening attack is desirable, as this will allow early intensive monitoring of these patients. Clinical assessment is unreliable in the crucial first 48 hours of an attack though certain signs (shock, abdominal mass and tetany) are informative.

A number of scoring systems using multiple laboratory criteria have been proposed of which Imrie's is widely accepted.

- Age > 55 years.
- WBC > 15×10^9/l.
- Glucose < 10 mmol/l.
- Albumin < 32 g/l.
- Urea > 16 mmol/l.
- PaO_2 < 8 kPa (60 mmHg).
- LDH > 600 i.u./l.
- AST > 200 i.u./l.

The presence of three or more of the above criteria within the first 48 hours indicates a severe attack (Ranson's criteria are essentially the same as above, but without the age criterion). A quicker assessment of severity can be made by abdominal paracentesis and examination of the fluid. A severe attack may be indicated by aspiration of more than 20 ml of free fluid irrespective of colour, dark free fluid or a dark lavage return. The combination of clinical assessment, multiple laboratory criteria and abdominal paracentesis will be accurate in identifying 75% of severe attacks.

Non-operative management

Repeated and careful clinical assessment of all patients during the first 24 hours is essential as the course of the disease is unpredictable during this time. A chest radiograph is mandatory as is estimation of arterial blood gases daily for the first 48 hours and oxygen should be administered by mask if there is hypoxaemia. Plain abdominal radiographs may show a sentinel loop, pancreatic calcification or calcified gallstones. Vital signs and urine output should be monitored hourly. The severely affected patient should be managed on the intensive care unit. Oral intake is withheld, so adequate fluid replacement, especially of colloid, is necessary. Energetic fluid replacement is the single most important therapeutic measure, since a large volume of protein-rich fluid is sequestered in the retroperitoneum. Volume replacement should be guided by central venous pressure measurement at the first sign of hypovolaemia (hypotension or low urine output). A large series showed an improved outcome in those given parenteral antibiotics. In a severe attack, parenteral nutrition will be necessary. Adequate pain control is important – an intravenous infusion of morphine or patient-controlled analgesia are both preferable to repeated intramuscular boluses. At present there are no specific non-operative measures that have been shown to improve the outcome in acute pancreatitis (e.g. antiproteases or peritoneal lavage). All patients require an abdominal ultrasound to exclude gallstones, and if the attack is severe, an early CT scan with intravenous contrast to assess pancreatic viability.

Complications

1. Systemic. The systemic response can vary from a mild fever to multi-organ failure in fulminant pancreatitis. The pathophysiological basis of this response is probably due to the release of cytokines and other inflammatory mediators that cause endothelial damage and capillary leakage in many organ systems. This can lead to refractory shock, where maintenance of the circulating volume can only be achieved by measurement of left atrial pressures (pulmonary capillary wedge pressures) to allow appropriate fluid replacement and inotrope administration. The lungs are commonly affected and respiratory failure occurs because capillary leak results in interstitial oedema. This is exacerbated by the presence of pain or an abdominal mass, both of which will promote sputum retention, atelectasis and pneumonia. Metabolic problems include hyperglycaemia and hypocalcaemia. Hypocalcaemia largely reflects the hypo-albuminaemia but calcium may be sequestered within intra-abdominal soaps. Calcium administration is only necessary if tetany occurs.

2. Local

- *Pseudocyst.* Peripancreatic effusions occur in up to 20% of cases but the majority of these resolve within 4–6 weeks. Pseudocysts are enzyme-rich fluid collections which arise in the region of the lesser sac from disruption of the pancreatic parenchyma. They have no epithelial lining but are surrounded by granulation tissue and may eventually develop quite well-defined capsules. They are generally detected by ultrasound or CT scanning but may present as an abdominal mass. They may be locally symptomatic, though the majority are not. Pseudocysts are more common in alcoholic pancreatitis than in gallstone pancreatitis

(15% versus 3%). Complications of pseudocysts can be severe, and include infection, major haemorrhage from erosion into the splenic artery, and obstruction of the duodenum, the gastro-oesophageal junction or rarely the common bile duct, if the far recesses of the lesser sac are involved. Haemorrhage and sepsis occur more frequently in gallstone-associated cysts and the incidence of these complications increases with the passage of time. Large, unresolving or symptomatic pseudocysts should be drained either percutaneously, or internally by cyst-gastrostomy.

- *Pancreatic mass, abscess and necrosis.* A pancreatic phlegmon is a clinical diagnosis confirmed on CT referring to a non-infected inflammatory pancreatic mass. The pancreas may become necrotic in part or wholly, and if infection supervenes, a pancreatic abscess may form. Infected necrosis becomes apparent early during the course of the attack (within two weeks) and produces a dramatic clinical picture with fever, deteriorating respiratory and renal function, painful abdominal mass and a leucocytosis. A necrotic pancreas may require extensive debridement, whilst the formation of a pancreatic phlegmon usually resolves. An abscess requires percutaneous or formal open drainage. All of these conditions are readily diagnosed by CT, particularly pancreatic necrosis which will not enhance following the injection of intravenous contrast unlike normal or recovering pancreatic tissue.

- *Colonic infarction.* This can occur if the blood supply is interrupted by extension of the extrapancreatic necrosis and may follow drainage of a pancreatic abscess. This is rare, but a functional obstruction at the level of the transverse colon is a familiar, though rare, complication or even presentation of acute pancreatitis.

- *Pancreatic fistula.* This results from external drainage of a pancreatic abscess or pseudocyst. Spontaneous closure usually occurs, unless there is distal pancreatic duct obstruction. Somatostatin or its synthetic analogues have been used with some success to reduce fistula output.

Surgery

1. ***Early ERCP.*** ERCP and sphincterotomy in patients with particularly gallstone pancreatitis results in significantly fewer major complications, however the urgent diagnosis of gallstones in acute pancreatitis can be difficult. There is a risk of excacerbating the attack, and emergency ERCP can be difficult to arrange.

2. ***Pancreatic necrosis.*** In a small proportion of patients a severe episode is evident from the outset or there is early deterioration despite full supportive measures. The major determinant of outcome in these cases is the prompt recognition of generalized pancreatic necrosis. In these patients surgery may be necessary to prevent sequential organ failure, sepsis and death. Surgery should be delayed for several days as this results in demarcation of necrotic tissue, while the patient is optimized on the intensive care unit, and allows for safe debridement at laparotomy (pancreatic necrosectomy). Following this the abdomen can be closed with large silicone tubes left in the cavity that can be irrigated postoperatively (closed drainage). Alternatively the abdomen is left open (laparostomy) but covered by moist packs should repeated re-exploration and debridement prove necessary, as is occasionally the case. Infected pancreatic necrosis, or abcess, requires drainage, either percutaneously or at

laparotomy. Drainage tubes are left in situ for irrigation with antiseptic or antibiotic solutions.

3. **_Preventative._**   Early cholecystectomy prevents recurrent episodes in patients with gallstones. Early cholecystectomy refers to surgery undertaken within two weeks after the onset of symptoms. Immediate surgery is associated with an increased incidence of postoperative complications, particularly an excacerbation of pancreatitis, while deferring operation to a subsequent admission may result in a 30–40% risk of another attack. Gallstones should be sought in all patients with acute pancreatitis, including those with alcohol-induced disease. ERCP is indicated after an episode of idiopathic pancreatitis, though a surgically treatable cause is rarely found.

Further reading

Poston GJ, Williamson RCN. Surgical management of acute pancreatitis. *British Journal of Surgery,* 1990; **77:** 5–12.

Kemppainen E *et al.* Early localisation of necrosis by contrast-enhanced comptuted tomography can predict outcome in severe acute pancreatitis. *British Journal of Surgery,* 1996; **83:** 924–929.

Farkas G *et al.* Surgical strategy and management of infected pancreatic necrosis. *British Journal of Surgery,* 1996; **83:** 930–933.

Related topic of interest

Chronic pancreatitis (p. 84).

ADRENAL TUMOURS

Christopher Lattimer, Nitin Gureja

Adrenal tumours are rare. Types of adrenal tumours present include:

- Adrenal adenoma.
- Adrenocortical carcinoma.
- Phaechromocytoma.
- Neuroblastoma.
- Incidentaloma.

Mesenchymal tumours may also present as adrenal tumours e.g. lipoma, lipomyosarcoma.

Adrenal adenoma

Adrenal adenomas can present with symptoms of:

1. Excess hormone production
   - Excess glucocorticoids causing Cushing's syndrome.
   - Excess mineralocorticoids causing Conn's syndrome.
   - Increased production of sex hormones producing feminizing or virilizing features.
2. Incidentally. Often found on imaging studies of the abdomen for unrelated pathology.
3. Non specific symptoms of abdominal pain, weight loss, and malaise.

Diagnosis consists of a careful history and examination, looking in particular for features suggestive of an endocrine disturbance, e.g. symptoms of polydipsia, polyuria, lethargy and muscle weakness (related to hypokalaemia); signs of Cushingnoid facies and habitus, hypertension, virilizing or feminizing features.

A 24-hour urine collection for cortisol and a positive low-dose dexamethasone test are diagnostic of Cushing's syndrome. Conn's syndrome (commonest cause being an adrenal adenoma) is diagnosed by an increased 24 hour urine excretion of potassium ions (>30 mmol), along with a high plasma aldosterone/renin ratio. An ability to lower plasma aldosterone and increase plamsa renin levels after captopril administration favours an adenoma as the cause of hyper-aldosteronism as compared to primary hyperplasia.

Iodocholesterol scintigraphy (using 131-iodomethyl norcholesterol) is also useful in differentiating an adenoma from hyperplasia and an adrenocortical carcinoma. In a carcinoma there is no uptake of NP-59, whilst in an adrenal adenoma there is uptake with suppression of the contralateral gland. In hyperplasia there is bilateral uptake of NP-59. Iodocholesterol scintigraphy is also useful in detection of any ectopic tissue. CT and MRI scanning are essential in detecting the adrenal mass, as well as in detecting the presence of any metastatic disease.

Adrenocortical carcinoma

Adrenocortical carcinoma is a rare carcinoma, with a bimodal peak. The first peak tends to be in patients under the age of 6, and the second peak in the 4th to 5th decade. Histologically the distinction between benign and malignant disease can be very difficult, and the single most reliable factor is the evidence of nodal disease and distant metastasis. It can histologically be very difficult to differentiate from renal cell carcinoma, but using vimentin stains (adrenal tumours staining positive), this is possible.

Surgical resection offers the best chance of cure, and this is best performed at the initial operation, with removal of all contiguous structures as deemed necessary at laparotomy.

Mitotane is the first line of chemotherapy, and acts by destroying normal and neoplastic adrenocortical cells. Approximately 1/3 of patients have a partial response to chemotherapy, usually occurring in the first 6 weeks of treatment.

In presence of metastatic disease, debulking of the tumour may alleviate symptomatic disease. Overall the 5-year survival rate is ~10.3%.

Phaechromocytoma

Phaechromocytomas are tumours arising from neuroectodermal cells of the adrenal medulla or extra-adrenal sites.

They are found in increased frequency in patients with hypertension, MEN 2a and MEN 2b syndromes, and von Recklinghausens's neurofibromatosis. Peak incidence is in the 4th and 5th decade.

The rule of tens applies to phaechromocytomas:

- 10% are bilateral.
- 10% are extra-adrenal.
- 10% are familial.
- 10% are multicentric.
- 10% are malignant.
- 10% occur in children.

The triad of headaches, palpitations and diaphoresis should arouse the suspicion of a phaechromocytoma. Other significant symptoms include hypertension, headaches, postural hypotension and tremors.

Diagnosis is confirmed by a 24-hour urine collection for VMA, metanephrine and catecholamines; with noradrenaline having the best sensitivity and VMA the best specificity for phaechromocytomas.

CT, MRI and MIBG are the imaging modalities used. CT has been shown to have a sensitivity of 85–90%, and a specificity of 70–100%. MIBG is similar to noradrenaline in structure, and is hence taken up by adrenergic tissue. MIBG scanning provides useful functional data on these tumours.

Treatment is by adrenalectomy, which can be performed by a midline, subcostal or transabdominal approach. Alternatively laparoscopy may be used if the disease is benign. Specific preoperative problems relating to surgery of phaeochromocytomas include massive hypertensive surge during tumour handling, hypotensive shock following tumour devascularization and hypoglycaemia. A week's pre-operative treatment with long-acting alpha-blocker phenoxybenzamine, combined with a beta-blocker if tachycardia develops, has reduced the operative mortality by controlling the catecholamine surges. Metyrosine (tyrosine hydroxylase antagonist) is also occasionally used pre-operatively. General anaesthetic induction is using inhaled gases e.g. isoflurane, to minimalize cardiac depressant effects. Adequate volume repletion is necessary, as often these patients are underfilled due to the increased vasoconstrictive state.

Neuroblastoma

These are aggressive tumours of childhood, common before the age of 3. Eighty percent are associated with a genetic abnormality on chromosome 1. They are unusual in that some have spontaneous regression.

Neuroblastomas often present with features of weight loss, lethargy and an abdominal mass. A nephroblastoma is the main differential diagnosis in this age group. They are diagnosed by elevated serum dopamine levels, and have an increased 24-hour urine vanillyl mandelic acid (VMA) and dopamine level.

CT scanning provides information on the extent of the disease, as well as staging the disease. Bone marrow aspirate is also used to stage the disease.

Surgery is indicated for stage I–II of the disease. Radiation and chemotherapy being used for Stage IV.

Incidentaloma

Since the increased use of CT scanning in medical practice there is a reported incidence of ~0.6–1.3% of finding an incidental mass in the adrenals. This poses obvious management difficulties as often the patients are entirely asymptomatic, and are being investigated for an unrelated pathology.

Recent review shows that of the incidentalomas found:

- 25.7% are cortical tumours.
- 4.7% are adrenocortical carcinoma.
- 4.1% were metastatic deposits.
- 0.06% are phaeochromocytomas.

A detailed history and examination, along with routine blood pressure measurements, and serum potassium should direct management. Routine 24-hour urine cortisol, potassium, VMA and metanephrine levels should also be recorded.

An adrenal tumour >6 cm on CT scan is very suggestive of malignant potential and hence surgery should be offered to the patient.

FNAC should only be used to assess the adrenal mass, once the 24-hour VMA screen has been completed and is negative to avoid the possibility of a hypertensive crisis. Seeding along the needle tract, as well as adrenal haemorrhage can occur, which limits the usefulness of this technique.

Further reading

Bravo EL. Evolving concepts in the pathophysiology, diagnosis and treatment of phaeochromocytoma. *Endocrinology Review*, 1994; **15:** 356.

Pommier RF, Brennen MF. Management of adrenal neoplasms. *Current Problems in Surgery*, 1991; **28:** 663.

Ross NS, Aron DC. Hormonal evaluation of the patient with an incidentally discovered adrenal mass. *New England Journal of Medicine*, 1990; **323:** 1401.

AIDS

Christopher Lattimer, Omar Faiz

Acquired immunodeficiency syndrome is becoming an increasing problem to the general surgeon. Current estimates of HIV infection range between 15 and 100 million infected cases world-wide. It is caused by infection with the human immunodeficiency virus (HIV) which suppresses cellular immunity rendering the host susceptible to opportunistic infections (*Pneumocystis carinii* pneumonia, cryptosporidium, CMV, HSV) and malignancies (Kaposi's sarcoma, lymphoma). HIV has been isolated from every body fluid including: blood, urine, tears, saliva, semen and cervical secretions. HIV belongs to the retrovirus family – characterized by the possession of the enzyme reverse transcriptase. This enzyme permits viral RNA to be transcribed into DNA and thence incorporated into the host genome. The CD4 molecule on T helper cells acts as the receptor for HIV and it is the progressive depletion of this cell line that leads to the clinical manifestations of AIDS. The most commonly used classification system for HIV is that of the Centers for Disease Control (CDC). This system sub-classifies HIV infection into the following groups: Group I (acute primary infection); Group II (asymptomatic infection); Group III (persistent generalized lymphadenopathy); and Group IV (symptomatic infection). Only symptomatic patients (Group IV) have the Acquired Immunodeficiency Syndrome (AIDS). Zidovudine (AZT), an inhibitor of reverse transcriptase, was the first therapy developed for HIV. It has demonstrated a survival advantage in patients with symptomatic HIV and is consequently widely used for this group[a]. The efficacy of AZT in the asymptomatic HIV+ve group has not been clearly established. Other inhibitors of reverse transcriptase, such as dideoxyinosine (DDI) and dideoxycytidine (DDC), have been used in patients unable to tolerate AZT but their clinical efficacy has not been fully evaluated. Surgical involvement is requested for HIV patients with anorectal complaints (40%), requests for venous access (20%), cutaneous manifestations of the disease (20%), abdominal pain, and requests for biopsy (20%).

Anal warts

Anal warts in AIDS patients tend to be aggressive, dysplastic and hard to eradicate. Topical podophyllin or 5% fluorouracil cream applied through a proctoscope is time consuming and often of little benefit. Diathermy is satisfactory for isolated warts but precise scissor excision of a bleb of raised skin is preferable for extensive warts to preserve the intervening skin bridges. Females should undergo regular cervical screening because of the associated risk of cervical cancer. There is good evidence that severe dysplasia may progress to carcinoma-in-situ and thence to squamous cell carcinoma. Human papilloma virus (HPV) subtyping and biopsy facilitates prediction of lesions that are likely to develop into invasive carcinoma. HPV subtype 16 is most often associated with severe dysplasia.

Anorectal disorders

Perianal sepsis and anal ulceration in AIDS patients is a common problem. The extensive differential diagnosis of conditions that can result in anorectal pathology in this patient group mandates the need for histological and microbiological analysis. Sphincter preservation is of utmost importance during all anal procedures as male homosexuals have a tendency towards incontinence and the diarrhoea associated with opportunistic colonic infections is often severe. Setons are recommended for most fistulae. Kaposi's sarcoma can resemble an ulcerated haemorrhoid, non-Hodgkin's lymphoma may present as a perianal abscess and squamous cell carcinoma may easily be mistaken for a small benign ulcer. Long-term cultures from an ulcer base may reveal *Mycobacterium avium intracellulare*. Viral cultures can detect CMV or acyclovir-resistant strains of HSV which can both cause extensive anal ulceration. Diarrhoea also encourages anal ulceration. Stool cultures for *Salmonella, Shigella, Campylobacter* and *Cryptosporidium* with microscopy for *giardia*, ova cysts and amoeba are mandatory. CMV can also be detected on rectal biopsy. Anal ulcers can be iatrogenic occurring in the region of a previous lateral sphincterotomy initially performed for an ulcer which was mistaken for a fissure. Inappropriate anal instrumentation or traumatic sexual injuries can result in severe sphincter injuries often necessitating permanent faecal diversion.

Abdominal pain

Gastrointestinal malignancies and opportunistic infections must be sought and excluded. CMV is the most common cause of abdominal pain in this group resulting in a wide range of conditions (oesophagitis, acalculous cholecystitis, sclerosing cholangitis, small bowel perforation, toxic megacolon, colonic perforation, GI haemorrhage and spontaneous splenic rupture). Kaposi's sarcoma and lymphoma may present with unremitting haemorrhage, small bowel obstruction, intussusception, perforation or mesenteric infiltration. Lymphadenopathy from *Mycobacterium avium intracellulare* or lymphoma can result in appendicitis or jaundice due to obstruction of the appendiceal ostium or porta hepatis respectively. Appendicectomy and colectomy are the commonest abdominal operations performed in this group. The decision to raise a colostomy is not undertaken lightly as they are rarely reversed. A platelet count is mandatory prior to any surgery since thrombocytopenia is common.

CMV retinitis

This condition occurs in 30% of AIDS patients and is the leading cause of blindness in this patient group. Treatment is usually with ganciclovir and maintenance therapy is usually required to prevent relapse.

Surgery

Operative mortality for emergency and elective surgery is high (30% for a routine open cholecystectomy). General anaesthesia results in depression of cell-mediated immunity and AIDS progression. Furthermore, the poor nutritional state of this patient group contributes to poor wound healing and susceptibility to further infection. Unfortunately, negative laparotomy is not too infrequent an event for an HIV patient with undiagnosed abdominal pain. The above factors have led to an increased use of diagnostic laparoscopy. However special precautions taken during laparoscopic procedures should include: the use of disposable ports; and deflation of the abdominal pneumoperitoneum into a closed system to prevent HIV contaminated aerosol escaping into the theatre environment. There is no documented evidence that aerosol transmission occurs[b]. The decision to undertake surgery is aided by patient staging according to their level of general immunity. A CD4 count greater than 500 indicates mild disease and implies appropriate operative treatment should not be withheld. In contrast, a CD4 count less than 500 indicates advanced disease and is associated with poor outcome.

Lymphadenopathy

Lymphadenopathy can be generalized during seroconversion or in the persistent generalized lymphadenopathy (PGL) state. Localized lymphadenopathy is usually attributable to infection or tumour. Open biopsy is rarely necessary since AIDS lymphadenopathy demonstrates non-specific reactive follicular hyperplasia and the diagnosis is better established by thorough clinical examination and a familiarity with the disease.

Cutaneous manifestations

Lymphoepithelial cysts are fluid-filled cutaneous lesions which are diagnosed by ultrasound. They are best obliterated by aspiration and tetracycline instillation. Individual cutaneous malignancies are treated as required.

Precautions

1. High risk groups. Homosexual males, intravenous drug abusers, haemophiliacs, sexual partners and children of the above as well as residents of sub-Saharan Africa represent the high-risk groups where certain additional measures (in addition to universal precautions) should be employed.

2. Surgeon protection. The surgeon is exposed to percutaneous (needlestick injuries) and mucocutaneous (eye splashes and glove perforation in the presence of abraded skin) infection when operating on this patient group. Investigators have attempted to calculate the lifetime risk to the surgeon and have yielded estimated lifetime cumulative risks between 0.12% and 50.0%[b]. However, figures reported to the Centers for Disease Control and Prevention up to 1997 revealed only six cases where surgeons were identified to have suffered possible occupational transmission[b]. The technique of double gloving is widely used by surgeons undertaking procedures with high associated transmission risk[b]. Studies suggest that double gloving significantly reduces blood exposure to the surgeons skin and thereby should decrease the mucocutaneous transmission risk[b]. Eye splashes are easily preventable by the use of eye-shields or goggles throughout surgery. A recent study that macroscopically and microscopically inspected surgeons eye-shields following surgery demonstrated blood spray contamination on 44% of the eye-shields tested. The surgeons wearing the eye-shields however only noticed the contamination in 8% of cases[a]. Given the above statistics, it would seem appropriate to endorse the use of double gloving and eye-shields for high-risk, or confirmed, cases of HIV.

3. Patient protection. Case numbers of patients who have potentially been infected by operative transmission from an HIV-positive surgeon are so small that it is impossible to ascertain the genuine risk. Surgeons are at present under no obligation to be tested for HIV.

Further reading

Flum DR, Wallack MK. The surgeon's database for AIDS: a collective review. *Journal of the American College of Surgery*, 1997 Apr; **184**(4): 403–412.

Megan J, Patterson M, Novak CB *et al.* Surgeons' concern and practices of protection against bloodborne pathogens. *Annals of Surgery*, 1998; **228**: 226–272.

Scott-Conner CEH, Fabrega AJ. Gastrointestinal problems in the immunocompromised host. A review for surgeons. *Surgery and Endoscopy*, 1996 Oct; **10**(10): 959–964.

Related topics of interest

Anorectal investigation (p. 28); Assessment of the acute abdomen (p. 41).

AMPUTATIONS

Nick Wilson

Most amputations are performed for lower limb ischaemia. Aggressive lower limb revascularization reduces the incidence of major amputation together with its attendant social and financial burdens and increases the ratio of below knee to above knee amputations. Where major amputation is unavoidable, the below knee level is preferable to the above knee procedure as subsequent mobility and prosthetic limb use are far superior. For most patients undergoing major amputation, the procedure itself is merely the beginning of a long process of rehabilitation, limb fitting and return to partial mobility. Even in those patients unlikely to walk again, the longest stump possible (commensurate with successful wound healing) will aid stability in a chair or bed and will facilitate transferring. Even after successful revascularization for critical ischaemia, some patients require minor amputations of a digit or possibly the forefoot. Wound healing may be delayed, but most patients attain a high level of mobility with minimal difficulty.

Indications

- End-stage unreconstructable atherosclerotic disease. Approximately 80–90% of all amputations are performed for ischaemic arterial disease.
- Buerger's disease.
- Diabetic microangiopathy and infection.
- Emboli.
- Trauma.
- Infection (gas gangrene, necrotizing fasciitis, septic arthritis, osteomyelitis).
- Soft tissue or bony malignancy.
- Malformations, deformities.
- Intractable ulceration.
- Painful paralysed limbs.

The ideal amputation stump

- Primary wound healing.
- No redundant tissue.
- Cylindrical stump.
- No pressure on suture line.
- Painless.
- Full extension and flexion in adjacent joints.

Complications

- Wound infection.
- Breakdown of suture line.
- Stump too long or too short.
- Bony spurs.
- Stump neuroma.
- Phantom pain.
- Causalgia.

- Muscle herniation.
- Deep vein thrombosis.
- Prosthesis chafing.

Postoperative wound care, physiotherapy and limb fitting

A firm stump bandage should be applied after wound closure and this should be left undisturbed for 5 days unless there are indications of wound infection or breakdown. Application of a temporary prosthesis in theatre with very early weight-bearing has largely been abandoned. Weight-bearing in a PAMaid (pneumatic postamputation mobility aid) may start at 5–7 days providing the stump is satisfactory. Physiotherapy to strengthen the upper and lower limb musculature should begin as early as possible. Care should be taken to prevent or improve flexion contractures in the hip and knee joints. Early referral to the regional limb-fitting centre should be made for measurement and fitting of a modular limb. Many elderly patients, particularly those with above knee amputations, will not use an artificial limb and are unsuitable for limb fitting.

Specific amputations

1. Toe and foot amputations.   A good blood supply is required to allow wound healing and patients most suitable for these distal amputations are those who have distal ischaemia following successful revascularization, diabetic patients with small vessel disease or localized infection and patients with small/medium artery disease (e.g. Buerger's disease). Toe amputations are usually performed through racket-shaped incisions, the 'handle' being used to divide bone and tendons proximal to the skin incision. Bone division should be through cortical bone to allow granulation tissue formation. Articular cartilage should not be left in the wound. A more extensive ray amputation may be indicated in diabetic patients to remove a toe with most or all of its metatarsal bone where there is deep infection.

Where all or most of the toes are non-viable, transmetatarsal amputation is indicated. Bone division is through the middle of the metatarsal shafts leaving a long plantar flap which is rolled up to leave a non-weight-bearing dorsal suture line.

Diabetic infection frequently calls for 'ad hoc' foot amputations where non-viable tissue is excised and deep infection is drained. The heel and other weight-bearing areas are retained if possible and once the infection has resolved the wound may be closed with primary suture or skin grafting.

2. Below-knee amputation.   Where major amputation is required, this level is preferable to through- or above-knee procedures. Many investigations (transcutaneous oxymetry, thermography, Doppler pressures, arteriography, plethysmography) have been assessed to predict the success of wound healing at this level, but none matches experience and the presence of bleeding from the skin flaps. The two techniques used are the long posterior flap (Burgess) and Robinson's skew flap employing equal anteromedial and posterolateral flaps. Both techniques result in similar rates of wound healing and mobilization.

3. Through-knee and Gritti-Stokes amputation.   Through-knee amputation is easy and quick to perform with equal lateral flaps and a posterior scar but leaves a large bulbous stump which causes difficulties with limb-fitting. Wound healing is frequently delayed in ischaemic disease. The Gritti-Stokes procedure is performed at the supracondylar level, leaving a longer stump than an above-knee amputation which provides good stability for the amputee in a chair or in bed. The fitting of an internal knee mechanism is difficult. The knee joint is disarticulated and the femur transected just above the condyles. The patella is cut to leave a flat posterior surface which is layed over the transected femur and may be wired in position. The patella tendon is sutured to the hamstrings.

4. Above-knee amputation.   Equal anterior and posterior flaps are fashioned with their upper ends at the level of bone section (12–14 cm above the knee joint line). Vastus lateralis is sutured to the adductors and the quadriceps are sutured to the hamstrings. This amputation is quick to perform and usually results in satisfactory wound healing, but many elderly patients fail to walk despite provision of carefully measured prosthesis.

5. Disarticulation at the hip.   This is used for malignant disease and infection and is rarely necessary for ischaemic disease. An anterior approach is made to the hip and the joint disarticulated. A long posterior gluteal flap is fashioned to cover the defect leaving an anterior suture line.

6. Hind-quarter amputation.   This amputation was devised to treat soft tissue and bony tumours of the pelvis, but is occasionally indicated for pelvic trauma. It is rarely used now.

7. Amputations of the upper limb.   Most of these amputations are performed for trauma, infection or tumour. Below the elbow, a stump of 15 cm allows the fitting of a prosthesis as does a stump of 19 cm from the shoulder above the elbow. Disarticulation at the shoulder joint or forequarter amputation are sometimes required for malignant disease.

Further reading

Campbell WB, Ridler BM. Predicting the use of prostheses by vascular amputees. *European Journal of Vascular Surgery*, 1996; **12:** 342–345.
Dormandy J, Heeck L, Vig S. Major amputations: clinical patterns and predictors. *Seminars in Vascular Surgery*, 1999; **12:** 154–161.

Related topics of interest

Critical leg ischaemia (p. 100); Vascular trauma (p. 356); Wounds: healing, closure and sutures (p. 364).

ANEURYSMS

Nick Wilson

An aneurysm is a localized dilatation of an artery. Cardiac and venous aneurysms are also described but will not be discussed. The significance of aneurysms lies in their tendency to rupture, thrombose or give rise to emboli.

Terminology

A true aneurysm involves all layers of the arterial wall and may be fusiform or saccular whilst a false aneurysm is formed by the compression of surrounding structures of an artery by blood escaping from a defect in its wall. Dissection of an aneurysm occurs when blood enters a tear in the diseased intima tracking down the wall splitting the media. A mycotic aneurysm develops when a bacterial (not fungal) focus locally infects an artery, weakening the wall. Alternatively, an established aneurysm may become infected. Periaortitis with thickening and dilatation of the aortic wall and a glistening white outer coat is known as an inflammatory aneurysm. The aetiology is unknown, but there is an association with retroperitoneal fibrosis.

Pathology

1. Degenerative. Most true aneurysms are degenerative (affecting the intima and media). Disordered connective tissue metabolism is the probable cause and abnormalities of matrix metalloproteinases have recently been implicated. Inhibitors of these enzymes are currently under investigation. Degenerative aneurysms contain a core of organized thrombus with a lumen through the middle.

2. Syphilis. Now an uncommon cause of aneurysm. The ascending aorta is affected and the adventitia and media are infiltrated by plasma cells and lymphocytes. Aortic valvular regurgitation and coronary osteal narrowing may also occur.

3. Collagen diseases. Marfan's syndrome, Ehler's-Danlos syndrome and pseudoxanthoma elasticum are rare conditions associated with the development of saccular or dissecting aneurysms.

4. Congenital aneurysm. Berry aneurysms occurring on the circle of Willis are caused by a congenital weakness of the arterial wall.

Abdominal aortic aneurysm

Aneurysms (aortic diameter ≥3 cm) occur most frequently in the abdominal aorta affecting 4% of the population (7% of males) aged 65–80 years. The prevalence is greatest amongst male hypertensives who smoke and appears to be increasing in Western countries, AAA accounting for 10 000 deaths per year in England. Approximately 20% of affected males have a first-degree relative with an abdominal aortic aneurysm. Extension above the renal arteries occurs in only 2%, but aneurysms of other vessels are commonly associated. Over 50% of people with an AAA remain asymptomatic and die of other causes with their AAA intact. A pulsating abdominal mass may be found by the patient or on routine medical examination. Rapid expansion or leaking of the aneurysm may give rise to severe back or abdominal pain and hypotensive shock. A pulsatile abdominal mass is classically found on examination, but the presentation may be obscure with atypical pain and no hypotension if the rupture is contained. Rupture is the principal complication of AAA, but thrombosis, distal embolization, and aorto-enteric and aortocaval fistulae occur rarely.

Ultrasound is the usual method of imaging following clinical aneurysm detection, but dynamic CT scanning and/or MRA are frequently required to determine the relationship to the iliac and renal arteries. Treatment of AAA is currently by surgical inlay prosthetic grafting, but endovascular repair (EVAR) is being evaluated. Elective surgery is associated with a 30 day mortality of 5%, complications usually arising as a result of concomitant cardiovascular disease. Following this period, however, life expectancy returns close to that of a healthy, age-matched population. Aortic rupture is fatal in approximately 80% of cases, surgery for rupture having a mortality of 45–65%. Small aneurysms (4–5.5 cm maximum diameter) are unlikely to rupture (1% risk per year), whereas the probability of rupture in an aneurysm measuring 5.5 cm or more is 10–15% per year and these should be repaired electively[b].

Ultrasound screening programmes to detect asymptomatic aneurysms (the majority) are currently being evaluated and pilot studies suggest an 85% reduction in rupture in screened subjects. The majority of aneurysms detected are small and require surveillance rather than treatment and this may have an adverse effect on quality of life.

Recently, EVAR techniques have been described involving the transfemoral introduction of an aortic prosthesis. Potential advantages include avoidance of an abdominal incision, no aortic cross clamping, improved cardiorespiratory, renal and gastrointestinal function and reduced hospital stay. Multinational registries indicate considerable difficulties with endoleaks (continued perfusion of the aneurysm sac), movement, failure and thromboembolic complications of prostheses such that 30% require revision or removal.

Thoracic and thoracoabdominal aortic aneurysm

These aneurysms are much less common than AAA and may present incidentally or with back pain and dyspnoea if expanding rapidly or dissecting. Repair should be considered if symptoms occur or if expansion occurs in an asymptomatic, fit patient. Surgery is associated with a considerable operative mortality and morbidity (particularly paraplegia and renal failure). Cardiopulmonary bypass is required for most thoracic aneurysm repairs. EVAR techniques are under investigation and have many potential advantages.

Iliac artery aneurysms

The common iliac (90%), internal iliac (9–10%) and rarely the external iliac (1%) arteries may be affected. They may occur in isolation or in conjunction with an AAA. They are rarer than AAA but are usually degenerative. False aneurysms can arise where there has been previous aorto-iliac surgery. They usually go undetected, but may give rise to symptoms attributable to pelvic organs or present as a pulsating pelvic mass. CT scanning is the most reliable imaging technique. Rupture is often the first indication and surgery for this complication has a higher mortality than that for AAA rupture. Common and external iliac artery aneurysms require exclusion and grafting, whereas internal iliac artery aneurysms can usually be ligated or possibly embolized if unilateral.

Femoral artery aneurysms

Femoral artery aneurysms may be true or false. True aneurysms often occur in conjunction with aneurysms at other sites (they affect 3–7% of patients with AAA). The common and superficial femoral arteries are usually affected. False femoral aneurysms affect 3% of groin anastomoses. Many femoral aneurysms are symptomless, but the presence of a pulsatile mass is common. Lower limb ischaemia caused by thrombosis, embolism or less commonly, rupture, occurs in about one third of patients.

Popliteal artery aneurysms

These are bilateral in 50% of patients and account for 70% of peripheral aneurysms. In over half of patients affected these aneurysms present with distal leg ischaemia caused by thrombosis or embolism. Less than 10% of presentations are for rupture. Thromboembolic distal ischaemia is ideally treated using thrombolysis, followed by aneurysm ligation and bypass. Large, asymptomatic aneurysms in fit patients should be repaired.

Axillosubclavian aneurysms

These aneurysms usually present as a mass in the supraclavicular fossa. Post-stenotic dilatation caused by a cervical rib may occur with symptoms of thoracic outlet syndrome. Distal embolization or thrombosis may occur, resulting in digital ischaemia or dense ischaemia of the forearm and hand. Treatment is by ligation and bypass with or without excision of cervical rib.

Carotid aneurysms

These account for less than 5% of peripheral aneurysms and are situated at the carotid bifurcation. They must be distinguished from tortuous and ectatic arteries. Patients may present with neurological symptoms as a result of embolization and treatment is by resection and replacement.

Visceral aneurysms

1. *Splenic artery.* These are the second commonest abdominal aneurysm comprising two thirds of all visceral aneurysms. They are four times commoner in women than in men and occur during childbearing years and in old age. They are usually symptomless, unless they rupture. Rupture is most likely during the third trimester of pregnancy. Treatment is by aneurysm excision and interposition grafting, ligation or splenectomy and should be considered if the aneurysm exceeds 3 cm diameter or during pregnancy.

2. *Hepatic artery.* These are one third as common as splenic artery aneurysms. They usually present with rupture into the biliary system causing biliary colic, obstructive jaundice and upper gastrointestinal haemorrhage. Treatment is by aneurysm excision and grafting if possible.

3. *Coeliac and mesenteric arteries.* These are rare and usually present with non-specific abdominal pain. Sometimes a mobile pulsatile mass is present. They are frequently mycotic. Resection and reconstruction should ideally be performed, but the collateral circulation will sometimes allow simple ligation.

4. *Renal artery.* These aneurysms are rare and are usually associated with hypertension. Rupture is unusual and most can be ignored.

Further reading

Scott RAP, Wilson NM, Ashton HA, Kay DM. Influence of screening on the incidence of ruptured abdominal aortic aneurysm: 5-year results of a randomised controlled study. *British Journal of Surgery*, 1995; **82:** 1066–1070.

Thompson MM, Sayers RD. Arterial aneurysms. In: Beard JD, Gaines P, eds. *Companion to Specialist Surgical Practice. Vol VII. Arterial Surgery.* London: WB Saunders 1998.

UK Small Aneurysm Trial Participants. Mortality results for randomised controlled trial of early elective surgery or ultrasonographic surveillance for small abdominal aortic aneurysms. *Lancet*, 1998; **352:** 1649–1655.

Related topics of interest

Critical leg ischaemia (p. 100); Intermittent claudication (p. 187); Renovascular surgery (p. 284).

ANORECTAL INVESTIGATION

Nick Lagattolla

Anorectal investigations comprise the objective measurement of the various components of anorectal function and their contribution to the normal state of anal continence. The results obtained may be applied to the accurate and objective diagnosis of anorectal disease, subsequent treatment, and the assessment of its effect.

Maintenance of continence

This is dependent upon a combination of factors.

1. Anal sphincters.   The internal anal sphincter (IAS) is a major determinant of flatus and faecal continence, providing as much as 80% of the pressure within the anal canal through tonic contraction. The IAS is under autonomic control with the parasympathetic system inhibiting, and sympathetic fibres stimulating contraction. The external anal sphincter (EAS) is comprised of voluntary striated muscle innervated by branches of the pudendal nerve. The IAS and EAS complex constitutes an effective muscular barrier to the inadvertent efflux of faeces.

2. Puborectalis and the anorectal angle.   The puborectalis muscle also plays an important role in faecal continence. This striated muscle, supplied by the S4 nerve root via the pudendal nerve, maintains an angle between the rectum and upper anal canal. Damage to puborectalis results in incontinence. The anorectal angle may function as a flap valve so that an increase in intra-abdominal pressure results in compression of the anterior rectal wall into the upper anal canal, thus occluding its lumen.

3. Intact rectal and anal sensation.   Distension of the rectum with faeces results in a sensation of filling which is an additional factor in continence. The receptors for this reflex are located in the musculature of the pelvic floor and also probably in the rectal wall itself. The existence of sensory receptors in the mucosa of the lower anal canal allows fine discrimination between flatus and faeces, which again contributes to the maintenance of faecal continence.

4. Other factors.   These include the capacious and compliant nature of the rectal reservoir and also the formation of bulky solid faeces.

Clinical investigations

1. Anal manometry.   Pressure measurements are taken from within the anal canal. The maximum squeeze pressure (MSP) refers to the highest recorded pressure at any site within the anal canal during maximal contraction of the pelvic floor, and reflects the activity of the EAS and thus of voluntary continence. The maximum resting anal pressure (MRP) is mainly an indicator of IAS activity. Anal manometry is a useful technique in studying continence and its disturbance, particularly after pelvic colorectal surgery (low anterior resections, ileo-anal pouch formation and sphincter repair procedures).

2. **Rectal sensation.** This is the subjective response of the patient as known volumes of air or water are introduced into a balloon that has been placed in the rectum, while rectal compliance is an objective measure of the response during rectal distension. Compliance is measured in units of volume/pressure over volumes up to a litre, depending on patient tolerance.

3. **Electromyography (EMG).** This technique allows an objective and physiological measurement of muscle denervation by recording the electrical activity in the puborectalis, EAS and IAS through appropriate placement of fine-wire electrodes. Thus EMG can map sphincter deficiencies, or, alternatively, locate the position of an ectopic sphincter.

4. **Endo-anal ultrasound.** This is a new technique that has emerged from modification of the endorectal ultrasound probe. The investigation is performed with the patient in the left lateral position and is relatively comfortable as compared to EMG. Images are taken from the upper, middle and lower anal canal and thus the entire sphincter complex is examined. Defects in the puborectalis, EAS and even IAS can be clearly visualized and localized. Additionally, the integrity of sphincter reconstruction procedures can be assessed.

5. **Defecating proctography.** This technique can reveal anatomical abnormalities such as rectal and anal intussusception, rectocele and megarectum, but its main application lies in the observation of the sequence of events in incontinence and rectal prolapse. Videoproctography and still radiographs are taken during rest, maximal contraction of the pelvic floor and defecation of a known volume of radio-opaque stool substitute introduced into the rectum. Anorectal angle, perineal and pelvic floor descent can be calculated from the still radiographs during videoproctography. The investigation can be integrated with puborectalis, EAS and IAS EMG together with anal manometry (dynamic integrated videoproctography).

6. **Colonic transit time.** Colonic transit is assessed by asking the patient to swallow radio-opaque markers of three different shapes on three consecutive mornings while fully active and off all laxatives. Plain abdominal radiographs are taken on the fourth and seventh days to assess the progress of the markers and hence calculate the transit time. The use of such studies is normally confined to the investigation of patients with intractable constipation in whom total colectomy is being considered.

Further reading

Bartolo DCC *et al.* Flap valve theory of anorectal incontinence. *British Journal of Surgery*, 1986; **73:** 1012–1014.

Related topic of interest

Anorectal sepsis and fissure (p. 30).

ANORECTAL SEPSIS AND FISSURE

Deya Marzouk

Anorectal abscesses

Aetiology

- Idiopathic in >80% of patients. These are thought to be secondary to infection in one of the 6–10 anal glands resulting in an intersphincteric abscess, which may extend in various directions (cryptoglandular hypothesis of Eisenhammer). These glands commonly ramify into the internal anal sphincter and can extend as far as the intersphincteric plane. They drain into the base of the anal crypts, i.e. at level of dentate line.
- Secondary to specific causes in 20% of patients. These may include IBD, especially Crohn's disease, local causes such as anorectal cancer, fissure, trauma or following anorectal surgery. AIDS patients are prone to develop opportunistic infections in the anorectal region.
- Pelvirectal abscesses are a special subset and many of these are secondary to diverticulitis, IBD or rarely tubo-ovarian sepsis.

Bacteriology

Bacteria isolated from these abscesses are either skin organisms such as *Staphylococcus epidermis* and *Staphylococcus aureus* or are gut organisms such as *Bacteroides fragilis*, *E. coli* or Enterococci. The main advantage of sending a specimen for culture and sensitivity from these abscesses is that isolation of gut flora makes a fistula very likely[a]. On the other hand culture of skin organisms usually mean there is no fistula.

Clinical features, diagnosis and classification

Patients usually present with **continuous** throbbing anal pain, painful defecation, tender swelling near the anus and anal discharge. Inspection of the anus and perianal area may disclose an obvious perianal (at anal margin) or ischiorectal (to one side of anus) abscess, which may be already discharging pus. Patients with intersphincteric, postanal or supralevator abscesses will show nothing on inspection, but digital rectal examination usually reveals localized tenderness. Patients with ischiorectal, postanal and supralevator abscesses may be febrile.

Suspicion of deep postanal or supralevator abscess with or without horseshoe extension calls for evaluation of anorectal anatomy by preoperative MRI or CT scan, but these should not delay operative drainage.

Delay in diagnosis may cause catastrophic damage to anal sphincters. Rarely these abscesses may be complicated by necrotizing fasciitis of the perineum and levator ani muscles especially in immunocompromised and diabetic patients[c].

Anorectal abscesses are classified into:

1. **Subcutaneous** (perianal) abscess (60%).
2. **Intersphincteric** abscess (5%).
3. **Ischiorectal** abscess (30%).

4. **Deep postanal** abscess (1%): This is rare and is located in the deep postanal space in the midline posteriorly. It is wedged inferior to the levator ani muscles and posterior and deeper to the external sphincter muscles. Patients usually complain of severe rectal pain, which may radiate to the lower back and buttocks and is frequently febrile. The pain may cause the patient to stop defecating. If it starts to drain into the rectum, pain may subside partly and the patient notices purulent anal discharge. Inspection of the anus and buttocks may reveal nothing. The diagnosis is clinched on bidigital examination (index in anal canal and thumb outside the external sphincter posteriorly). This reveals exquisite posterior rectal tenderness and may suggest the presence of a horseshoe or supralevator extension.

5. **Supralevator** abscess (2%): These usually present with deep-seated pelvic and buttock pain as well as fever. Examination reveals a tender mass above the levator muscles. Most patients have inflammatory bowel disease, although a minority is secondary to complicated trans-sphincteric fistula or a high extension from an intersphincteric fistula.

Treatment of anorectal abscesses

All patients need examination under anaesthesia (EUA) and incision-drainage of the abscess. It is mandatory to send a specimen from the pus to look for gut organisms (as this indicates a high possibility of a fistula). All swabs culturing gut organisms indicate the need for a subsequent EUA after 6 weeks.

Anal fistulae are present in 40–50% of patients with perianal abscesses and most patients with other types. Fistulotomy is only done if a fistula is encountered easily. Probing oedematous infected tissues may actually create an internal opening converting an abscess into a fistula.

It is advisable to drain ischiorectal abscesses by an incision close to the anal margin, so that should the patient require subsequent fistulotomy, he or she is not left with a wound extending far laterally which needs longer time to heal.

1.   Role of a second EUA (looking for a fistula).   This is indicated in all those with gut flora organisms, usually 7 to 10 days after the initial incision and drainage of the abscess.

2.   Treatment of supralevator abscess.   Treatment depends on the aetiology of fistula. Drainage should be into the rectum in cases secondary to pelvic sepsis (external drainage creates a high anal fistula). On the other hand supralevator abscesses thought to be secondary to trans-sphincteric fistulae (identified by an internal opening at the level of the dentate line or external openings) should be drained via the perineum (internal drainage creates a high anal fistula) in addition to managing the primary fistulous tract. Ocassionally a supralevator abscess is secondary to a blind superior tract from an intersphincteric fistula. These are identified by an internal opening at the dentate line with a tract running superiorly and almost parallel to the rectal lumen to the supralevator abscess. The latter should be drained to the rectum (external drainage via the perineum leads to an extrasphincteric fistula).

Anal fistulae

Aetiology

- Most anal fistulae result from pyogenic anorectal abscesses.
- Some are secondary to specific causes such as Crohn's, TB or carcinoma.
- Rarely they are secondary to actinomycosis or lymphogranuloma venerum.

Clinical features and diagnosis

The most frequent symptoms are discharge, pain and swelling. Discharge tends to occur intermittently, while swelling and pain are usually associated with abscess formation, when the external opening is closed.

Clinical examination may reveal the presence of one or more external openings, discharge and soiling of underclothes. Bidigital examination (placing the index finger inside the anal canal and the thumb on the outside) may reveal the induration of the tract and occasionally the induration of the internal opening. Goodsall's rule is useful in determining the possible location of the internal opening based on the location of the external opening, although exceptions occasionally occur.

Goodsall's rule: When the external opening lies anterior to a transverse line between ischial tuberosities, the internal opening tends to be located radially. Conversely when the external opening lies posterior to this plane and those >3 cm from anal verge usually open internally in midline posteriorly.

All patients must have rigid sigmoidoscopy to exclude inflammatory bowel disease and neoplasia.

Radiological assessment is limited to selected cases, if clinical assessment is difficult (e.g. in cases of complex or recurrent fistulae). MRI scan of the anal canal and perianal area can be invaluable in delineating the anatomy of these fistulae.

Final assessment is done intraoperatively by initial examination under anaesthesia, using anoscopy to search for the internal opening as well as probing using malleable probes. Injection techniques using methylene blue, indigo carmine, milk and hydrogen peroxide may also help to locate elusive tracts.

Anal fistulae always have a primary tract (see below), but may also have an associated abscess cavity and/or a secondary tract or tracts. Some of these secondary tracts may be in the form of horseshoe extensions. Successful treatment depends on identification and dealing with all these tracts during surgery.

Classification

Anal fistulae have been traditionally classified according to the location of the internal opening into low (below puborectalis), high (at or just above puborectalis) and anorectal (rectum). Sir Alan Parks classified them according to the location of the primary tract into: intersphincteric, transsphincteric, extrasphincteric and suprasphincteric fistulae.

1. Intersphincteric.   Primary internal opening is on the dentate line, runs through the internal sphincter and then between internal and external sphincters to open on the perineal skin. It may have a secondary high blind tract or rarely a second opening upwards higher than the dentate line.

2. *Transsphincteric.* Primary internal opening is on the dentate line, runs through both the internal and external sphincters into the ischiorectal fossa and then to perineal skin. It may have secondary tracks horizontally (horseshoe) or blind vertical secondary tracks (infra- or supralevator).

3. *Suprasphincteric.* Primary internal opening is on the dentate line, runs through the internal sphincter and then upwards intersphincterically and discharges through the levator ani into the ischiorectal fossa and then perineal skin. The tract curves above the puborectalis sling.

4. *Extrasphincteric.* The internal opening is above the levators and the track runs external to the external sphincter. This type may be secondary to pelvic sepsis (diverticulitis, Crohn's disease), rectal trauma, and rectal Crohn's disease. It may also be secondary to development of a secondary supralevator tract in a transsphincteric fistula.

Treatment of non-specific anal fistulae

Treatment strategy consists of drainage of pus collections during the acute stage (abscess) and eradication of all fistula tracts with maximum preservation of sphincter muscles soon afterwards.

1. *Fistulotomy with or without sphincter repair.* Fistulous tracts may be eradicated by excision or coring, but this is rarely practised nowadays as laying open of tracts with curettage of blind tracts and cavities often achieve similar results with better preservation of continence[b]. Laying open of fistulous tracts often means partial division of sphincter muscles. Division of any of the sphincters threatens continence, however this is more so with division of the external sphincter and certain with division of the puborectalis. If a substantial part of the external sphincter is divided, it is often advisable to combine this with partial sphincter repair (repair of the uppermost part of divided sphincter) after thorough curettage of the tract's infected granulation tissue.

Other methods. These include coring out the tract and closure of internal opening (simple closure or using mucosal advancement flap) and/or sphincter repair.

Setons. A seton is a length of suture material (prolene, nylon or rubber sling) used to traverse the fistulous tract. It may be used when the fistula tract encircles > 30% of sphincter complex or when local sepsis or fibrosis preclude coring out, sphincter repair and raising of advancement flap.

These are of two types: loose setons and tight setons. Loose setons are used to drain pus or allow staged division of fistula (laying open the lower half, passing a seton around the upper half and dividing it at a second operation after healing of the lower half). Tight setons are used to progressively cut through the sphincters.

It is important when using a tight seton to lay open track outside sphincters, divide the perineal skin overlying the encircled tissue as well as the internal sphincter, so that the seton encircles mainly the external sphincter (or part of it), otherwise excessive fibrosis result. Tightening of seton is only started after sepsis has settled completely (usually 3 weeks post-operatively) every 1–2 weeks.

2. *Drainage of postanal abscess and horseshoe fistulae.* Treatment is challenging. The traditional treatment of deep postanal abscesses and the almost inevitable horseshoe extension has been laying open of the primary tract in the midline posteriorly, as well as secondary horseshoe extension laterally. This results in a large gaping wound that needs months to heal. More often, however, the primary posterior midline tract is laid open, with coring out of other external openings and curettage of secondary tracts. This may be combined with drainage of individual secondary external openings. The latter approach markedly reduces healing time[c].

Alternatively, an incision is made 2 cm posterior to the anal verge in the midline and deepened to adequately deroof the postanal space. This is combined with enlarging the internal opening at the dentate line in the middline posteriorly, division of the internal sphincter and skin to the first incision and a tight seton is applied around the external sphincter to progressively divide it over the succeeding 3–4 weeks. This may be combined with separate stab incision to deroof lateral horseshoe extensions.

Anal fissure

Anal fissure is a longitudinal tear in the anal canal anoderm (area between dentate line and anal verge). There are two types: acute and chronic fissures. Inadequately treated acute fissures may become chronic. Acute fissure is a superficial tear with no induration and no associated skin tag. Chronic fissure is a deeper tear extending down to (and exposing) the internal sphincter and is usually associated with fibrosis, external skin tag (sentinel pile) at the lower end and internal anal polyp at the upper end. It rarely extends beyond the dentate line. Fissures are located in the posterior midline in 99% of men and 90% of women. Most of the rest are located in the anterior midline (some are lateral or even multiple).

Aetiology

The vast majority of fissures are idiopathic. Fissures are rarely secondary to specific causes, such as Crohn's disease, leukaemia or TB.

The aetiology of idiopathic fissures is still incompletely understood. It was traditionally thought to be secondary to a tear of the anoderm from the passage of hard faeces. It is also rarely seen following transanal surgical procedures or forced anal intercourse.

More recently, anal fissures are thought to be ischaemic in origin. The blood supply to the posterior midline anoderm seems to be less dense than elsewhere in the anal canal in most people[b]. High internal sphincter pressure (spasm) associated with a fissure, further reduces the perfusion of the posterior commissure, causing rest pain and ulceration (non-healing).

It is possible that fissures are initiated by one event (resulting in the tear to the anoderm) and then maintained by ischaemia induced by sphincter spasm. A vicious cycle of pain – internal sphincter spasm – ichaemia – poor healing – chronicity sets in.

Clinical features and diagnosis

The most prominent symptom is pain **during and after defecation** (75–100% of patients). Equally frequent is bleeding per rectum, which is always bright red in colour and on the surface of motion. Other symptoms include anal discharge and pruritus ani. Symptoms of chronic anal fissure are typically cyclical with periods of acute pain followed by temporary healing, only to be succeeded by further acute pain.

Examination usually suggests or confirms the diagnosis. Most fissures lie in the midline posteriorly or anteriorly. Fissures that lie laterally should raise strong suspicion of a specific cause. Gentle parting of buttocks usually reveals the mucosal tear in acute fissures. It is not necessary or possible to examine patients with acute fissure digitally. However, if an acute fissure cannot be seen on parting the buttocks, one has to consider the possibility of alternative causes of acute anal pain and it is justifiable to attempt gentle digital examination to exclude intersphincteric and postanal abscesses. If this causes any pain, it should be terminated and either the patient is treated as an acute fissure and reviewed soon afterwards or examined under a short anaesthetic if there is doubt about the diagnosis.

Chronic fissures are often less painful and most patients can be examined digitally (advisable to exclude anal canal cancer). These chronic fissures are usually indurated and there may be associated skin tags (sentinel pile) and anal polyps. Rarely long-standing chronic fissures may result in anal stenosis.

Investigations

Endoanal ultrasound and anal canal manometry are only needed in patients thought to be at high risk of incontinence following lateral sphincterotomy. These include patients with history of imperfect continence, clinically weak sphincters and women who had third degree tears during labour.

Treatment of idiopathic fissures

Many acute fissures heal spontaneously without medical intervention[c]. Those patients who present to doctors tend to have more severe pain and warrant active treatment. The aim of treatment is to abolish internal sphincter spasm. This leads to rise in anoderm blood supply and healing of fissures. This may be accomplished by dividing the internal sphincter surgically or pharmacologically by GTN cream. Acute fissures often respond to conservative measures, while a substantial proportion of chronic fissures eventually need surgery.

1. Conservative medical treatment. This consists of avoidance of constipation, increasing consumption of vegetables, fruit and whole grain bread as well as warm sitz baths. Topical local anaesthetic creams may also be useful. This regime heals more than 80% of acute fissures within 2–3 weeks[b].

2. Topical glyceryl trinitrate (GTN) 0.2% treatment. Relaxation of internal sphincter may be mediated physiologically by nitrous oxide. This explains response to GTN cream, which acts as a nitrous oxide donor. GTN 0.2% cream is used twice daily for 8–12 weeks. Initial healing rates were reported to be up to 90%. Long-term controlled studies showed that it probably succeeds in only 50–60% of cases[a]. The major side effect with GTN is headaches, which occur in half or more of patients and may be severe necessitating stoppage of treatment in 15%[b]. Poor tolerance or poor compliance with GTN treatment often contributes to fissure nonhealing. Some fissures which initially heal with GTN recur (30–40%) and require further treatment. It is thus important for patients to be made aware that treatment is likely to take some months to be effective, may need repeating and may be associated with headaches. Despite these shortcomings, it is a worthwhile first line of treatment in many if not all patients.

3.   *Internal lateral sphincterotomy.* This remains the gold standard surgical treatment. It results in healing of 96% or more of all fissures[b]. It can be done by an open technique or by a closed technique (in the latter the anus is gently stretched by a Parks retractor and the intersphincteric plane is defined and a fine blade is introduced in this plane to divide the internal sphincter). The major disadvantage of lateral sphincterotomy is that it may result in continence defects in up to 11% in the immediate postoperative period (usually incontinence to flatus). This may be permanent in about 1% of patients[c].

The incidence of continence defects seems to correlate with the length of the sphincterotomy cut in the internal sphincter. It may be advisable to limit the extent of the sphincterotomy to the length of the fissure rather than extending to or above the dentate line (tailored or measured lateral sphincterotomy)[b]. Some of these patients with continence defects may be amenable to internal sphincter repair subsequently.

Internal lateral sphincterotomy may be combined with excision of external skin tag and anal papilla. Excision of the fissure itself is rarely necessary, unless edges are very fibrosed and likely to hamper healing or if biopsy is required to exclude anal canal carcinoma or specific causes of fissures.

4.   *The role of anal dilatation (gentle anal stretch).* Maximum anal dilatation (Lord) is no longer used, because of the high risk of incontinence, it leads to internal sphincter fragmentation and occasionally may also cause external sphincter defects. Even gentle 2 or 3 finger dilatation is no longer accepted as appropriate treatment of fissures, again because of the uncontrolled disruption of the internal anal sphincter. The latter is only acceptable in patients in whom an EUA reveals sphincter fibrosis making distinction of internal and external sphincters impossible[c].

5.   *Other methods.* Advancement V–Y flaps is rarely used, when anal canal pressure is low or in recurrent fissures despite bilateral internal sphincterotomy at 3 and 9 o'clock. Botulinum A toxin injection has also been tried in treatment of anal fissures, but experience is scanty. Posterior internal sphincterotomy may result in the so-called 'keyhole' deformity with a higher tendency to leakage than lateral sphincterotomy[c]. St Marks dilators are seldom used these days. They may be lubricated with local anaesthetic cream and inserted up to its hilt for 1 minute, twice daily in some mild chronic fissures (without skin tags) with fair results.

Treatment of fissures secondary to specific diseases

In the vast majority of these patients, pain is not a prominent symptom and they can be adequately treated medically as outlined above. In particular patients with

Crohn's disease (especially when it affects the rectum) should not have lateral sphincterotomy because of the risk of non-healed wounds. Surgery is reserved for patients who develop anorectal sepsis and fistulae arising from the base of the fissure and should consist of drainage of pus mainly.

Further reading

Altomare DF, Rinaldi M, Milito G *et al*. Glyceryl trinitrate for chronic anal fissure – healing or headache? Results of a multicenter, randomized, placebo-controled, double-blind trial. *Diseases of Colon and Rectum*, 2000; **43**: 174–179; discussion 179–181.

Garcia-Aguilar J, Belmonte Montes C, Perez JJ, Jensen L, Madoff RD, Wong WD. Incontinence after lateral internal sphincterotomy: anatomic and functional evaluation. *Diseases of Colon and Rectum*, 1998; **41**: 423–427.

Lund JN, Scholefield JH. Aetiology and treatment of anal fissure. *British Journal of Surgery*, 1996; **83**: 1335–1344.

Philips RKS, Lunniss PJ. In: Philips RKS and Lunniss PJ, Eds. *Anal Fistula: Surgical Evaluation and Management*. 1st edition. London, Chapman & Hall Medical. 1996.

ANTIBIOTICS AND BACTERIAL RESISTANCE

Nick Lagattolla

Antibiotics are the most commonly prescribed pharmaceutical. They have vital roles in both the treatment of specific infections, and the prophylaxis of infection, particularly in surgical practice. Unfortunately, antibiotics are overprescribed. Bacteria develop resistance to antibiotics through exposure to antibiotics with only partial activity, combined with an innate ability to adapt. Newer generations of antibiotics are continually being developed to combat bacterial resistance.

Antibiotics in common surgical practice

1. Penicillins. These are bactericidal, and there are four groups. Benzylpenicillin (penicillin G) was the first discovered, and is administered parenterally. The oral form is phenoxymethylpenicillin (penicillin V). This is active against most Gram-positive cocci, though *Staphylococcus aureus* has developed many resistant strains, and Gram-positive bacteria, including *Clostridium tetani* and *Clostridium welchii*, and *Bacillus anthracis*.

Penicillinase-resistant penicillin molecules include flucloxacillin, which is highly active against *Staphylococcus aureus*. The broad-spectrum penicillins include ampicillin, amoxycillin and co-amoxiclav, which is the latter combined with the beta-lactamase inhibitor clavulanic acid. The spectrum is augmented to include many Gram-negative bacilli, though not pseudomonas. However, the carboxypenicillin ticarcillin, and the ureidopenicillins azlocillin and piperacillin, are active against pseudomonas. Some of these antipseudomonal penicillins are also available with clavulanic acid to further the spectrum.

2. Cephalosporins. This important group of antibiotics are bactericidal, structurally similar to the penicillins, and may be termed beta-lactams. Three generations are recognized. The spectrum of all of these is very broad and similar for each drug. The first generation has given rise to the favoured oral cephalosporins, including cephalexin, cephadroxil and cephradine. The second gereration gave rise to the popular cefuroxime, which is greatly favoured in surgical practice for both prophylaxis and treatment. An oral version is available. The third generation includes cefotaxime, ceftriaxone and ceftazidime, and all are delivered parenterally.

Newer related antibiotics in this group include aztreonam, a mono-bactam, which is active against Gram-negative aerobic bacteria, but not against Gram-positives. The carbopenems include imipenem and meropenem, which have particularly broad spectrums.

3. Aminoglycosides. These are bacteriocidal and highly active against some Gram-positive and many Gram-negative organisms, particularly bacilli, though not all are anti-pseudomonal. The exceptional activity against Gram-negative bacilli has to be offset against potentially severe ototoxicity and nephrotoxicity which mandate the monitoring of plasma levels. Gentamicin is the most commonly used. It may only be given parenterally, but may still be the antibiotic of choice in severe systemic infections of unknown aetiology, to cover a variety of organisms causing endo-carditis and Gram-negative septicaemia. Neomycin is used topically; orally it obliterates bowel flora, as it is non-absorbed and highly bacteriocidal.

4.   Metronidazole.   This is an important anti-anaerobic antibiotic with excellent activity against *Bacteroides fragilis*. The widespread use of this agent in the 1970s resulted in an appreciable reduction in mortality and morbidity following bowel surgery. It has an important role in the prophylaxis against and the treatment of any intra-abdominal bowel-related infection. It is also active against many protozoa and is indicated in giardiasis and entamoeba infections.

5.   Tetracyclines.   These are bacteriostatic and have little to do with surgical practice, though it is important to note that a wide variety of atypical organisms are susceptible. These include chlamydiae, rickettsiae, mycoplasma, and borrelia which is responsible for Lyme disease. Doxycycline has good penetration into prostatic tissue, and is thus often used to treat chronic prostatitis.

6.   Macrolides.   This group includes erythromycin which has a spectrum very similar to penicillin, and is thus used as an alternative to penicillin in allergic patients. It has activity against a variety of bacilli including legionella, chlamydia, *Corynaebacterium diphtheriae* and mycoplasma, and is thus often the treatment of choice in atypical pneumonias. It is active against campylobacter and may be used to treat the bloody diarrhoea resulting from this infection. However, erythromycin may cause gastrointestinal side effects, and the newer clarithromycin and azithromycin result in less disturbances.

7.   4-Quinolones.   This group includes ciprofloxacin, which has a broad spectrum including Gram-negative and Gram-positive bacteria, especially Gram-negative bacilli. It is particularly indicated in respiratory, gastrointestinal and genito-urinary infections.

Development of antibiotic resistance

Resistance can signify that a bacterium has developed tolerance to an antibiotic, or that it has developed enzymatic activity against an antibiotic. Resistance can super-vene by mutation of a bacterium, particularly in response to prolonged antibiotic treatment, ineffectual dosage, or persistent infection within an impenetrable focus despite antibiotic therapy. Examples of tolerance include urinary tract Gram-negative bacillus infections and resistance to nalidixic acid. Enzymatic resistance is best shown by the beta-lactamase (penicillinase) producing *Staphylococcus aureus* that render many strains resistant to penicillin, a characteristic that happily strepto-coccus species have not mastered.

Resistance may be transferred from one resistant organism to a non-resistant organism by the transfer of gene packages conferring drug resistance. This can arise from the action of bacteriophages, or by transfer of R-plasmids, which contain extra-chromosomal genetic material, which are transferred freely between coliform bacteria usually found in the gut.

Apparent resistance may occur if a site becomes infected by an already-resistant organism during the treatment of an infection from a sensitive organism. This is termed superinfection. Importantly, resistance may occur in a single bacterial strain simultaneously to a wide variety of antibiotics, resulting in so-called multi-resistance.

Methicillin-resistant *Staphylococcus aureus* (MRSA) and other resistant organisms

MRSA is the most prevalent of the multiply resistant bacteria. It is a frequent colonizer of asymptomatic individuals, but may result in severe focal and systemic infections, which are life-threatening. Treatment where necessary is usually parenteral vancomycin. Once present in a ward environment, it is difficult to eradicate. Measures to control include isolation of suspected cases as well as known cases, utilization of disposable garments and masks, and topical antisepsis. Measures to eradicate may amount to the temporary cessation of all clinical work and extensive general disinfection and cleaning. However recurrent outbreaks are common.

Vancomycin-resistant enterococcus (VRE) outbreaks occur in a similar fashion to MRSA, often on specialized surgical and medical units, and are dealt with by isolation of cases, and institution of standard precautionary measures.

The organism responsible for the STD gonorrhoea is virtually totally sensitive to penicillin and its derivatives; however a resistant strain is identified as penicillinase-producing nesseria gonnorrhoea (PPNG), named after the mode by which it has attained resistance. Strains of pneumococcus and meningococus have also developed penicillin resistance, rendering this an innapropriate first-line treatment.

Further reading

Review

Condon RE, Wittmann DH. The use of antibiotics in general surgery. In: *Current Problems in Surgery.* Wells A, Ed. 1991.

Metanalysis

Song F, Glenny A-M. Antimicrobial prophylaxis in colorectal surgery: a systematic review of randomized controlled trials. *British Journal of Surgery*, 1998; **85:** 1232–1241.

ASSESSMENT OF THE ACUTE ABDOMEN

Nick Lagattolla

The acute abdomen is a vague term referring to any condition causing abdominal pain of recent onset. Most causes reside within the abdomen, however there are exceptions. Pain may result from epigastric pain in inferior myocardial infarction or basal pneumonia. Conversely, abdominal pathology may present outside the abdomen, for example shoulder tip pain from subdiaphragmatic irritation by free blood (Kehr's sign) or pus, or inner thigh pain from an obturator hernia (Howship-Romberg sign).

History

1.   Origin of pain.   It is essential to elicit a history from patients with an acute abdomen. In many inflammatory and obstructive conditions, pain is first experienced around the midline. This reflects the embryological origin of the diseased viscus, with pain from foregut structures referred to the epigastrium, midgut structures to the umbilicus and hindgut structures to the suprapubic area. This visceral pain is often poorly localized and colicky. An inflammatory process progressing through the bowel wall to involve the serosa causes local peritonitis, and the pain becomes constant and localized to the site of the inflammation.

2.   Colicky and constant pain.   The obstruction of a hollow viscus causes an intermittent cramping pain known as colic. This represents overactivity of the viscus in an attempt to relieve the obstruction: for example, obstructed small bowel, a midgut structure, causes central abdominal colic.

Obstruction of the ureters by calculi results in pain that radiates from the loin to the groin. The pain has very severe colicky exacerbations, though there is also a constant background ache. A similar pain in the loin suggests renal stones. The gallbladder and pancreas are foregut structures and thus biliary colic and acute pancreatitis are usually experienced in the epigastrium. The pain often radiates to the back in pancreatitis, and to the right hypochondrium in biliary colic.

Localized sepsis or peritonitis results in a constant pain in that area. The patient will have systemic signs of sepsis. Generalized peritonitis results from the presence of free intraperitoneal irritant fluid, such as pus, gastric juice, bile or blood. This causes a constant and severe generalized pain. Retroperitoneal haemorrhage also results in a severe constant pain, though this is experienced in the back rather than in the abdomen. Retroperitoneal haemorrhage often occurs to one side or in the iliac fossa, causing pain in the loin or groin respectively. This is a source of diagnostic confusion between leaking abdominal aortic aneurysms and renal or ureteric colic.

3.   Associated symptoms.   Vomiting occurs early and prominently in small bowel obstruction, but may not occur at all in colonic obstruction. Distension occurs in both small and large bowel obstruction. Vomiting may occur in association with severe abdominal pain, including ureteric colic and acute pancreatitis. An alteration in bowel habit or the passage of blood per rectum suggests colonic pathology.

Gynaecological symptoms must be sought in young women with acute abdominal pain. Missed menstruation with recent vaginal bleeding points to an ectopic pregnancy. Pains that are bilateral and inguinal plus the presence of a vaginal discharge point to salpingitis. Urinary frequency and dysuria suggest a lower urinary tract infection, and if associated with rigors and loin pain then an acute pyelonephritis is likely.

4. Past medical history. Small bowel obstruction with prior abdominal surgery suggests adhesion obstruction. Previous episodes of peptic ulceration, acute diverticulitis, biliary colic, or known chronic pancreatitis may prompt the diagnosis of recurrence of that disorder.

Examination

The patient is examined for tachycardia, pyrexia and hypotension. The presence of pallor, jaundice and lymphadenopathy is noted. Tachypnoea may signify an acidosis. The patient may be dehydrated from vomiting, as assessed by inspecting the tongue or feeling the turgidity of the skin. Cool and clammy peripheries suggest hypovolaemic shock, whilst warm peripheries and hypotension suggest endotoxaemia.

1. Abdominal inspection. A rigid abdomen from underlying peritonitis fails to move with respiration. Pain from an inflamed viscus may be reproduced on coughing. Masses may be visible such as pulsating abdominal aneurysms, retroperitoneal haematomas, hernias or tumours. The groins and scrotum are inspected for strangulated hernias. Old scars are noted. The abdomen may be distended.

2. Abdominal palpation. The acute abdomen is usually associated with tenderness. An exception occurs in acute mesenteric infarction which often causes exceptional pain but few signs. Localized tenderness suggests an inflamed viscus. If the inflammation involves the serosa, localized peritonitis is present, and pain will be felt if the examining hand is quickly released from the tender area. This represents rebound tenderness. This can be very painful and the sign should not be repeatedly elicited. A gentler method for eliciting rebound is percussion of the abdomen.

If the inflammation spreads to involve the parietal peritoneum, the patient will exhibit involuntary rigidity of the abdominal wall caused by reflex muscular tensing. Diffuse rigidity occurs if there is a generalized peritonitis. The patient appears unwell, with tachycardia, fever, hypotension or endotoxaemia. In a patient with no systemic signs but apparent rigidity on palpation, the rigidity is likely to be entirely voluntary and not true reflexic rigidity. Rigidity is often termed guarding.

3. Bowel sounds. In peritonitis these are often reduced or absent. Bowel obstruction causes increased, often tinkling sounds. The abdomen is distended in obstruction, and if one looks carefully, peristaltic waves may be seen coursing over the abdomen, particularly in small bowel obstruction.

Radiology

Small bowel and colonic obstruction is readily differentiated, as small bowel has numerous transverse folds (valvulae conniventes) that course around the entire circumference of the bowel, while colon has wide sacculations (haustrae). Multiple air–fluid levels occur on erect abdominal films in a 'step pattern' in small bowel obstruction. Colonic obstruction with an incompetent iliocaecal valve results in small bowel dilatation. If some colon is dilated, the obstruction must be colonic.

Free intraperitoneal gas indicates a perforated gas-containing hollow viscus. This is commonly caused by perforated peptic ulcers. The gas is seen under one or both hemidiaphragms, but up to 20% of patients with perforated peptic ulcers, and most patients with colonic perforations, do not have it. Free gas may also be seen between loops of bowel, such that both sides of the bowel wall are visible on a plain X-ray. This is known as Rigler's sign and may be the only clue of a colonic perforation.

Blood tests

FBC and U&E are requested. Arterial blood gases are performed if acute pancreatitis is suspected, or in any patient with suspected metabolic disturbance or renal failure. Serum amylase must be requested to exclude acute pancreatitis. In all cases, blood must be sent for group and save if there is any possibility of the patient undergoing surgery.

Immediate management

The severely unwell patient with an acute abdomen must be resuscitated fully and reassessed frequently. I.v. fluids, antibiotics and analgesia will settle many patients, and allow a clearer picture to emerge. The patient ought to be catheterized, and a central venous catheter placed via the internal jugular route. The immediate 'blind' operation of such patients results in a high mortality. Patients with severe acute pancreatitis for example frequently present in this fashion, and conservative treatment, rather than surgery, is required. If surgery later becomes necessary, then the additional resuscitation performed will be of benefit.

Special investigations

Peritoneal lavage with estimation of the amylase and red and white blood cell counts of the peritoneal fluid may be performed in cases where the diagnosis is in doubt. Laparoscopy is frequently performed in younger women presenting with lower abdominal pain, as the ovaries, uterine tubes or uterus are far more often the origin of lower abdominal pain than the appendix. Sometimes the cause of an acute abdomen remains obscure. If the clinical picture warrants it, the ultimate investigation for acute abdominal pain is a laparotomy.

Further reading

Reviews

Clain A. The acute abdomen. In: Clain A (ed.) *Hamilton Bailey's Demonstrations of Physical Signs in Clinical Surgery*. Briston Wright, 1986; 294–330.

de Dombal FT. Acute abdominal pain. *Surgery*, 1990; **82:** 1967–1971.

Patterson-Brown S, Vipond MN. Modern aids to clinical decision-making in the acute abdomen. *British Journal of Surgery*, 1990; **77:** 13–18.

Related topics of interest

Acute appendicitis (p. 4); Acute pancreatitis (p. 8); Aneurysms (p. 24); Common paediatric conditions (p. 96); Crohn's disease (p. 103); Diverticular disease (p. 116); Gallstones and their complications (p. 130); Intestinal obstruction (p. 190); Peptic ulceration (p. 255).

BENIGN BREAST DISEASE
Nick Wilson

Benign conditions of the breast are commoner than malignant disease. They present with a lump, pain, nipple retraction or nipple discharge and are frequently difficult to differentiate from malignant disease.

Congenital abnormalities

*1. **Absence of a breast.*** Complete absence of a breast and nipple (amastia) is accompanied by pectoral muscles aplasia or hypoplasia in 90% of cases. Breast hypoplasia (amazia) is commoner, and minor asymmetry quite normal. Breast construction, augmentation and/or reduction of the contralateral side may be required. Isolated a*bsence* of a *nipple* is very rare.

*2. **Accessory breasts and nipples.*** This is caused by failure of full regression of the primitive breast line. Supernumary nipples are present in 1–5% of people, but accessory breasts are less common. Treatment is by excision.

Developmental disorders

*1. **Excessive breast enlargement.*** Minor degrees of breast enlargement frequently occur in infancy, and before puberty. Uncontrolled juvenile hypertrophy usually occurs in the absence of endocrine abnormalities. Histological examination reveals proliferation of periductal connective tissue and ducts but not lobules. Breast reduction may be required.

Male breast enlargement (gynaecomastia) occurs in neonates, puberty (30–70% of boys) and old age. It is benign and usually regresses spontaneously. Occasionally, subcutaneous mastectomy is necessary. Pathological gynaecomastia can be induced by hypogonadism, hormone-secreting neoplasms, hepatic and renal disease and drugs (spironolactone, cimetidine, digoxin, metoclopramide, cytotoxics).

*2. **Fibroadenoma.*** These are probably developmental anomalies rather than benign neoplasms. They occur between 15 and 40 years, accounting for 15–20% of all discrete breast masses. They are firm, smooth, mobile and may be multiple. Clinical diagnosis is frequently wrong and FNAC or excision biopsy are advisable. Following diagnosis by FNAC, the fibroadenoma may be observed or removed. A few will gradually increase in size. Giant fibroadenoma (>5 cm diameter) are usually excised. Malignant change occurs occasionally (1 : 1000).

Disorders of cyclical change and involution

*1. **Cyclical mastalgia.*** This affects premenopausal women and is characterized by marked premenstrual breast nodularity and discomfort affecting the outer quadrants. There may be excessive prolactin release or abnormal sensitivity of breast tissue hormone receptors. FNAC, biopty or trucut biopsy are advisable to exclude malignancy. Histological changes include cyst formation, fibrosis, adenosis and epitheliosis. Mammography should be performed in women over 35. Reassurance, simple analgesia and a firm bra usually help. Linoleic acid (oil of evening primrose) is sometimes beneficial. Occasionally, danazol, bromocryptine or tamoxifen are required, but side effects occur in 30% of patients. Rarely, mastectomy or subcutaneous mastectomy with prosthetic replacement is justified.

2. Cystic disease. Palpable cysts occur frequently in women approaching the menopause. They present as discrete, smooth breast lumps. Hormonal profiles appear normal and the cause is unknown. Aspiration should be attempted. Yellow/green/brown fluid is obtained which should only be sent for cytological examination if evenly blood-stained. Ultrasound and mammography should be performed in women over 35 prior to aspiration. Persistence of a mass following aspiration, repeated refilling of a cyst and blood-stained aspirate with cytological abnormalities are indications for excision biopsy. Cysts associated with breast cancer are commoner in postmenopausal women and should be investigated. Repeated multiple cyst formation can be treated with danazol.

Infective disorders

1. Mastitis neonatorum. Neonatal breast enlargement may be complicated by infection and abscess formation. Antibiotics may help in the early stages, but if fluctuation develops, incision and drainage is necessary.

2. Lactational breast abscess. This is commonest in the first month after delivery and is caused by *Staphylococcus aureus, Staphylococcus epidermidis* or a *Streptococcus* entering through a cracked nipple. The breast becomes tense, inflamed and tender. Antibiotics can resolve the infection if given early. Repeated aspiration of pus and antibiotics may be successful, but frequently, incision and drainage is necessary. Providing no antibiotic harmful to neonates is used, lactation using both breasts may continue.

3. Non-lactational abscess. Most result as a complication of periductal mastitis, but should be distinguished from an inflammatory cancer by FNAC. Repeated aspiration with antibiotics may be attempted if the overlying skin is normal, otherwise incision and drainage are required. Mammary duct fistula may be a complication.

4. Tuberculosis, syphilis, actinomycosis. Rare. Tuberculosis usually spreads by lymphatics from regional lymph nodes or directly from a rib. An axillary or breast sinus is strongly suggestive. Treatment is by appropriate antituberculous chemotherapy. A syphylitic chancre may occur on the nipple with axillary lymphadenopathy. Syphilis and actinomycosis are treated with penicillin or other appropriate antibiotics.

Inflammatory disorders

1. Periductal mastitis. Women in their early 30s are affected. Smoking is an important factor. Mastalgia, nipple discharge, nipple retraction and peri-areolar inflammation are prominent. The main ducts are surrounded by polymorphs, giant cells and epithelioid cells, but are not dilated. Treatment is by antibiotics, but abscess or mammary duct fistula may follow.

2. **Duct ectasia.**   Duct dilatation occurs with an intermittent clear, cheesy or blood-stained discharge or nipple retraction. This affects older women. Cytology reveals benign changes only and duct thickening and coarse calcification may be seen on mammography. A persistent discharge can be treated by microdochectomy, or duct excision.

3. **Mammary duct fistula.**   Most follow periductal mastitis but may result from biopsy of a periareolar mass or incision and drainage of a non-lactational breast abscess. The nipple is usually indrawn. Fistulotomy or fistulectomy are frequently successful, but total duct and fistula excision may be required.

4. **Fat necrosis.**   A dense fibrous scar forms causing skin tethering and retraction, mimicking a carcinoma. In the early stages, haemorrhage can usually be seen, with fat liquefaction and surrounding inflammation. A history of trauma is often lacking. FNAC or excision are required to exclude carcinoma.

Benign neoplasms

1. **Duct papilloma.**   These are common and may be multiple. They present with a blood-stained nipple discharge. Treatment is by microdochectomy or total duct excision if there is multiple duct discharge.

2. **Lipoma.**   These are common, but may be confused with the soft fatty mass that sometimes surrounds a carcinoma.

3. **Granular cell myoblastoma, leiomyoma, chondroma, chondrolipoma, myxoma.**   All are rare and must be distinguished from carcinoma.

Miscellaneous

1. **Non-cyclical breast pain.**   No cause is usually found, but malignancy, costo-chondritis and periductal mastitis should be excluded. A firm bra and simple analgesia provide relief.

2. **Fibromatosis.**   Benign proliferation of myelofibroblasts. Behaves like desmoid tumours. A variant, nodular fasciitis affects the pectoral fascia.

3. **Haematoma.**   Follows FNAC, trucut biopsy, trauma or anticoagulation.

4. **Amyloid.**   Rare.

5. **Intramammary lymph node.**   Common. Enlarge in response to local or general causes.

6. **Silicone granulomas.**   Silicone used in breast augmentation may escape from the silastic capsule inducing the formation of granulomata and foreign-body giant cells. The prosthesis envelope can induce fibrous capsule formation.

7. **Galactocele.**   Encysted milk collection. Treated by aspiration.

8. **Mondor's disease.**   Superficial thrombophlebitis of veins overlying the breast. Usually self-limiting.

9. **Sebaceous cyst.**   Common on the skin overlying the breast.

10. *Eczema of the nipple.* A biopsy is frequently necessary to differentiate this from Paget's disease. Nipple erosion, unilateral site and an associated mass suggest Paget's disease. May signify underlying periductal mastitis or duct ectasia or may be local or part of generalized eczema.

11. *Nipple adenoma.* Ulceration of nipple. Remove by wide excision.

Further reading

Dixon JM, Mansel RE. The breast. In: Burnand KG, Young AE (eds). *The New Aird's Companion in Surgical Studies (2nd Edn)*. London: Churchill Livingstone, 1998: 631–663.

Related topic of interest

Breast cancer (p. 57).

BLADDER OUTFLOW OBSTRUCTION

Christopher Lattimer, Adrian Simoes

The pathology may be neuropathic due to the failure of the sphincters to relax in harmony with detrusor contraction or due to obstruction from bladder neck hypertrophy, BPH, urethral stricture, urethral calculus, meatal stenosis or a tight phimosis.

Urethral stricture

'Once a urethral stricture always a urethral stricture'. This adage still holds good. Pharaohs even took dilators with them to their burial chambers for the after life. The causes are numerous:

Insult	Urethral site	Mechanism
Catheter	Penoscrotal junction	Pressure necrosis
		Paraurethral gland sepsis
Perineal injury	Bulbar	Crush injury
Pelvic fracture	Membranous	Prostatic displacement
		Shear injury
Infection	throughout	Gonorrhoea
		Chlamydia
BXO	Meatal	Fibrosis
Chemotherapy	throughout	Chemical urethritis
Instrumentation	throughout	Iatrogenic
		Masturbation

Presentation

Depending on the degree and length of narrowing and the detrussor compensation the symptoms will vary. The symptoms are indistinguishable from bladder outflow obstruction due to any other cause. The finding may include thickening of the corpus spongiosum and a palpable bladder in patients who go into either chronic or acute on chronic retention.

Diagnosis

In those who present with retention failure to catheterize urethrally may suggest the possibility. Flow rate and abdominal ultrasound will indicate bladder outflow obstruction. The diagnosis is comfirmed on flexible/rigid cystoscopy or an ascending urethrogram.

Management

The management depends on the site, extent and degree of narrowing.

1.   Urethral dilatation.   This is the traditional way of opening up the stricture by using graded metallic or flexible dilators.

2.   Internal urethrotomy.   Using the optical urethrotome the stricture is incised open under vision. This technique has replaced urethral dilatation and to keep the stricture open urethrotomy may need to be followed by regular dilatation preferably by the patient.

3.   Urethroplasty.   When the above procedures fail then urethroplasty is undertaken using skin or buccal mucosa. The skin may be used as a split or full thickness graft and may be free or on a pedicle.

Benign prostatic hyperplasia

Benign prostatic hyperplasia (BPH) is increasingly common with age and is present in an estimated 50% of men over the age of 60 years and in nearly 88% by the age of 88 years. This is a histological diagnosis and is due to the hyperplasia of the periurethral glands in the transitional zone of the prostate. This enlargement causes varying degrees of obstruction to the flow of urine and leads to a group of symptoms categorized as lower urinary tract symptoms (LUTS). The extent of the prostatic enlargement may not be directly proportional to the degree of bladder outflow obstruction nor to the amount of symptoms. The clinical definition of BPH is therefore a combination of LUTS, palpable benign prostatic enlargement and urodynamic evidence of bladder outflow obstruction.

Presentation

Patients may have no symptoms and are found to have a palpable bladder due to chronic retention of urine and occasionally in post-renal obstructive renal failure. LUTS can be divided into two groups: obstructive symptoms associated with voiding which are hesitancy, poor stream, straining, prolonged micturition, post-micturition dribbling and a feeling of incomplete emptying, and irritative symptoms associated with filling which are frequency, nocturia and urgency. Patients may also present with acute retention, heamaturia and urinary tract infections.

Diagnosis

Physical examination of the abdomen will indicate a palpable or percussable bladder and digital rectal examination will assess the prostate. Patients are evaluated by using a validated symptom scoring system such as the International Prostate Symptom Score (I-PSS) and a Quality of Life Score due to urinary symptoms. Routine investigations include urinalysis, renal function estimation and PSA. Uroflowmetry and ultrasound of the urinary tract with assessment of post-micturation volume will suggest the degree of bladder outflow obstruction and in equivocal cases cystometry may be required to prove a high pressure low flow picture. A post-void volume of over 100 ml usually indicates significant obstruction. In certain cases cystoscopy and transrectal ultrasonography may be required to rule out any urethral or bladder pathology and to assess the size and morphology of the gland and to take biopsies.

Management

The choice of therapy depends on the severity of symptoms, the impact on quality of life and the complicating effects of bladder outflow obstruction. Surgical intervention is indicated for urinary retention which has failed a trial of voiding without the catheter, recurrent urinary tract infections, renal failure, recurrent gross haematuria, bladder stones and failure of other modalities of management which are as follows:

1. *Watchful waiting*

2. *Pharmacotherapy:*

- *Phytotherapy.* In recent years the use of plant extracts (Saw Palmetto) have become popular[c].
- *α-adrenergic antagonists.* These agents block the action of noradrenaline on the prostatic smooth muscle to cause relaxation and thereby better emptying of the bladder.
- *5α-reductase inhibitor.* Finasteride blocks the enzyme 5α-reductase which inhibits the conversion of testosterone to dihydrotestosterone. This reduces intracellular activity and brings about a decrease in the prostatic volume.

3. *Minimally invasive procedures.* These are mostly experimental and have not yet found their way into clinical practice and include prostatic stents, balloon dilatation of the prostate, electrovapourization, endoscopic laser ablation of the prostate (ELAP), high-intensity focused ultrasound (HIFU), transuretheral microwave thermotherapy (TUMT), transuretheral needle ablation (TUNA).

4. *TUIP/TURP.* Transuretheral resection of the prostate is the gold standard. For small glands, incision of the prostate may be used to open up the prostatic urethra.

5. *Retropubic prostatectomy* is an open procedure and is considered when the gland is large. It is also indicated if there is an additional pathology requiring intervention, e.g. a bladder calculus.

Neuropathic bladder

Neuromuscular dysfunction of the urinary tract has proved difficult to describe as no two neural lesions result in the same type of dysfunction no matter how similar the anatomic lesion. The International Continence Society has created a simple and function-based classification, which takes into consideration detrusor behaviour, striated sphincter competence and bladder sensations. Broadly two main types of neuropathic bladder conditions are described depending on the site of lesion in relation to the sacral micturition centre. In lesions above the sacral micturition centre the sacral reflex arcs remain intact. The inhibitory effect of the higher centres causes the bladder to be spastic while the sphincter activity varies depending on the site of the lesion. Common lesions responsible are cerebrovascular accidents, dementia, multiple sclerosis, tumours, inflammatory conditions and spinal cord lesions. This spastic neuropathic bladder is characterized by reduced bladder capacity, involuntary detrusor contractions, high intravesical voiding pressures, bladder wall hypertrophy, spasticity of pelvic striated muscle and autonomic dysreflexia. Autonomic dysreflexia is a condition associated with cervical spinal cord injury which is characterized by hypertensive blood pressure fluctuations, bradycardia and sweating. This can be triggered by catheterization, mild overdistension of the bladder or dyssynergic voiding. Neuropathic bladders caused by lesions at or below the sacral micturition centre are again caused by a variety of conditions. They include traumatic lesions, neuropathies, anterior horn damage due to poliovirus or herpes zoster, disc herniations and iatrogenic factors such as radiation or surgery. These lead to flaccid neuropathic bladder characterized by large capacity, lack of voluntary detrusor contractions, low intravesical pressure, mild hypertrophy of the bladder wall and decreased tone of the external sphincter. The diagnosis of a neuropathic bladder depends on the clinical history and physical (including neurologic) examination, radiological imaging, video urodynamic studies, cystoscopy and neurologic studies (EMG, evoked potentials). The aims of treatment are to restore low-pressure activity to the bladder in order to preserve renal function, continence and control infection.

Further reading

Barry MJ, Fowler FJ Jr., O'Leary MP, Bruskewitz RC, Holtgrewe HL, Mebust WK, Cockett AT. The American Urological Association symptom index for benign prostatic hyperplasia. *Journal of Urology*, 1992; **148:** 1549–1557.

Emberton M, Neal DE, Black N, Fordham M, Harrison M, McBrien MP, Williams RE, McPherson K, Devlin HB. The effect of prostatectomy on symptom severity and quality of life. *British Journal of Urology*, 1996; **77:** 233–247.

Oesterling JE. Benign prostatic hyperplasia. Medical and minimally invasive treatment options. *New England Journal of Medicine*, 1995; **332:** 99–109.

BLOOD TRANSFUSION

Christopher Lattimer, Chris Perera

There are two main landmarks in blood transfusion which have allowed many major operations to be successfully performed. Firstly, the discovery of ABO isoagglutinins in 1901 by Landsteiner marked the development of safe blood transfusion. Secondly, the addition of acid-citrate-dextrose (ACD) from 1943 provided anticoagulant activity and nutrition for the red cells which resulted in a dramatic increase in the shelf life of stored blood. The main indications for transfusion of blood and its components are to replace acute blood loss, treat anaemia and to correct any disorders of haemostasis.

Replacement

Red cell transfusions are used to augment the delivery of oxygen in the hope of avoiding the deleterious effects of oxygen debt. The ideal replacement fluid in rapid haemorrhage is red cells in saline-adenine-glucose-mannitol (SAG-M). These additives provide the nutrition and preserve the shape of the red cells. Large amounts of crystalloid and colloid solutions dilute blood and its clotting factors and could impair coagulation and the oxygen-carrying capacity. In adults, blood losses up to 1 litre can be replaced by crystalloids/colloids, but larger losses should be replaced with blood. Therapy for rapid blood loss should be directed primarily toward the arrest of haemorrhage. Neat packed cells have a high viscosity and are not indicated in the acute situation as the sole replacement fluid. Blood substitutes like the synthetic perfluorocarbons (PFCs) and modified haemoglobin solutions (polyhaemoglobins) did not gain popularity in clinical practice.

Anaemia

Transfusion is rarely indicated when the Hb concentration is greater than 10 g/dl and is almost always indicated when it is less than 6 g/dl, especially when anaemia is acute.

Whether intermediate Hb concentrations (6–10 g/dl) justify or require red cell transfusion should be based on the patient's risk for complications of inadequate oxygenation.

The use of a single Hb 'trigger' for all patients and failure to consider all physiological and surgical factors affecting oxygenation are not recommended.

Correction of anaemia is vital if ischaemic events like angina, claudication, transient ischaemic attacks and gut ischaemia is present or anticipated.

Haemostasis

The major bleeding problems that accompany surgical disease occur in patients on warfarin, heparin or aspirin, in those patients with disseminated intravascular coagulation (DIC), and in patients with haemophilia, liver disease, thrombocytopenia and hypersplenism. Heparin is easily reversed with protamine sulphate. Warfarin is reversed by intramuscular vitamin K, which takes at least 24 hours to work. FFP is required for emergency reversal. Regular prothrombin estimations are still required because the half-life of warfarin is much longer than that of FFP. Aspirin prolongs the bleeding time by interfering with platelet function. The aim of treating DIC is to correct the underlying surgical problem (usually sepsis). Component therapy (platelets, clotting factors) is given on the advice of a haematologist. A low fibrinogen count indicates the need for cryoprecipitate.

Infection

The following infections can be transmitted by blood transfusion:

Viral	Bacterial	Protozoal
Hepatitis B	Syphilis	Malaria
Hepatitis C	Brucellosis	Chagas disease
Hepatitis D	Contaminants	Babesiosis
HIV		
CMV		
Epstein–Barr		

Hepatitis

1. Hepatitis B. All donors are routinely screened for HbsAg. Infection still occurs because of the undetectable concentrations of antigen present at the beginning and the end of an acute infection. Ten per cent of all infected patients develop chronic hepatitis. All patients requiring multiple transfusions and all health-care workers should be vaccinated against Hepatitis B.

2. Hepatitis C. This virus was successfully cloned in 1989. It was responsible for the majority of cases of post-transfusion hepatitis even before routine HbsAg testing. This incidence has fallen over the recent years. Fifty per cent of infected patients develop chronic hepatitis and 10% of patients cirrhosis or hepatoma.

3. Hepatitis D (delta agent). This virus uses HGBsAg as its coat and cannot exist without HbsAg. This is fortunate because screening for HbsAg is all that is required to exclude the virus.

Human immunodeficiency virus

HIV can be transmitted by cellular elements and by plasma. In the UK, most infections occur in haemophiliacs treated with clotting factors but these can now be virus inactivated. Modern testing and self-exclusion questionnaires have reduced the risk of HIV transmission to an estimated 0.0002% per unit of blood. The risk of transmission is extremely low because there is only a 3 week time span during which the donor is infected but the test is not positive.

Cytomegalovirus

Immature neonates, immunosuppressed patients and pregnant mothers seronegative for CMV are all susceptible to CMV infection. In these groups blood must be filtered to remove the leucocytes, which transmit the intracellular virus.

Glandular fever

The Epstein–Barr virus is not screened for because in most cases the donor's anti-bodies protect against infection and the majority of recipients have high levels of antibodies already in their circulation.

Malaria

In areas where malaria is endemic, a course of antiprotozoal therapy is usually prescribed along with the transfusion. In non-endemic areas, travellers who have recently resided in an endemic area are excluded from donation.

Autologous predonation

Autologous predonation of blood for elective surgery began in 1960 and is now widespread in Europe and the USA. The method avoids the cost of extensive screen-ing used for homologous blood. It also prevents immunosuppressive and allergic reactions, and is acceptable to some Jehovah's witnesses. Donation criteria consist of:

1. *Haemoglobin.* This should be greater than 11 g/dl.

2. *Infection.* Active infection is a contraindication.

3. *Blood loss.* Procedures where this is expected like vascular or cardiothoracic operations.

4. *Cardiorespiratory disease.* If severe (unstable angina, left main coronary stenosis, myocardial infarction within the last 6 months), donation is ill advised.

The minimum accepted haemoglobin level for surgery is around 9 g/dl. A unit is taken each week, 500 ml of saline are infused to maintain the intravascular volume and 200 mg of ferrous sulphate is started. Two to four units of blood predeposited in this way, especially in the polycythaemic arteriopath, would nearly always result in a haemoglobin of greater than 10 g/dl prior to surgery. Blood is screened for HIV, hepatitis and syphilis, and grouped. 'Cross-over' for use on other patients is prohib-ited. The use of erythropoietin, given prior to predeposit, and the method of cryo-precipitation using hydroxyethyl starch (blood can be stored over 10 years and thawed for immediate use) can increase the amount of blood predonated. Should there be much blood loss at the time of surgery, the haemopoietic system will already be primed to function at an increased rate of manufacture.

Intraoperative autotransfusion

Intraoperative autotransfusion decreases the need for homologous transfusion and thus the risk of transmissible disease. It is indicated in cardiothoracic surgery, trauma and aortic surgery, where major blood loss is often expected, and involves the retrieval of blood shed during an operation and its subsequent reinfusion into the patient.

1. *Solcotrans.* This passive system of retrieval was introduced in 1980. It consists of a polycarbonate container with an inner bag attached to a low-pressure suction system. When full this is inverted and any unwanted air is trapped. Reinfusion occurs by gravity through a 40 μm filter. It is insufficient to have anticoagulant only in the reservoir; the patient must be fully systemically heparinized.

2. **Cell saver system.** This system is an active process which involves centrifugation and cell washing. It can be used in the non-heparinized patient.

Relative contraindications to intraoperative autotransfusion include its use in putative curative cancer resection (although peritoneal-venous shunting for malignant ascites does not encourage pulmonary metastasis), contamination with faecal material and in the HIV patient (risk to health-care worker). The concurrent use of collagen haemostats is an absolute contraindication.

Transfusion immunomodulation

Modulation of immunological behaviour by perioperative transfusion was first noted in 1973 when renal allograft survival was enhanced in patients receiving over 10 units of blood. Over 70 publications exist examining the deleterious effects of blood transfusion on colonic, prostatic, breast, renal and lung cancers. With most tumours, the literature is divided but the balance of evidence points towards perioperative transfusion being detrimental to colonic and prostatic cancer patients. The data should be interpreted with caution as the biological behaviour of the tumour determining the need for tranfusion may be more aggressive and due to the observation that blood loss and blood donation are themselves immunosuppressive. The components of blood (red cells, white cells or plasma proteins) thought to be detrimental have not been fully established but studies using packed cells instead of whole blood and white cell filters are in progress.

Further reading

Carson JL, Duff A, Berlin JA *et al.* Effect of anaemia and cardiovascular disease on surgical mortality and morbidity. *Lancet,* 1996; **348:** 1055–1060.

Carson JL, Duff A, Berlin JA *et al.* Perioperative blood transfusion and postoperative mortality. *Journal of the American Medical Association,* 1998; **279:** 199–205.

Hebert PC, Wells G, Blajchman MA *et al.* A multicentre, randomised, controlled clinical trial of transfusion requirements in critical care. *New England Journal of Medicine,* 1999; **340:** 409–417.

McLelland B. Perioperative red cell transfusion: evidence, guidelines and practice. *Vox Sanguinis,* 1998; **74** (supplement 2): 3–10.

Weiskopf RH, Viele MK, Feiner J *et al.* Human cardiovascular and metabolic response to acute, severe, isovolaemic anaemia. *Journal of the American Medical Association,* 1998; **279:** 217–221.

Related topics of interest

BREAST CANCER

Nick Wilson

This is the commonest cancer amongst women, affecting 1 in 13 and resulting in 25000 new cases and 15000 deaths per year in the UK. The incidence rises rapidly to 200/100000 women/year by age 45 and continues to rise into old age. One per cent of breast cancers occur in men. The severity of the problem in the UK has led to a government directive that all women suspected of having breast cancer must be offered an outpatient appointment within 2 weeks of referral.

Nulliparous women in developed countries are at increased risk of breast cancer whereas women who have their first child young and breast feed are protected. Modern low dose oral contraception does not seem to increase the incidence of breast cancer. Predisposing factors include oestrogen exposure unopposed by progesterone, hyperoestrogenism, family history of premenopausal breast cancer, saturated dietary fats and previous benign atypical hyperplasia. Two important breast cancer genes (*BRCA1* – chromosome 11 and *BRCA2* – chromosome 17) are associated with inherited breast cancer which accounts for about 5% of cases, but environmental factors seem more important.

Pathology

It is very difficult to define the cell of origin of most tumours and the WHO classification divides tumours into those derived from epithelial cells and those derived from connective tissues.

Epithelial tumours	• Non-invasive:	Ductal carcinoma-in-situ (DCIS)	3–5%
		Lobular carcinoma-in-situ (LCIS)	1%
	• Invasive:	Invasive ductal carcinoma (not otherwise specified NOS)	80–90%
		Invasive lobular	1–2%
		Mucinous, medullary, papillary	rare
		Tubular, secretory, apocrine	rare
	• Paget's disease		2%
Mixed connective tissue/epithelial			
Miscellaneous/unclassified			

Non-invasive pathology is increasingly common in screening-detected tumours. Lobular carcinoma-in-situ is uncommon as is ductal carcinoma in situ (DCIS) in isolation. This is much commoner in combination with invasive ductal cancers. DCIS is premalignant. Invasive ductal tumours (NOS) form the majority of breast cancers although most are undifferentiated and cannot easily be classified morphologically. Lobular, medullary, mucinous, etc. are specific differentiated forms of invasive cancer that can sometimes be identified. Their differentiation gives them a better prognosis than the NOS group. Pagets disease indicates an underlying invasive or intraduct carcinoma. Phylloides tumours are the commonest group in the mixed connective tissue and epithelial group. Their behaviour is difficult to predict, but a high mitotic rate, atypia and infiltration indicate local reccurrence after simple excision.

Invasion of the regional axillary lymph nodes has an adverse effect on prognosis with a 5-year survival of less than 20% where more than five lymph glands are involved[b]. Other markers of poor prognosis are vascular invasion, tumour multi-centricity and poor differentiation. The content of oestrogen receptor protein in the primary tumour is useful for indicating the response to endocrine therapy and for prognosis.

Staging

The TNM and Manchester systems are commonly used. Tumours up to T2 N1 M0 (stage 2) are termed 'Early breast cancer' and are potentially curable. Tumours beyond this stage are advanced.

The TNM classification of breast cancer

Primary tumour = T		Nodes = N
Tis	Carcinoma-in-situ/Pagets	N1 Ipsilateral axillary (mobile)
T1	≤ 2 cm	N2 Ipsilateral axillary (fixed)
T2	> 2 cm but < 5 cm	N3 Ipsilateral int mammary nodes
T3	> 5 cm	
T4a	Chest wall extension (fixed)	Metastases = M
T4b	Dermal extension (ulcer,	
	peau d'orange)	M0 None
T4c	Both 4a and 4b	M1 Distant (lung, liver, other nodes)
T4d	Inflammatory cancer	

Clinical features

- Firm, irregular, painless lump. May be fixed to skin or muscle.
- Pain (10%).
- Axillary/supraclavicular lymph node involvement.
- Recent nipple retraction and/or bloody discharge.
- Paget's disease.
- Peau d'orange
- Signs of metastatic disease (weight loss, ascites, jaundice, CNS signs)
- Asymptomatic presentation following screening.

Investigations

1. Mammography.   Used for investigating symptomatic patients and for screening. 80–95% accurate, but less accurate in young, dense breasts.

2. Ultrasound.   Demonstrates cystic disease. Colour flow duplex mode may distinguish abnormal tumour circulation. Often used to guide FNAC or core biopsy for smaller lesions.

3. Fine needle aspiration cytology (FNAC).   Simple and quick, 95% accurate.

4. Trucut or biopty gun biopsy.   For lumps larger than 2 cm diameter a tissue core can be obtained under local anaesthesia for histological examination.

5. Excision biopsy.   This is performed where other investigations have failed to define the lump. Proceeding to a more extensive procedure after frozen section analysis is not recommended.

6. Wire-guided biopsy.   Impalpable suspicious lesions identified at mammography are localized by insertion of a wire under screening control. A core of breast tissue around the wire is then excised surgically. A radiograph of the specimen is taken to ensure total excision of the abnormality.

7. Chest X-ray, Bone scan, CT scan, MRI scan.   Helpful in defining the extent of metastatic disease.

Control of local disease

1. Surgery.   In patients without systemic disease, local surgery may be curative, but most patients have occult micrometastases. A mobile tumour with or without axillary lymph nodes (T1–3, N0–1, M0) is generally operable. Prospective trials indicate no difference in 5–10-year survival rate of patients undergoing mastectomy or breast conservation (lumpectomy, wide local excision, quadrantectomy) and radiotherapy, but the local recurrence rate in the latter group is slightly higher[a]. Mastectomy with axillary clearance results in 5 year recurrence rates of 4% and 8% in node-negative and node-positive patients respectively. It is not yet clear if there are differences in longer-term survival (10–25 years) between radical surgery and conservation. Subcutaneous mastectomy is indicated for prophylactic mastectomy in women at high risk of breast cancer.

Palliative mastectomy with or without local adjuvant treatment may be necessary to control advanced local disease.

Anxiety and depression accompany mastectomy in many women, but breast conservation does not protect against this, many women fearing the possiblity of residual or recurrent disease.

2. Management of the axilla.   Failure to treat the axilla does not confer a worse prognosis, node involvement being an expression of poor outcome rather than a determinant. Recently the technique of sentinel lymph node biopsy has gained popularity to avoid unnecessary axillary clearance in patients with node-negative disease. At the procedure to remove the primary tumour the area is injected with a vital blue dye and a radiocolloid (technetium 99m sulphur colloid). A small axillary incision is made and the first nodes to drain the tumour are identified by direct vision (stained blue) and a hand-held gamma detector. The nodes are excised and examined histologically. If this is clear of tumour no further axillary procedure is deemed necessary. If the nodes are positive axillary clearance is undertaken as a separate procedure. The technique has high accuracy and low morbidity[b]. In node-positive patients level III axillary clearance (removal of all axillary nodes including apical nodes) has a long-term local recurrence rate of under 2%. Arm swelling affects less than 5% of women providing the axilla is not irradiated. Radical axillary irradiation effectively prevents node recurrence, but brachial plexus neuropathy occurs in 0.5–1.0%.

3. Radiotherapy. Radiotherapy is necessary after breast-conserving surgery to reduce local recurrence rates[a]. Overall survival is not improved, but aggressive radiotherapy causes excess long-term mortality from other tumours and ischaemic heart disease. Chest wall radiotherapy is unhelpful in patients undergoing modified radical mastectomy, and axillary irradiation should not be performed if level III axillary clearance has been performed. Chest wall and axillary radiotherapy are usually the treatment of choice in advanced, inoperable tumours.

4. Breast reconstruction. Reconstruction probably does not interfere with the detection of tumour recurrence and restores appearance to near normal. Techniques include the placement of an implant with or without prior tissue expansion, and latissimus dorsi and rectus abdominis myocutaneous flaps which result in extensive scarring and possible complications (infection, flap necrosis, late capsule formation). Considerable asymmetry is the norm and nipple reconstruction is often unsatisfactory. The reconstruction can be performed combined with the original mastectomy or as a secondary procedure at a later date.

Control of systemic disease

1. Radiotherapy. Provides excellent palliation of metastases, particularly of bone.

2. Chemotherapy. Reduces the 10-year probability of death by 10% in younger, premenopausal women with early breast cancer[a]. Cyclophosphamide, methotrexate and fluorouracil (CMF) given for 6 months is a typical regimen. The benefit is independent of menopausal status, oestrogen receptor status or the use of tamoxifen[a]. A short course of chemotherapy in a fit patient may temporarily control advanced or inoperable disease.

3. Hormonal treatment. Tamoxifen used for at least 2 years at a dose of 20 mg/day reduces the 10 year probability of death by 17%, together with reduced local recurrence rates[a]. This benefit is most apparent in older women, and seems independent of menopausal and oestrogen receptor status.

4. Oophorectomy, ovarian irradiation, LHRH agonists. In women under 50 with early breast cancer ovarian ablation significantly improves long-term survival[a]. It is useful in advanced, metastatic disease to induce regression or delay spread. If no response is obtained, second-line agents (aminoglutethamide, progestagens) can be used.

Pain relief and counselling

Oral opiates, non-steroidal agents, radiotherapy and steroids (for cerebral involvement) should be used liberally when the disease advances and symptoms develop. Drainage of effusions and ascites may be beneficial. Councelling and contact with a hospice are helpful in the late stages of disease.

Breast screening

Evidence that breast screening reduces mortality from breast cancer in women in New York, Holland and Sweden has resulted in the UK breast screening programme offered to women aged 50–64. No clear survival advantage has yet been seen in the UK, although more early tumours are being detected and treated. A considerable increase in work load has resulted and women are unecessarily alarmed when mammograms are falsely positive.

Treatment of high-risk groups

Studies are underway to examine the protective effect of tamoxifen in patients at high risk of developing breast cancer by virtue of their family history.

Further reading

Dixon JM, Mansel RE. The breast. In: Burnand KG, Young AE (eds). *The New Aird's Companion in Surgical Studies (2nd Edn)*. London: Churchill Livingstone, 1998: 631–663.

Early Breast Cancer Trial Lists Collaborative Group. Tamoxifen for early breast cancer: an overview of the randomised trials. *Lancet*, 1998; **351**: 1451–1467.

Early Breast Cancer Trial Lists Collaborative Group. Polychemotherapy for early breast cancer: an overview of the randomised trials. *Lancet*, 1998; **352**: 930–942.

Early Breast Cancer Trial Lists Collaborative Group. Favourable and unfavourable effects on long-term survival of radiotherapy for early breast cancer: an overview of the randomised trials. *Lancet*, 2000; **255**: 1739–1740.

Krag DN, Harlow S, Weaver D, Ashicaga T. Radiolabelled sentinel node biopsy: collaborative trial with the national cancer institute. *World Journal of Surgery*, 2001; **25**: 823–828.

Related topics of interest

Benign breast disease (p. 45); Screening (p. 293).

BURNS

Christopher Lattimer, Omar Faiz

Burn injuries often result in profound physical and metabolic insult. Those most at risk include alcoholics, epileptics, drug addicts and the mentally handicapped. Children under six are most liable to scald injuries from bath water, hot drinks and kettle spills. The mortality associated with severe burn injury reaches 90% in patients: with >40% surface area burns; over 60 years of age; and those with concomitant inhalation injury[a]. Treatment involves an aggressive approach, with close collaboration between the intensivist, plastic surgeon and microbiologist, to curb mortality from fluid loss and sepsis.

Fluid replacement

A burn results in a substantial loss of fluid, protein, blood and heat. The percentage of total body surface area burnt (%TBSA), and consequently the severity of the injury, is estimated from the Wallace *Rule of Nines* chart. One per cent of the patient's TBSA is represented by the palmar surface area of the subject's hand. Adults suffering a burn greater than 15% surface area, or children greater than 10%, require admission and fluid resuscitation. The *Muir and Barclay* regime calculates fluid replacement requirement during the first 36 hours. Each of the six time periods requires an equal volume of fluid replacement in addition to normal requirements.

Period	1	2	3	4	5	6
Duration (hours)	4	4	4	6	6	12

$$\frac{\text{Surface area burnt (\%)} \times \text{weight (kg)}}{2} = \text{Requirement (ml/Period)}$$

This formula is only a guide which must be adjusted according to regular measurement of haemoglobin, haematocrit, electrolytes and urinary output. Another regime commonly used is the *Parkland formula* which suggests an approximate guide to fluid resuscitation over the first 24 hours of 4 ml/kg of body weight/% area of surface burn. Severe burn injuries predispose to a generalized increase in vascular permeability (including ARDS) with a concomitant decrease in cardiac output. The latter changes have been attributed to the release of inflammatory mediators, such as IL-6 and TNFα, and the humoral response to burn injury. It was previously believed that crystalloids exacerbate the latter complications and should be avoided. In consequence, albumin has been the mainstay of resuscitation for major burn injuries. Recently, systematic reviews have raised doubts over the safety of colloid resuscitation (particularly albumin) and a universal protocol for acute fluid resuscitation in burn injuries is yet to be agreed[a].

Analgesia

Intravenous morphine is the most appropriate analgesic and can be administered from a patient-controlled analgesia system. Cool water (uncovered ice is harmful) is an effective analgesic for smaller burns and has been demonstrated to reverse tissue damage[b]. Rectal paracetamol is useful for pyrexia in children.

Sepsis

Burnt surfaces provide an excellent culture medium for bacteria. Colonization is rapid and the associated immunosuppression with large burns makes septicaemia a common complication. Staphylococcal, Pseudomonas and Candida organisms are the commonest wound offenders. Severely burnt patients should be isolated and barrier nursed. Intravenous antibiotics are required for septic episodes (including: septicaemia, pneumonia, UTI or cellulitis) but should *never* be administered prophylactically as this practice favours colonization with resistant strains thereby complicating the treatment of established infections. Signs of sepsis can be subtle as core temperature is often elevated in severely burnt patients. These may include: changes in clinical condition or mental status; either elevation or depression of the white cell count (WCC); acidosis; hypoxia; thrombocytopenia or hyperglycaemia. Regular cultures of the urine, sputum, wound and blood are taken to determine appropriate antibiotic therapy.

Nutrition

All burns require high-energy dietary supplementation to facilitate healing. In severely burnt patients basic metabolic rate can double leading to severe catabolism. Fine-bore nasogastric feeding should be used for patients with large burns as it can deliver essential nutrition, as well as bolstering the gut mucosal barrier to infection. Parenteral feeding lines present a high risk of infection and are consequently best avoided. A dynamic ileus, acute gastric dilatation and stress (Curling's) ulceration frequently follow major burn injuries and prophylactic measures should be taken to avoid them.

Open or closed therapy?

Burns of the face and perineum as well as all superficial burns should be treated by exposure. A dry eschar discourages bacterial colonization and often separates spontaneously after two weeks. Closed treatment involves covering the burn with Vaseline gauze and leaving the inner layers undisturbed for 10 days. Burns are often covered with topical silver sulfadiazine – an agent with broad antibacterial activity. All closed treatments moisten the eschar thereby preventing spontaneous separation. Surgical debridement under general anaesthesia is consequently required.

Surgery

The surgical approach depends upon the extent and depth of the burn. A general guide to depth identification is tabulated below.

Depth	Sensation	Blistering	Colour	Healing
Superficial (First degree)	Painful	Often	Pink	Regeneration
Deep dermal (Second degree)	Analgaesic	Occasional	White/yellow	Repair
Full thickness (Third degree)	Anaesthetic	None	Grey/olive	Contraction

Superficial burns heal by regeneration from undamaged keratinocytes in hair follicles, sebaceous glands and sweat glands. Deep dermal burns mostly heal by repair but are capable of some regeneration from the deeper situated sweat glands. The latter burns are treated by tangential excision (shaving) using a skin graft knife between the third and fifth day to preserve the deeper dermis that would otherwise die. This occurs as the interface between viable and non-viable tissue deepens from the time of injury due to thrombosis of the surrounding microcirculation. Grafts take well on this prepared surface. The application of temporary synthetic skin substitutes may also be used for superficial and dermal burn injuries where spontaneous healing is possible. Their use has been shown to significantly reduce healing time[b]. Full thickness burns require excision and skin cover. If small (1–2 cm), the surrounding skin can be sutured directly over the defect. Full thickness burns over the face, palms and pressure areas or over denuded perichondrium, periosteum or paratenon require full thickness skin cover. Larger defects are covered with allogenic meshed split skin grafts. In extensively burnt patients the paucity of available donor sites complicates management.

Escharotomy

Deep circumferential burns of the chest or limbs require urgent relieving incisions (escharotomies) to prevent respiratory or vascular compromise.

Inhalation injuries

Inhalation injuries are suspected from the appearance of facial oedema, singed nasal hair and oropharyngeal carbon staining along with stridor and bronchospasm. Inhalation injury comprises three main mechanisms which commonly occur together. These include: carbon monoxide (CO) poisoning; airway heat injury; and inhalation of toxic gases released from the incomplete combustion of synthetic materials such as plastic furnishings, paints and fabrics. Treatment comprises: airway maintenance (occasionally emergency tracheostomy); humidified oxygen; and bronchodilators. CO levels should be monitored in the patient with suspected inhalation injury.

Electrical burns

Electrical burns are usually much deeper, and more extensive than the skin wounds might suggest. Current flows preferentially along nerves, muscle and blood vessels as the latter present less resistance than the skin. The current is transferred into heat energy in vivo with resultant protein denaturation and tissue destruction.

Arrhythmias, compartment syndrome and myoglobinuria complicate electrical burn injuries and require early and aggressive treatment. Wounds should be debrided early and may require subsequent excision of necrotic tissue prior to eventual grafting.

Acid/alkalis burns

Acid burns damage tissues by *coagulative necrosis* and alkaline burns (e.g. cement) damage by, more prolonged, *colliquative necrosis*. Treatment of chemical burns consists of immediate immersion in running water until wound pH has returned to normal. This process can take several hours with alkaline burns.

Aftercare

Severe burn injury patients often require multiple plastic surgical procedures for scar revisions and release of skin contractures. Unfortunately, rehabilitation can take years and, due to hypertrophic scarring, total cosmetic resolution is often not achieved. This can have a profound psychological impact on the patient and highlights the need for counselling as part of the rehabilitation process.

Further reading

Cochrane Injuries Group Albumin Reviewers. Human albumin administration in critically ill patients: a systematic review of randomised controlled trials. *British Medical Journal*, 1998; **317:** 235–240.

Muller MJ, Herndon DN. The challenge of burns. *Lancet*, 1994; **343**(8891): 216–220.

Robson MC *et al*. Prevention and treatment of postburn scars and contracture. *World Journal of Surgery*, 1992; **16:** 87.

Related topics of interest

Fluid replacement (p. 127); Multiple organ failure (p. 227); Nutrition in the surgical patient (p. 233).

CALF PUMP FAILURE AND VENOUS ULCERATION

Nick Wilson

The calf pump failure syndrome comprises dermatological and subcutaneous changes developing after any condition impairing calf pump function (varicose veins, DVT). The prevalence of venous ulceration (the end-point of calf pump failure) is 0.1–0.25%, and 40–60% of such patients have post-thrombotic changes[c]. Milder calf pump failure is much commoner. The annual cost of treating venous ulcers in the UK is £230–400 million[c].

Pathophysiology

Calf pump failure occurs because of an inability to reduce superficial venous pressure during exercise as a result of one or more of the following:

1. Valvular incompetence

- Deep vein reflux (post-thrombotic or non-thrombotic).
- Communicating vein reflux.
- Superficial vein reflux (varicose veins).

2. Outflow tract obstruction

- Post-thrombotic.

3. Muscle pump failure

- Primary (neuromuscular disorders).
- Secondary (ankle stiffness).

The underlying pathological events are varicose veins, post-thrombotic damage to the deep and/or communicating veins and non-thrombotic deep vein incompetence. The effects of these factors are countered by poorly understood phenomena that protect tissues against venous hypertension (the fibrinolytic capacity of the skin and subcutaneous tissues), many patients who have poor calf pump function never developing the syndrome.

Theories proposed to explain the effects of calf pump failure on microcirculation:

- Stasis (venous stasis causing desaturation and tissue hypoxia – disproven).
- Arteriovenous shunts (no evidence).
- Fibrin cuff and pericapillary oedema imparing gas exchange.
- The white cell theory (activated white cells release toxic metabolites – unproven).

Clinical presentation

The clinical features are:

- Aching.
- Venous claudication.
- Swelling.
- Varicose veins.

- Incompetent communicating veins.
- Pigmentation.
- Eczema.
- Lipodermatosclerosis.
- Atrophie blanche.
- Ankle stiffness.
- Ulceration.

Ulceration is the end-point of the calf pump failure syndrome. Lipodermatosclerosis is frequently present before an ulcer develops, and local trauma is often an initiating factor. Post-thrombotic ulcers are usually intractable, and even when healed often recur.

Investigation

1. Anatomical and functional assessment
- Define anatomy of any varicose veins. Duplex ultrasound/varicograms if necessary.
- Ascending phlebography. Demonstrate post-thrombotic damage, incompetent communicating veins. Both legs should be investigated.
- Duplex ultrasound. To detect significant deep vein reflux (30–60% of patients).
- Plethysmography or foot vein pressure measurement to determine efficiency of calf pump.
- Femoral vein pressure measurements. If bypass surgery considered for iliac vein occlusion. A rise of 10 mmHg or more indicates significant iliac vein obstruction.

2. Prothrombotic screen
- Including FBC, antithrombin III, proteins S, C, plasma fibrinogen, lupus anticoagulant.

3. Differential diagnosis of leg ulcers
- Doppler ankle pressure (arterial disease/ulcer).
- Urinalysis/blood glucose (diabetic ulcers).
- ESR/rheumatoid serology (rheumatoid or arteritic ulceration).
- VDRL/TPHA (syphilitic ulceration – rare).
- Skin biopsy (malignant ulcers).
- Sickle cell test (sickle cell ulcers).
- Self-inflicted (dermatitis artefacta).

Treatment

Most treatments are palliative.

1. Compression and elevation. Prolonged elevation reduces venous pressure at rest, relieving most symptoms and healing almost all ulcers. Graduated compression reduces the transmural venous pressure by increasing the surrounding tissue pressure. Class III elastic stockings exert 30–40 mmHg pressure at the ankle and lower pressures (20–30 mmHg) at the knee. Below-knee stockings are prescribed for all patients and should be worn continuously when the patient is out of bed.

2. **Superficial and communicating vein reflux.** Where superficial and/or communicating vein incompetence contributes to calf pump failure, high saphenous ligation and stripping should be performed. Division of incompetent communicating veins is highly successful at preventing ulcer recurrence in limbs with non-thrombotic deep veins. This is now performed using the technique of subfascial endoscopic perforating vein surgery (SEPS) in preference to open surgical techniques[c].

3. **Deep vein obstruction.** Bypass surgery. Anatomical and functional obstruction must be demonstrated. Only 2% of patients are suitable.

The Palma procedure is used for unilateral iliac vein obstruction, and the Warren–Thayer bypass for femoral vein occlusion. The five-year patencies are 80% and 55%, respectively[c]. Inferior vena caval occlusion may be bypassed with ePTFE graft if conservative methods fail. Patency rates are 70–90% up to 1 year after implantation[c]. Very few patients are suitable for these procedure.

4. **Deep vein reflux.** There must be evidence of significant deep venous reflux demonstrated by duplex ultrasound and calf pump function tests.

Direct valve repair (valvuloplasty) to tighten floppy valve cusps and indirect valvuloplasty to compress the valve sinus with a collar restoring cusp apposition can be used in patients with non-thrombotic deep vein reflux.

Valve transposition which employs anastomosis of incompetent superficial femoral veins to valve-bearing segments of either long saphenous or profunda femoris veins has not proved durable.

Valve autotransplantation has become the most widely practised form of valve replacement. A valve-bearing segment of the axillary vein is resected and transplanted into either the femoral or popliteal veins. Patients are encouraged to continue wearing graduated compression stockings and anticoagulants are given for a short period.

Few patients are suitable for these procedures and the long-term benefits remain unclear.

Ulcer healing

1. **Graduated compression.** Layered graduated compression bandaging remains the most useful treatment for healing venous ulcers, the various different bandages and topical agents available offering no demonstrable benefit. Compression should be the highest at the ankle and be maintained for 1–2 weeks. Bandaging techniques such as the Charing Cross 4- layer system have been developed to achieve this and generally comprise an inert inner layer, elastic compression and weaker elastic protective outer layer. Bandages and dressings should ideally reduce pain, be non-allergenic, prevent ulcer desiccation, and be easy to change, while remaining inexpensive.

2. **Pharmacological agents**
- Fibrinolytic agents. Reduce lipodermatosclerosis but do not heal ulcers.
- Hydroxyrutosides. May reduce oedema and discomfort.
- Prostaglandins. Prolonged infusion may improve ulcer healing.
- Methylxanthines. Oxypentifyline may speed ulcer healing.

3. *Ulcer excision and skin grafting.*   When ulcers fail to heal with compression bandaging, split skin grafting should be considered. The ulcer base should be tangentially excised and meshed split skin grafts applied immediately or after a few days dressing when the granulation tissue has started to form.

Indefinite use of class 2 or 3 graduated compression hosiery is usually recommended to prevent recurrence after ulcer healing.

Further reading

Browse NL, Burnand KG, Lea Thomas M. *Diseases of the Veins: Pathology, Diagnosis and Treatment.* London: Edward Arnold, 1988.

Related topic of interest

Deep vein thrombosis (p. 113); Varicose veins (p. 346).

CARCINOMA OF THE BLADDER

Adrian Simoes

Histologically carcinoma of the bladder can be categorized as transitional cell carcinoma, squamous cell carcinoma and adenocarcinoma. Transitional cell carcinoma is the commonest form (90%) in the UK and USA, but squamous cell carcinoma which is associated with chronic infection and inflammation may account for nearly 70% in areas where schistosomiasis is endemic, such as Egypt. Four to 10% of patients with bladder TCC may develop TCC of the upper tract which is also lined by the transitional cell urothelium up to the renal pelvis. Forty per cent of upper tract TCC patients are known to develop bladder TCC and hence need cystoscopic surveillance.

Transitional cell carcinoma (TCC)

Incidence

TCC is three times more common in males than females. It is the fourth commonest cancer and the eight commonest cause of cancer death in males. TCC may be superficial in 70–75% cases and behave in a benign manner or may be invasive in 20–25%. Carcinoma-in-situ is seen in about 10%.

Aetiology

A number of environmental carcinogens have been implicated in its development and they are 2-naphthylamine, benzidine, 4-aminobiphenyl, dichlorobenzidine, orthotolidine, phenacetin and cyclophosphamide. Occupations involving printing, dyeing, hairdressing, tanning, rubber and coal therefore carry an increased risk. Smoking is a recognized cause with a two- to five-fold increase in risk along with increase in the recurrences, stage and grade as compared to non-smokers. The correlation is stronger with bladder cancer than lung cancer.

Presentation

Patients usually present over the age of 40 with painless haematuria, recurrent urinary tract infections or irritative lower urinary tract symptoms. Asymptomatic microscopic haematuria is regarded as a part of the spectrum of painless haematuria. Advanced disease is associated with systemic symptoms due to ureteric obstruction causing loin pain, pyelonephritis and renal failure. Local invasion results in pain and metastases cause chest pain, cough, bone pains and pathological fractures.

Investigations

Urinalysis and cytology will detect haematuria, infection and exfoliated malignant cells. Imaging in the form of ultrasound and intravenous urography may reveal lesions as well as obstruction of the upper urinary tract. The bladder is examined by performing a rigid or flexible cystoscopy. Once the disease has been diagnosed using histology, grade and pathological stage, further imaging in the form of CT scan, Chest X-ray and bone scan may be necessary for staging.

Staging

Tumour cells are graded as well, moderate or poorly differentiated on histology depending on the degree of anaplasia. TNM staging is as follows:

pTis   carcinoma-in-situ
pTa   papillary non-invasive lesion arising from epithelium
pT1   lamina propria invasion
pT2a   superficial muscle invasion
pT2b   deep muscle invasion
pT3a   perivesical tissue invasion (microscopically)
pT3b   perivesical tissue invasion (macroscopically)
pT4   extravesical invasion.

N0   No regional lymph node metastasis
N1   Metastasis in single lymph node 2 cm or less in greatest dimension
N2   Metastasis in a single lymph node more than 2 cm but not more than 5 cm in the greatest dimension, or multiple lymph nodes none more than 5 cm in greatest dimension.
N3   Metastasis in a lymph node more than 5 cm in greatest dimension

M0   No distant metastasis
M1   Distant metastasis

Management

1. *Superficial disease.* Most superficial pTa and pT1 disease can be completely resected and approximately 40% of such patients will have no further recurrences. The rest will suffer recurrences and some of these will progress to a higher stage. It is therefore necessary to follow up these patients with regular cystoscopies, which depending on the grade and number of recurrences, may be for a 10-year tumour free period or life long. Factors suggesting progression of the disease include large or multiple tumours, high-grade lesions, tumours associated with CIS or severe dysplasia. Intravesical chemotherapy with mitomycin or epirubicin are used to prevent frequent and numerous recurrences. Intravesical immunotherapy with BCG is found to be superior in controlling recurrences and is used in those cases not responding to intravesical chemotherapy. Radical cystectomy may be indicated for uncontrollable high-grade disease. Photodynamic therapy using a photosensitizing drug followed by panvesical laser therapy is still an experimental treatment modality.

2. *Carcinoma-in-situ.* CIS may be primary when it exists on its own or secondary when it presents alongside a concomitant or previous TCC. CIS has a high rate of progression to invasive muscle disease and may spread to lymph nodes without progressing to muscle invasion. It therefore needs to be adequately eradicated with surgical resection and adjuvant intravesical chemotherapy and immunotherapy. BCG immunotherapy is reported to bring about a complete remission in 75% cases with repeated courses. In the fit patient radical cystoprostatourethrectomy may be indicated for relapse.

3. *Invasive TCC.* The mainstay of treatment is either radical cystectomy or radical external beam radiotherapy. Multi-drug chemotherapy is also used and there is a trend of late to organ sparing, thereby combining radiotherapy and chemotherapy. After a radical cystectomy urinary drainage is achieved with either an ileal conduit, orthotopic bladder reconstruction using small bowel, ileocaecal segment or large bowel, or by creating a continent stoma using Mitrofanoff's principle. The appendix, ureter, fallopian tube or plicated bowel may be used to create a neourethra for catheterization.

Squamous cell carcinoma

Comprises 5–10% of bladder cancer in developed countries. It is usually invasive with nodular infiltrating growth pattern and has a poor prognosis. The treatment of choice in the fit patient is radical cystectomy.

Adenocarcinoma

Adenocarcinoma accounts for about 2% of bladder cancers. They arise from the urachal remnant of the allantois and are solitary, high grade and ulcerative in nature and sited at the dome of the bladder. The non-urachal tumours are those associated with bladder extrophy. The prognosis is generally poor but one may get away with a partial cystectomy if diagnosed early.

Further reading

Cohen SM, Shirai T, Steineck G. Epidemiology and etiology of premalignant and malignant urothelial changes. *Scandinavian Journal of Urology and Nephrology*, 2000; **205** suppl: 105–115.

Herr HW. Natural history of superficial bladder tumours: 10 to 20 year follow-up of treated patients. *World Journal of Urology*, 1997; **15**: 84–88.

Thurman SA, DeWeese TL. Multimodality therapy for the treatment of muscle-invasive bladder cancer. *Seminars in Urologic Oncology*, 2000; **18**(4): 313–322.

CARCINOMA OF THE PROSTATE

Adrian Simoes

Prostate cancer is an important and increasing public health problem. It is the third commonest cause of cancer death in developed countries after lung and large bowel cancers. It is probably the commonest cancer with the highest incidence seen in blacks in the USA.

Incidence

It is rare before the age of 40 and the incidence increases with age. Autopsy studies show that it is present in 40% at 50 years of age to 80% by age 80. Many prostate cancers are not life threatening and hence more men die with the disease than from it. However some progress rapidly and there is intense pressure on investigative methods to identify these lesions.

Presentation

Prostate cancers present with symptoms of bladder outflow obstruction, local invasion of surrounding organs to cause haematuria, haematospermia, renal failure due to ureteric obstruction or perineal pain and from distant bony and lymph metastases. The bony metastases are typically osteosclerotic in nature and involve the axial skeleton to cause pain, pathological fractures and spinal cord compression. With increased awareness asymptomatic cases may be detected by PSA (prostate-specific antigen) testing, digital rectal examination (DRE), transrectal ultrasound (TRUS) of the prostate and as an incidental finding after TURP.

Diagnosis

The diagnosis is based on DRE, PSA and TRUS. It is confirmed by TRUS-guided prostatic trucut biopsies. PSA elevation is the most predictive single test for the presence of prostate cancer but is not necessarily diagnostic of prostate cancer. To improve its diagnostic ability research continues in the following areas: age-specific PSA, PSA velocity, PSA density and ratio of free to total PSA and new markers.

Pathology

Ninety-five per cent of prostate cancers are adenocarcinomas, 85% are multifocal and 80% arise in the peripheral zone. PIN (prostatic intraepithelial neoplasia) represents the putative precancerous end of the morphologic continuum of cellular proliferation within the prostatic ducts, ductules and acini. PIN predates carcinoma by 10 years or more and is often found in close proximity to adenocarcinomas.

Staging

Local staging accuracy by rectal examination can be improved by TRUS and MRI. CT scan or MRI are considered equal in assessing pelvic and abdominal lymphadenopathy. A radioisotope bone scan is the most sensitive method of detecting bone metastases and accompanying plain skeletal radiographs may be necessary to exclude false-positive bone scan results. A combination of local disease extent, PSA and the Gleason grade on biopsy histology is useful in predicting the probability of organ-confined disease.

UICC (Union Internationale Contre le Cancer) TNM staging

T1   Not palpable nor visible on imaging
   a   < 5% in TURP specimen
   b   > 5% in TURP specimen
   c   identified by needle biopsy due to raised PSA.

T2   Confined within the prostate
   a   one lobe
   b   both lobes

T3   Locally advanced tumour
   a   extracapsular extension
   b   seminal vesicle invasion

T4   Tumour fixed or invades adjacent structures

N1   Regional lymph node metastasis

M1   a   non regional lymph node
   b   bones
   c   other sites

Screening

Population-based screening for prostate cancer cannot be justified at the present time due to lack of knowledge about its natural history, the absence of an accurate diagnostic test and the lack of data from randomized trials on the effectiveness of current therapy for localized disease.

Treatment

1. **Localized disease.**   There exist three conventional treatment modalities.
- *Active monitoring.* This policy involves regular follow-up using DRE, PSA testing and TRUS to monitor the cancer and check its progression so as to intervene. It is considered appropriate in older patients with low-volume, well-differentiated tumours particularly in the presence of other significant co-morbidity.
- *Radical prostatectomy.* Radical removal of the prostate with the seminal vesicles, the obturator and internal iliac group of lymph nodes with attempts at preserving the cavernous neurovascular bundle. The procedure can be performed via the retropubic or perineal approach, as well as laparoscopically. Though the results of randomized control trials comparing various modalities of treatment are still awaited, many urologists believe that it offers the best results in younger men who have at least 10-year life expectancy, organ-confined disease and no significant co-morbidity. Complications include erectile dysfunction, and incontinence of urine.
- *Radical radiotherapy.* Radiotherapy offers an advantage in patients who are not suitable either due to co-morbidity or evidence of extraprostatic extension of disease and the results are comparable to surgery. Conventional external beam

radiotherapy and conformal radiotherapy is used. Lately brachytherapy has been gaining popularity whereby radioactive implants (Iodine 125 or Palladium 103) are placed in the prostate.

2. *Locally advanced disease.* Hormonal treatment and or external beam irradiation is used to achieve palliation.

3. *Metastatic disease.* Androgen deprivation is the mainstay of treatment for metastatic disease and can be achieved by medical castration, androgen blockade, maximal androgen blockade and surgical castration. Medical castration is achieved by administering LHRH agonists like goserelin (Zoladex®) as depot subcutaneous injections on a monthly or 3-monthly interval. These initially stimulate the release of pituitary gonadotrophins and then inhibit it thereby causing an initial rise in testosterone followed by reduction to castrate levels. Hence in those men in whom this peak in testosterone may cause worsening of symptoms such as cord compression or ureteric obstruction, anti-androgens need to be administered before the initiation of LHRH agonists. Oestrogens, like stilboestrol, by its negative feedback also causes medical castration but has become unpopular due to serious cardiovascular side-effects. Androgen blockade is brought about by blocking the binding of dihydrotestosterone to its receptor. These antiandrogens are grouped as steroidal or non-steroidal. The steroidal anti-androgens also have a central action to suppress gonadotrophin release. Surgical castration is achieved by means of either total or subcapsular bilateral orchidectomy. Five to 10% of androgens are produced by the adrenals and hence maximal androgen blockade can only be achieved by adding anti-androgens to a patient who has been either medically or surgically castrated.

Palliation

Palliation of painful bony metastases is achieved with adequate analgesia and external beam radiotherapy to the painful sites or by bone-seeking isotopes. Second line hormone therapy and chemotherapy may be indicated in hormone refractory disease.

Further reading

Newling D. Advanced prostate cancer: immediate or deferred hormone therapy? *European Urology*, 2001; **39** Suppl 1: 15–21.

Potter SR, Partin AW. Prostate cancer: detection, staging, and treatment of localized disease. *Seminars in Roentgenology*, 1999; **34**(4): 269–283.

Walsh PC. Radical prostatectomy for localized prostate cancer provides durable cancer control with excellent quality of life: a structured debate. *Journal of Urology*, 2000; **163**(6): 1802–1807.

Wolfe ES, Wolfe WW Sr. Discussion of the controversies associated with prostate cancer screening. *Journal of the Royal Society of Health*, 1997; **117**(3): 151–155.

CEREBROVASCULAR DISEASE

Christopher Lattimer

Stroke is the third leading cause of death in developed countries and a major cause of morbidity. Although hypertension and embolization from cardiac causes are major causes for stroke, between 17% and 24% of ischaemic strokes are due to carotid artery disease. The North American Symptomatic Carotid Endarterectomy Trial (NASCET) and the European Carotid Surgery Trial (ECST) have both demonstrated clear benefits of carotid endarterectomy in patients with severe stenosis by the prevention of stroke. Trials are now evaluating carotid angioplasty and stenting as an alternative to surgery.

Pathology

Atherosclerosis is the most common pathology of carotid artery disease. It occurs almost exclusively within 2–3 cm of the carotid bifurcation. Transient neurological events are the main symptoms that occur in patients and these may precede a stroke. Symptoms are usually due to plaque degeneration, with the release of platelet, cholesterol or thrombotic emboli, but are occasionally due to cerebral hypoperfusion. Fibromuscular dysplasia is a rare cause that occurs predominantly in young women. Medial hyperplasia is the underlying pathology that occurs in a segmental fashion. This is observed radiologically by a beaded appearance of the vessels. Other rare causes include arteritis (temporal artery, lupus erythematosus, polyarteritis nodosa, Takayasu's disease), trauma, irradiation injury and aneurysmal disease (atherosclerotic, syphilitic, fungal or following trauma).

Clinical examination

The common carotid artery is evaluated by a carotid impulse on palpation and a bruit on auscultation. It is important to recognize that the internal carotid artery is usually not palpable in the neck and may be occluded despite the presence of a good neck pulsation. The presence of radial and superficial temporal pulses should be noted and any delay between both sides recorded. Blood pressure should be taken in both arms to evaluate any potential proximal disease. The presence of rubeosis or a reduced intraoccular pressure (occuloplethysmography) may indicate hypoperfusion secondary to a carotid stenosis or occlusion. The presence of retinal cholesterol emboli confirms an embolic cause.

Diagnosis

All patients presenting with transient ischaemic attacks should have a duplex examination of their carotid arteries. This will establish the degree and site of the stenosis, indicate the level of the bifurcation and determine the heterogeneous nature of the plaque. Heterogeneous plaques are potentially unstable and more likely to give rise to symptoms[c]. A peak systolic velocity of greater than 1.25 m/s with marked spectoral broadening indicates a significant stenosis. Stenoses greater than 50% should be treated[(b)]. A duplex report is occasionally all that is required before intervention however most surgeons will evaluate the disease further:

- Intra-venous digital subtraction arteriogram (IVDSA). Infrequently performed due to the large doses of contrast required and the sub-optimal quality of the images produced.
- Intra-arterial digital subtraction arteriogram (IADSA). Arch studies are more invasive but give very good images using high pressure injection and state-of-the-art equipment. Selective four vessel catheterization is the gold standard in image quality but has a small (<1%) risk of stoke.
- MRI is the least invasive technique. It gives detailed information on all four extracranial vessels as well as the intracerebral circulation and the patency of the circle of Willis. It may however overestimate the degree of stenosis. Cerebral infarcts, too small to be noticed on CT scanning, are also identified. MRI is also better than CT at distinguishing haemorrhagic from ischaemic lesions. Space occupying lesions and other intracerebral pathology can be excluded.
- Cerebral reactivity studies. These tests indicate the cerebral reserve by measuring the response of the intracranial vessels and cerebral circulation (usually with transcranial Doppler) to an ischaemic challenge (usually CO_2). Its use is in evaluating whether patient symptoms are due to cerebral ischaemia or embolization.

Referral to a neurologist is desirable if the aetiology of the patient's symptoms remain unclear.

Carotid endarterectomy

Carotid endarterectomy is indicated in patients with transient ischaemic events or amaurosis fugax when the ipsilateral carotid artery is confirmed as responsible. This operation is also indicated for symptomatic non-stenotic atherosclerotic ulcers and in symptomless patients with a high grade stenosis, as prophylaxis against stroke prior, after or most frequently with cardiac by-pass surgery. The benefits of endarterectomy for asymptomatic patients with critical or severe stenosis are yet to be determined and multicentre trials are in progress to clarify this controversy (Asymptomatic Carotid Surgery Trial, ACST). An endarterectomy itself can cause a stroke in 1–4% and patients should be made aware of this risk. There are several techniques available:

- Intra-operative shunting. The use of a Pruitt or Javid bypass shunt during the operation reduces cerebral ischaemia time. Measurement of the carotid 'stump pressure', middle cerebral flow patterns on trans-cranial Doppler or an awake patient may help in deciding whether a shunt is necessary. Shunts can, however, cause intimal damage beyond the endarterectomized region and increase the complexity of the surgery and as such are used selectively by some surgeons.
- Patch angioplasty reconstruction. Meta-analysis of randomized controlled trials indicate that patches have a powerful advantage over primary closure in terms of peri-operative carotid occlusion, peri-operative stroke and >50% restenosis

at 1 year[a]. Obligatory primary closure is no longer recommended. The ideal patch material has yet to be determined.

- Eversion endarterectomy. The results are comparable with standard carotid endarterectomy[b]. The plaque is separated from the arterial wall by dividing the internal carotid at its origin, eversion and reattachment.

- Local anaesthetic. Deep cervical blocks allow carotid endarterectomy under local anaesthesia. This is considered the ultimate intra-operative monitoring modality. The surgeon should be experienced in rapid shunt placement should this be required.

- External carotid endarterectomy. This is an important collateral supply to the brain and internal carotid artery and forms part of a standard carotid endarterectomy. Its occlusion can produce stroke. Isolated endarterectomy of the external carotid artery is occasionally performed in patients with common occlusion when a reduced collateral contribution from this artery is considered significant in the production of symptoms.

- Carotid bypass. Revascularization distal to a common carotid occlusion can be performed with a subclavian to ICA bypass, an axillary to ICA bypass or a superficial temporal to middle cerebral bypass. These are highly specialized techniques indicated in a small minority of symptomatic patients.

Intraoperative monitoring

Intra-operative duplex scanning, completion arteriography and transcranial Doppler (TCD) of the middle cerebral artery are the most frequently used methods to assess the surgical technique of carotid endarterectomy. These methods may detect intimal flaps, dissection, spasm and residual disease, correction of which could improve the clinical outcome.

Follow-up

The majority of patients should receive anti-platelet medication, either aspirin or clopidogrel (both, 75 mg once per day) before and after carotid surgery. The benefits of these drugs in reducing recurrent symptoms and in preventing restenosis is, however, marginal. Any effect on mortality is due to a reduction in cardiac-related deaths. Hypercholesterolaemia must be controlled and patients must stop smoking.

Restenosis

The introduction of non-invasive methods of detection, like occuloplethysmography and duplex, has increased the incidence of this condition from 1–4% to 6–37%. Restenosis within 2 years is usually due to myointimal hyperplasia and thereafter due to recurrent atheroma. Revision surgery is indicated for patients who present with symptoms but the literature is divided as to whether a repeat operation is of benefit in symptomless patients. This has led several centres to discontinue routine postoperative surveillance by duplex. Symptomless patients with recurrent stenosis are marginally more likely to develop symptoms than those with a symptomless primary stenosis, however, revision surgery is technically more difficult with an increase in morbidity and stroke rates.

Carotid angioplasty/stenting

The Carotid and Vertebral Artery Transluminal Angioplasty Study (CAVATAS) has increased awareness in using angioplasty as a less invasive alternative to surgery in treating carotid stenosis. Although very rare, distal and intracranial stenoses can now be reached. Plaque remodelling and stabilization is the proposed mechanism by which this technique works. Initial results indicate equivalent results of surgery vs angioplasty (10% stroke rates), however this study has been criticised on two counts.

- Patients were not randomized on an intention-to-treat basis.
- The stroke rates were unacceptably high in the surgery group reflecting the treatment of high-risk patients.

The considerable amount of particulate microembolization that is detected by transcranial Doppler during angioplasty, the high stroke rate and the disregard of the external carotid artery has led many vascular surgeons not to recommend this approach.

Cerebral protection

Devices are now available which can prevent distal embolization. The PercuSurge GuardWire™ system has a balloon on the end of a catheter which occludes the ICA distal to the stenosis whilst the angioplasty/stenting is performed. The ICA is then flushed clean before the balloon is deflated. The MedNova NeuroShield™ consists of an umbrella which catches micro-emboli whilst maintaining cerebral flow. The Parodi Anti Emboli Catheter (PAEC) relies on flow reversal in the ICA during angioplasty. Early results are promising, however the placement of protection devices are not without risk and can cause stroke.

Carotid body tumours

These are slow growing and usually benign. They are the commonest non-chromaffin paraganglia tumours and may be bilateral. Also known as the 'potato tumour' they are situated at the carotid bifurcation and splay these vessels apart as they grow. The vessels are often embedded in and surrounded by the tumour. They are very vascular deriving most of their blood supply from the ECA. Removal requires generous exposure to avoid vessel and cranial nerve injury. Emergency arterial repair and shunting may be necessary in a small number of patients.

Further reading

Burnard KG, Lattimer CR. Intraoperative duplex scanning and completion DSA in the assessment of carotid endarterectomy. In: Greenhalgh RM (ed.) *Vascular Imaging for Surgeons*. London: W.B. Saunders, 1995; 129–139.

Greenhalgh RM (ed.). *Vascular and Endovascular Surgical Techniques*. London: W.B. Saunders, 2001.

Lattimer CR, Burnand KG. REVIEW: Recurrent Carotid Stenosis after Carotid Endarterectomy. *British Journal of Surgery*, 1997; **84**: 1206–1219.

Related topics of interest

Vascular imaging and investigation (p. 350); Vascular malformations and tumours (p. 353).

CHEST TRAUMA

Nick Wilson

Chest injuries may be blunt or penetrating. Blast injuries frequently involve a combination of these. Fewer than 15% of chest injuries require surgery. Tube thoracostomy, blood or fluid replacement, oxygen therapy and analgesia are the mainstay of treatment in most patients. Hypoxia is the final common pathway of most chest injuries and all patients should receive oxygen at an FIO_2 of at least 0.85.

Treatment approach

Primary survey, resuscitation, secondary survey and definitive care are undertaken as described in *Trauma management* (p. 328).

Specific chest injuries

1. ***Uncomplicated rib fracture.*** A common injury. Pain impedes respiration facilitating retention of secretions, atelectasis and infection, particularly in those with pre-existing respiratory disease. Injury to the upper ribs (1–3) usually implies a severe injury. Ribs 4 to 9 sustain the majority of injuries. Localized pain, tenderness and crepitus indicate a fracture. An erect CXR must be performed to identify associated injuries rather than to accurately identify fractures. A short course of non-steroidal analgesics may be given if not contraindicated. Alternatively, local infiltration of the fractures with bupivicaine or thoracic epidural may be necessary.

2. ***Simple pneumothorax.*** Lung laceration caused by blunt or penetrating injury is the most common cause. Air in the pleural space results in lung collapse and a consequent ventilation perfusion mismatch. Reduced hemithorax movement, dyspnoea, hyper-resonance and reduced breath sounds are usually detected. An erect CXR will show the collapsed lung, but needle aspiration will establish the diagnosis if the patient is in extremis. Pneumothorax associated with other injuries should be treated using an intercostal tube drain inserted via the fourth or fifth intercostal space. General anaesthesia, ventilation and air transport should not be undertaken until a drain has been inserted.

3. ***Open pneumothorax.*** Most penetrating wounds close themselves, but large defects may persist causing a sucking chest wound and impairing ventilation. The defect should be covered by a large occlusive dressing (taped on three sides to create a flutter valve, allowing air to escape during expiration) until surgical closure can be performed.

4. ***Tension pneumothorax.*** A one-way valve effect occurs allowing air to pass into the pleural space either from the lung or through the chest wall. The lung collapses and the mediastinum is displaced towards the opposite hemithorax further impairing ventilation and impeding venous return. Dyspnoea, cyanosis, tracheal deviation, hyper-resonance, absent breath sounds and raised venous pressure are the cardinal signs. Immediate decompression should be performed by inserting a needle

into the second intercostal space in the midclavicular line. A formal intercostal tube drain should be inserted as soon as possible.

5.   Flail segment.   This occurs where multiple rib fractures allow an island of chest wall to move independently of the rest of the chest wall. The free-floating segment moves paradoxically, reducing the efficiency of the chest wall excursion in expanding and deflating the lung. More important, however, is the injury to the underlying lung which is the more potent cause of hypoxia. Dyspnoea, poor chest movement, the identification of a segment moving paradoxically and crepitus of rib or cartilage fractures are the physical signs. A CXR may show multiple fractures. Patients with flail chest often compensate adequately in the first 24–48 hours and then rapidly develop respiratory failure. Treatment includes adequate analgesia, oxygen therapy, intravenous fluids (avoid overhydration). Intercostal tube drainage may be necessary if there is a co-existent pneumothorax. Ventilation may be necessary if respiratory failure supervenese.

6.   Haemothorax.   Massive haemothorax (blood loss >1500 ml) occurs following disruption of major intrathoracic vessels, usually by a penetrating wound; poor respiratory movement, dullness to percussion, absent breath sounds and shock are prominent. An erect CXR is required to detect even the presence of large volumes of blood. Pneumothorax may co-exist. Intravenous lines for transfusion are necessary and a large bore intercostal drain is placed to drain the dependent areas of the thorax. Continuing blood loss of 200–300 ml/h necessitates thoracotomy. Wounds medial to the nipple or the scapula indicate possible mediastinal trauma.

7.   Pulmonary contusion.   Localized oedema may result from blunt trauma, but widespread pulmonary oedema may also occur in response to primary lung injury in the presence of normal cardiac filling pressures (ARDS). The alveolar transudate impedes gas exchange resulting in respiratory failure. Ventilation may become necessary, especially in those with pre-existing pulmonary disease, impaired consciousness, other concomitant injuries and multisystem organ failure.

8.   Tracheobronchial tree injuries.   Penetrating tracheal injuries are often associated with oesophageal, carotid and jugular injuries and require prompt surgical exploration and repair. A major bronchial injury is unusual and often fatal. Patients present with haemoptysis, surgical emphysema and pneumothorax. A persisting large air leak after intercostal tube drainage suggests bronchial injury. Surgical repair is necessary in most patients.

9.   Cardiac tamponade.   This usually results from a penetrating injury. Physical signs include hypotension, raised venous pressure, muffled heart sounds and pulsus paradoxus. Pericardiocentesis should be attempted but open pericardiotomy and arrest of haemorrhage may be required.

10.   Aortic rupture.   Aortic rupture is the most common cause of death following major trauma and usually occurs at the ligamentum arteriosum or the aortic root. In survivors a thin layer of adventitia persists and a contained haematoma extends into the mediastinum. A CXR showing a widened mediastinum is often the first indication, and CT scanning should be performed to confirm the diagnosis. Immediate surgical repair is necessary.

11. *Myocardial contusion.* Blunt trauma, especially to the left chest wall, is the usual mechanism. Premature ventricular contractions, ST segment changes, sinus tachycardia and right bundle branch block may be evident on the ECG and sudden dysrhythmias may supervene. Serum troponin levels may indicate myocardial damage.

12. *Oesophageal injury.* Penetrating trauma (usually by instrumentation) is the commonest injury, but forceful ejection of gastric contents into the oesophagus with the glottis closed may lead to oesophageal rupture (Boerhaave's syndrome). Mediastinitis and empyema follow and are usually fatal. Left haemothorax/pneumothorax without rib fracture or the presence of mediastinal air suggest, and Gastrografin swallow confirms the diagnosis. Tube drainage and antibiotics with subsequent direct surgical repair of the defect should be undertaken if possible.

13. *Diaphragmatic rupture.* Blunt trauma, usually to the abdomen, causes large radial tears leading to immediate herniation and respiratory embarrassment. Over 90% are on the left. Penetrating injuries produce small defects that do not usually cause immediate herniation. The diagnosis is frequently missed, but the CXR may reveal viscera in the chest. Surgical repair is necessary.

Further reading

ATLS Core Handbook. American College of Surgeons, Chicago, 1993.

Goldstraw P. The chest wall, lungs, pleura and diaphragm. In: Burnand KG, Young AE (eds) *The New Aird's Companion in Surgical Studies (2nd Edn).* London: Churchill Livingstone, 1998; 553–585.

Goldstraw P. The mediastinum. In: Burnand KG, Young AE (eds) *The New Aird's Companion in Surgical Studies (2nd Edn).* London: Churchill Livingstone, 1998; 615–630.

Related topic of interest

Trauma management (p. 328).

CHRONIC PANCREATITIS

Nick Lagattolla

Chronic pancreatitis may be defined as repeated episodes of inflammatory pancreatitis combined with evidence of structural damage to the pancreas. The damage usually starts in the duct system, and is characterized by ductal stenoses, which are frequently multiple with dilated portions in between. The prevalence of this condition is approximately 3/100 000.

Aetiology

The vast majority of cases of chronic pancreatitis result from alcohol, though the exact mechanism remains obscure. The anatomical abnormality of pancreas divisum accounts probably for more cases than is generally thought. This is due to the persistence of the embryological ductal drainage of the ventral and dorsal pancreatic portions. The dorsal part comprising the bulk of the pancreas remains drained by what in the normal pancreas becomes the smaller accessory duct of Santorini. The ventral pancreatic bud, which rotates to form the lower part of the pancreatic head and uncinate process, freely drains through a wide duct, which should join the main duct of Wirsung allowing free drainage of the major dorsal portion of the pancreas. Gallstones passing repeatedly through the lower portion of the common bile duct can damage the pancreatic duct and result in not only acute pancreatitis, but chronic pancreatitis. Any cause of acute pancreatitis may result in chronic pancreatitis if there are repeated episodes, or if damage to the pancreatic ductal system results.

Clinical examination

The symptoms are pain, in 95% of patients, which is usually epigastric and possibly radiating to the back, and weight loss, which is usually marked and clinically evident. The pain may be severe and protracted and patients can become reliant on opiate analgesics for relief. Less common symptoms include steatorrhoea, jaundice or symptoms of diabetes mellitus. A raised amylase is not a reliable indicator of chronic pancreatitis, as the exocrine pancreas is very often damaged to such an extent that the production of amylase is limited. Even in acute attacks occurring in chronic pancreatitis, the amylase is rarely raised significantly. Eighty per cent of sufferers are male, and most are middle aged.

Investigations

Endoscopic retrograde cholangiopancreatography (ERCP) is the only method to establish the diagnosis of chronic pancreatitis with certainty. This endoscopic procedure is performed under sedation as an out-patient. A side-viewing gastroscope is passed into the duodenum, and the ampulla of Vater is cannulated via a side arm through which contrast is injected. X-rays are taken which show both the biliary tree and pancreatic duct. In the realms of chronic pancreatitis, ERCP is a diagnostic tool rather than therapeutic.

Plain abdominal radiographs may demonstrate small flecks of calcification in the head and body of the pancreas. This is highly suggestive of chronic pancreatitis. The calcification may also be seen on CT scanning. Pancreatic cysts are common in chronic pancreatitis, and these may be visualized by ultrasound, CT, and, if they communicate with the ductal system, by ERCP.

The function of the exocrine part of the pancreas may be tested by means of pancreatic function tests such as the pancreolauryl test. This comprises an oral dose of a compound that is intestinally absorbed and excreted in the urine only after, and proportional to, the action of pancreatic enzymes.

Conservative treatment

The principles of managing chronic pancreatitis are to treat any identified underlying cause, to control the pain, to supplement pancreatic exocrine function, and to correct any anatomical abnormality that is amenable to surgery. Most cases are managed conservatively. If severe pain is a feature, then potent analgesics are required. An unfortunate complication of many opiate analgesics is spasm of the sphincter of Oddi at the duodenal papilla, and this may aggravate pancreatic duct obstruction. Pethidine causes less spasm than other opiates and is thus the drug of choice, but it is not as effective an analgesic as most other opiates, and patients may resort to using vast amounts. More lasting pain relief may be achieved with a coeliac ganglion block. However, tolerance may arise, and it may need to be repeated. Transthoracic splanchnotomy has also been advocated. Various oral pancreatic enzyme supplements are available and should be prescribed, although pain is not affected by this treatment.

Surgical treatment

The role of surgery is limited in chronic pancreatitis but is quite well defined. Mostly, the aims of surgery are to reduce pain but should not be attempted until less invasive means of pain control have been tried. If surgery is planned, anatomical abnormalities (cysts, stenoses, dilatated ducts) may be corrected.

1. Relief of obstruction. Any obstruction at the ampulla of Vater, such as a benign or malignant tumour, should be resected. If there is a cyst obstructing the duct, this should be bypassed as a cystjejunostomy or cystgastrostomy. Cystic dilatation of the duct of greater than 1 cm as a result of downstream obstruction may be treated by pancreatojejunostomy.

2. Pancreatic resection. If the duct system is too narrow to bypass, and pain persists despite all conservative measures, and if the patient is fit for major surgery, then the last option is to resect the pancreas. In order to preserve as much of the remaining pancreatic function as possible, a pancreatic resection should be limited in benign disease. Thus, if the distal pancreas is diseased and the head is normal, then a distal pancreatectomy is performed. If the head is abnormal, then a pancreaticoduodenectomy (Whipple's procedure) is performed, preserving the distal pancreas and reanastomosing the duct with the jejunum. If there is no discernible normal tissue worth preserving, or if there has been a previous pancreatic resection, then a total pancreatectomy is performed. This is complicated surgery, with up to 5% mortality, and a high incidence of complications such as pancreatic or duodenal fistula. Diabetes will ensue. The results are reasonable, however, with up to 75% of patients pain free and 15% improved as a result of surgery. 10% remain unchanged.

3. Pancreatic cysts and pseudocysts. Rarely, pancreatic cysts may become complicated by infection or may compress the extrahepatic biliary tree giving rise to jaundice, or compress the splenic vein causing left-sided or sectoral portal hypertension. Haemorrhage into a large pancreatic cyst is rare, but is life threatening. All these complications require surgery, which must be immediate to arrest haemorrhage if present. The cyst is decompressed, and this is best done by internal drainage to the stomach or jejunum. Percutaneous drainage of pancreatic cysts sounds an attractive proposition, but may be fraught with problems. Generally, if a cyst is found not to be communicating with the pancreatic duct system on ERCP, then percutaneous drainage may be performed. However, should a cyst be of proportions that require decompression, then an internal drainage may be a better option. If a cyst is seen to be communicating with the duct system, then attempts at percutaneous drainage can result in a distressing pancreatic fistula.

Further reading

Reviews

Bornman PC, Russell RCG. Endoscopic treatment for chronic pancreatitis. *British Journal of Surgery*, 1992; **79**: 1260–1261.

Bornman PC, Beckingham IJ. Chronic pancreatitis. *British Medical Journal*, 2001; **322**: 660–663.

Grace PA, Williamson RCN. Modern management of pancreatic pseudocysts. *British Journal of Surgery*, 1993; **80**: 577–581.

Russell C. Chronic pancreatitis. *Surgery*, 1992; **10**: 247–250.

Observational study

Stapleton GN, Williamson RCN. Proximal pancreatoduodenectomy for chronic pancreatitis. *British Journal of Surgery*, 1996; **86**: 1433–1440.

Related topics of interest

Acute pancreatitis (p. 8); Nutrition in the surgical patient (p. 233); Pancreatic cancer (p. 248).

CLINICAL GOVERNANCE

Christopher Lattimer, Prakash Sinha

Practising to a high standard has always been central to the ethos of all caring medical professionals. Continuing medical education, training, meetings, peer reviews and in recent years introduction of clinical audit were all changes which sought to make quality a more explicit part of health care. Historically there was no relationship between improvement delivered by the health system, each health organization and individual practitioners. Clinical and managerial approaches to quality tended to be pursued separately.

The government's white paper on the National Health Service (NHS) in England outlined a new style of NHS to redress this imbalance. It presented each health organization with a duty to maintain standards and improve quality.

Definition

Clinical governance is a system through which NHS organizations are accountable for continuously improving the quality of their services whilst safeguarding high standards of care by creating an environment in which excellence in clinical care will flourish.

Proposal

This will require practitioners as well as professional and statutory bodies to accept responsibility for maintaining standards within local NHS organizations. The Government will require every NHS trust to embrace 'Clinical governance' so that quality is at the core of their responsibilities as organizations and of each of their staff.

A quality organization will ensure that:

- Quality improvement processes (e.g. clinical audit) are integrated in the organization.
- Leadership skills are developed at a team level.
- Evidence-based practice is in day-to-day use.
- Good practice, ideas and innovations (which have been evaluated) are systematically disseminated.
- Clinical risk reduction programmes are in place.
- Adverse events and near misses are detected, openly investigated (no blame culture) and the lessons learned applied.
- Lessons for clinical practice are learned from complaints made by patients and staff.
- Poor clinical performance is recognized at an early stage and corrected.
- All professional development programmes reflect the principles of Clinical Governance.
- The quality of data collected to monitor clinical care is of a high standard.
- Sufficient funds, finance and infrastructure are made available to support all the above.

Team approach

The Chief Executive is ultimately accountable for this duty of quality on behalf of the board. A designated clinician (Medical Director) will lead and face the challenge of leadership and accountability by creating a new organizational culture in which education and research are valued, good practice is shared, multidisciplinary team work is the norm and patients and carers are actively involved.

The National Institute for Clinical Excellence (NICE) will set standards and the Commission for Health Improvement (CHI) will inspect local clinical governance arrangements.

For the individual practitioner these changes will mean:

- Playing a part in the organization's assessment of its present capacity for quality improvement.
- Working within the team to look at the strength and weaknesses of the services they deliver and propose ways for improvement.
- Leading and participating in quality improvement activities.
- Awareness of best practice guidelines from NICE and other sources and adopting them as part of individual practice development.
- Involving staff and patients in the planning of service improvements.
- Taking a full part in continuing professional development programmes.

Evidence and good practice

Accessing and appraising evidence is an essential clinical skill. Clinical decisions or health policy should no longer be based on opinion alone.

The NHS research and development programme is partially responsible with the production and marshalling of the evidence needed to inform clinical decision making and service planning. Unfortunately the local infrastructure to support evidence-based practice is not always in place (e.g. information technology to access specialist databases such as the Cochrane collaboration, Medline).

Presenting evidence and access to it is a necessary condition for adopting new practices. The field of behaviour change among health professionals is also developing an evidence base, through which strategies such as input from a respected colleague, academic detailing, individual audit and feedback are needed.

Clinical governance also addresses how good practice can be recognized in one service and transferred to others.

Poor performance

Poorly performing staff are a risk to patients and the organization. Though few in number, their existence is important to the standing of the NHS in the eyes of the public. The controversy generated can lead some to believe that the sole purpose of clinical governance is to sort out a small minority of problem doctors. The introduction of revalidation and appraisal by the General Medical Council has signalled a change away from a reluctance to do anything that might be seen as criticism of a fellow professional. Local professional regulation and 'Clinical Risk Management' are in place to tackle this appropriately. The test will be whether poor performers can be dealt with in a sympathetic manner which, while correctly putting the protection of patients first, will also deal fairly with experienced and highly trained professionals.

Poor performance will be rapidly investigated and, where necessary, corrected. This can be achieved five ways:

1. Health Authorities could call in the NHS Executive Regional Offices when an NHS Trust fails to deliver against the Health Improvement Programme.
2. NHS Executive Regional Offices could investigate if there is a question over compliance with their statutory duties.
3. The Commission for Health Improvement could be called in to investigate a problem.
4. Primary Care Groups could change their local service agreements if NHS Trusts fail to deliver.
5. The Secretary of State could remove the NHS Trust Board.

Retraining programmes are being developed for poorly performing doctors. The evidence they work remains controversial.

Data quality
There have been substantial failings in the completeness of vital clinical data. A renewed commitment to the accuracy, appropriateness, completeness, and analysis of healthcare information will be required if judgements about clinical quality are to be made and the impact of clinical governance is to be assessed.

Audit
Audit is best defined as a systematic process by which a group of professionals review a current system, identify possible weaknesses in that system, make alterations in practice and monitor whether the standard of practice has improved. The aim is to provide an efficient cost-effective service with improvement in the quality of patient care, avoidance of complications and a smooth running, well-managed department. In short, quality assurance at individual level, firm level and department level.

Clinical risk management
This is about reducing risk to patients and is central to quality care. Every clinical situation needs to be assessed so that risks are avoided in the first place. All staff have a responsibility to minimize clinical risk. There should be a clear clinical reporting system in place and there should be a culture of openness so that we can learn from our mistakes.

National Institute for Clinical Excellence (NICE)
NICE was set up as a Special Health Authority on the 1st April 1999 to provide the NHS (patients, health professionals and the public) with authoritative and reliable guidance on current 'best practice'. This will cover health technologies and the clinical management of specific conditions. It will be based on robust research findings as well as clinical effectiveness and will be distributed to clinicians and patients in a form that will be useful on a day-to-day basis. It will make sure that best practice is spread across the whole country and end the lottery of postcode healthcare.

Commission for Health Improvement (CHI or CHIMP)

CHI was set up as a statutory body to offer an independent guarantee that local systems to monitor, assure and improve clinical quality are in place. It will support local development and 'spot-check' the new arrangements. Where local action is not able to resolve problems, the commission will be able to intervene to investigate and identify the problem. The members are drawn from the professionals, NHS, academics and patient representatives.

Evidence-based practice

Evidence-based practice is defined as an approach to healthcare that promotes the collection, interpretation and integration (into clinical practice) of clinician observed and research derived evidence.

Revalidation and appraisal

All doctors on the General Medical Council register must be able to demonstrate that they remain fit to practice. Each practitioner will be required to submit a personal portfolio to include details of their achievements, professional development, audit activity and shortcomings. Regular interviews will assess how each person may improve their individual performance and service to the trust.

Further reading

Department of Health. *A First Class Service – Quality in the New NHS*. London: Department of Health, 1998.

Department of Health. *Clinical Governance Quality in the New NHS*. London: Department of Health Service Executive, 1999.

Secretary of State for Health. *The New NHS: Modern and Dependable*. London: Department of Health, 1997.

COLORECTAL CARCINOMA

Nick Lagattolla

This is the second highest cause of cancer deaths in men after lung cancer, and the third highest in women, after breast and lung cancer. Annually 20 000 deaths result, and the incidence appears to be rising. The peak incidence occurs between 65–75 years, but no age group is immune. Five per cent of colorectal carcinoma occurs below the age of 30, and it has occurred in children.

Pathology

Forty-five per cent occurs in the rectum and 25% in the sigmoid colon, 20% occurs in the caecum. Ten per cent occurs throughout the rest of the colon, in order of frequency in the ascending and transverse colon, splenic flexure, descending colon and hepatic flexure. Synchronous carcinomas are present in 2–5% of cases.

Macroscopically the carcinoma is usually either polypoidal or ulcerating. The latter is prevalent in the rectum, whilst larger polypoidal carcinomas are mostly found in the right colon. Ulcerating carcinomas often spread circumferentially to cause an annular stricturing tumour. Other morphological types are also seen, including colloidal and plaque-like carcinomas.

Colorectal carcinoma spreads preferentially via the lymphatics and via the portal blood to the liver. Transcoloemic metastasis and ascites may occur in advanced stages.

Predisposition

A total of 70–80% of all colorectal carcinoma arises as a result of the polyp–cancer sequence from sporadic colonic adenomas. This requires multiple steps, from initial adenomatous polyposis coli (APC) gene mutation, through various oncogene mutations, including k-ras, DCC and cytochrome p53. Specific familial tendencies towards colorectal carcinoma have been identified, including familial adenomatous polyposis coli (FAP), arising from a germline mutation in the APC gene, hereditary non-polyposis colonic cancer (HNPCC or Lynch-type) and hereditary flat adenoma syndrome. These together account for about 4% of all colorectal carcinoma. Long-standing ulcerative colitis also predisposes to dysplastic colonic epithelium and malignancy. Other colorectal carcinomas may occur in familial clusters.

Presentation

1. *Alteration in bowel habit.* Rectosigmoid carcinomas usually present with a recent alteration in bowel habit, more frequently tending towards constipation, but sometimes towards loose motions. Carcinomas of the right colon are less likely to present in this way as flow of semi-solid ileal content is less readily impeded than the solid motions of the left side of the colon. However, diarrhoea can occur in right-sided colonic carcinomas.

2. *Bowel obstruction.* The rectum is a capacious structure and rectal carcinoma rarely obstructs. Annular carcinomas elsewhere frequently obstruct. If the ileocaecal valve is incompetent, loops of small bowel will distend, and symptoms may develop slowly. If the ileocaecal valve is competent, then a closed loop obstruction results, with gross caecal distension carrying a high risk of perforation and faecal peritonitis. Caecal carcinomas can obstruct the terminal ileum. Obstructed colonic carcinomas carry a worse prognosis than a similar staged non-obstructing carcinoma.

3. Bleeding. Left-sided carcinomas often present with the passage of dark blood per rectum. This symptom must raise suspicion of underlying colonic malignancy in any patient, and should never simply be put down to minor anorectal conditions such as haemorrhoids. Up to 30% of patients presenting with rectal bleeding have a colonic carcinoma or polyp. Because of the distance from the anus, right-sided carcinomas are less likely to present with overt blood loss per rectum. However, occult bleeding occurs, and anaemia is a very common presentation of caecal carcinoma.

4. Fistula. Colovesical fistula may occur presenting with recurrent urinary tract infection. Rectovaginal fistula is a distressing complication of locally advanced rectal carcinoma. A transverse colonic carcinoma may result in a gastrocolic fistula causing faecal vomiting.

5. Perforation. Faecal peritonitis will result from the spontaneous perforation of colonic carcinoma, which is most likely to occur in right-sided colonic tumours.

Investigation

- Careful rectal examination and rigid sigmoidoscopy is mandatory in those with rectal bleeding. Over 50% of all colorectal carcinoma will be within the range of an examining digit or sigmoidoscope. If a rectal carcinoma is encountered, its location, circumferential spread and distance from the anal verge, mobility and the relationship to the levator ani will determine the choice of operation to be undertaken.
- Barium enema is requested to confirm a lesion seen at sigmoidoscopy, or demonstrate carcinomas out of reach of the sigmoidoscope. It will detect any synchronous carcinoma or coexistent polyps, which occur in up to 30% of cases. Patients with a colonic obstruction may have an unprepared barium enema to confirm the site of obstruction (bowel preparation in colonic obstruction may result in colonic perforation).
- Colonoscopy should also ideally be performed to confirm a histological diagnosis. Synchronous carcinomas will also be identified and polyps may be snared and removed.
- Liver ultrasound will detect metastases although, if present, this should not deter surgery to remove potentially obstructing or bleeding carcinomas. Solitary hepatic metastasis or metastases confined to a single lobe may be treated by hepatic resection, CT scan will exclude liver metastases, and show local infiltration of the primary.
- FBC, group and save, U&E and liver function tests are requested. Anaemia is corrected by transfusion.
- Pre-operative carcinoembryonic antigen is requested if estimation of this will form part of the postoperative follow-up.

- Arrangements are made to admit the patient to the ward at least 1 day prior to the proposed date of surgery for a full bowel preparation. This usually amounts to fluids only and two sachets of picolax on the day before surgery. If endo-rectal surgery is planned, a rectal washout is performed on the morning of surgery.

Dukes' staging

Colorectal carcinoma is usually staged according to Cuthbert Dukes' classification (Care: various modifications of this are in use).

- Dukes A is carcinoma confined to the bowel wall and does not penetrate through it.
- Dukes B is carcinoma penetrating the bowel wall to involve the serosa or extrarectal tissue.
- Dukes C carcinomas have lymph node metastases. (If the highest resected lymph node is clear of metastasis, this is Dukes C_1 and if involved it is Dukes C_2.)
- Hepatic metastases has been termed stage D, although this is not part of Dukes' original staging.

The value of Dukes' staging lies in prognosis. The 5-year survival in Dukes A carcinoma is 95%, in Dukes B it is 70% and in Dukes C it is 50%. TNM staging is more complicated and comprehensive, and may be of greater scientific value.

Treatment

1. Curative resection. In the absence of hepatic involvement, which can be assessed intraoperatively by careful palpation of the liver, the objective of colonic resection for carcinoma is to achieve a cure. This requires the draining lymph nodes to be excised, and necessitates the interruption of the arterial blood supply as proximally as is feasible. The level at which the arterial supply to the colon is taken governs the extent of the colonic resection. It is important, however, to ensure that the bowel ends to be anastomosed and their adjacent mesentery must have a visibly adequate arterial blood flow. If this is not so, then the doubtful segment is resected further until the bowel is indisputedly viable.

- *Right hemicolectomy.* This is performed for carcinomas from the caecum to splenic flexure. Ileo-colic anastamoses have a reduced incidence of breakdown compared to colo-colic anastomoses.
- *Left hemicolectomy.* This is undertaken for carcinomas of the sigmoid and descending colon.
- *Anterior resection of the rectum.* Carcinomas of the rectum may be resected as low as the level of the levator ani. The requisite clearance from tumour is 1–2 cm. Low colorectal anastomoses may be hand-sewn or stapled. CoPo-anal anastomoses may be fashioned transanally.
- *Abdomino-perineal excision of the rectum.* If a low anterior resection of the rectum is not technically possible, the rectum and anus are excised, and a permanent left iliac fossa end colostomy is fashioned. The patient will have been counselled by the stoma therapist preoperatively, and the optimal location for the stoma will have been marked.

2. *Emergency bowel resections.* Obstructing carcinomas from caecum to the splenic flexure are best treated by (extended) right hemicolectomy with primary anastomosis. Resecting all the proximal obstructed colon avoids potential anastomotic dehiscence resulting from proximal faecal loading, and avoids an anastomosis involving obstructed colon. This is a one-stage procedure.

Obstructing carcinomas of the rectosigmoid may be treated by subtotal colectomy and ileorectal anastomosis. Hartmann's procedure, resection of the tumour, oversewing of the distal end or formation of a mucous fistula, and formation of a left iliac fossa end colostomy, is an alternative. Should the primary tumour be difficult to resect, or the patient be too unwell to have a resection, or if the operator is inexperienced, a simple proximal loop colostomy can be fashioned. This is followed by a staged resection of the obstructing carcinoma and eventually by closure of colostomy, as a three-stage procedure.

Perforated carcinomas of the sigmoid may be dealt with by Hartmann's operation.

3. *Palliative surgery.* Resection of a colonic carcinoma should be undertaken even if liver metastases are detected to avoid continued bleeding and bowel obstruction. The resection can be limited. If a carcinoma is unresectable, a bypass may be fashioned to avoid obstruction.

In unresectable rectal carcinoma, local symptoms may be controlled by endoscopic transanal resection (ETAR) using a technique identical to that used for transurethral resection of the prostate. Expanding metal stents have also been used. Radiotherapy may be of help if pain results from invasion of pelvic structures.

Adjuvant therapy

Postoperative chemotherapy regimens are based on 5-fluorouracil. It is not offered in Duke's stage A where a surgical cure is achieved, but offers a proven survival benefit in Duke's stage C. The value in Duke's stage B remains unknown, though this is being addressed by the current QUASAR trial. Controversies exist over the optimal duration of chemotherapy, mode of delivery, newer agents and combinations.

Pre-operative radiotherapy to a bulky or locally advanced rectal carcinoma often results in a reduction in size and facilitating resection. Post-operative radiotherapy is of unproven value in these groups unless there is unclear residual disease.

Follow-up

Unfortunately, symptomatic recurrence of colorectal carcinoma is very rarely curable. Therefore if follow-up is intended, it should be designed to detect primarily asymptomatic disease. The exact form of follow-up, and whether it is cost effective on a large scale, is the subject of continued debate.

Metachronous carcinomas occur in 2–5% of patients. Regular review in the outpatient clinic is usual to monitor for a new lesion or a recurrence. A rise in carcinoembryonic antigen above pre-operative levels may indicate disease progression. Liver function blood tests and hepatic ultrasonography should be performed at intervals. Digital rectal examination and sigmoidoscopy must be performed to detect anastomotic recurrence. Further episodes of rectal bleeding require barium enema or colonoscopy. Yearly colonoscopic follow-up is mandatory for those with multiple or recurrent polyps or multiple carcinomas but not in those with advanced disease. Colonoscopy every two years is advocated for those who have had fully resected solitary carcinomas.

Further reading

Golligher J. *Surgery of the Anus, Rectum and Colon, 5th Edn.* London: Ballière Tindall, 1984.
Midgley RS, Kerr DJ. Colorectal cancer. *Lancet*, 1999; **353:** 391–399.
Mini Symposium – Large Bowel Cancer. *Current Practice in Surgery*, 1993; **5:** 181–201.

Related topics of interest

Gastrointestinal polyps (p. 142); Intestinal obstruction (p. 190); Ulcerative colitis (p. 331).

COMMON PAEDIATRIC CONDITIONS

Nick Lagattolla

Inguinal hernia

This is common, particularly amongst boys, and frequently associated with maldescent of the testis. The hernial sac lies within the spermatic cord. They may contain bowel, and they readily strangulate, and should be repaired as soon as they are discovered. A strangulated inguinal hernia is managed conservatively. The child is sedated and put into bed with a head-down tilt. The majority will reduce and surgery can be planned for the next operating list. The child must be re-examined after 4 hours. If reduction has not occurred, the hernia must be explored urgently. A patent processus vaginalis presents as a hydrocele.

Congenital hypertrophic pyloric stenosis

Pyloric stenosis affects four in one thousand births. This presents with projectile vomiting, and affects boys more often than girls. In one in seven cases, there is a family history of the condition, mostly on the maternal side. It typically presents in the sixth week of life, though with modern methods of diagnosis and a high degree of suspicion, cases are being identified at younger ages. The child should be admitted under a medical paediatric team for investigation. If vomiting has been persistent, the infant may be dehydrated, hypokalaemic or alkalotic. The child is given a 'test feed' whilst simultaneously being palpated in the right upper quadrant. Prior to vomiting, a palpable 'tumour' may be felt (the hypertrophic pylorus). This should be confirmed by ultrasound, which is the optimal method of investigation. A barium meal also demonstrates pyloric stenosis. Pyloric stenosis is treated by Ramstedt's pyloromyotomy.

Undescended testes

Undescended testes are present in 40% of full-term male births. The proportion is higher in pre-term births. Most will come to lie in the scrotum, but in 2% the testes remain in the incorrect position. It is more common on the right, and in 20% it is bilateral.

If the testis has not entered the scrotum at 1 year of age, it is highly unlikely to do so. Undescent of the testis comprises incomplete descent and maldescent. Incompletely descended testes lie at some point between the retroperitoneum and the neck of the scrotum, having stopped at some point along their normal developmental descent into the scrotum. They usually lie in the vicinity of the internal inguinal ring, where they are impalpable. Maldescended testes take up an ectopic position. Ectopic testes are most commonly in the superficial inguinal pouch, immediately lateral to the external inguinal ring, where they may be easily palpated. Other positions include perineal, femoral, or at the base of the penis. Ectopic testes may be pulled into abnormal sites by extrascrotal gubernacula, the so-called gubernacular 'tails of Lockwood'.

Complications of testicular maldescent include torsion of the testis, loss of seminiferous function and infertility, and a risk of developing seminoma of the testis, which may be as much as 40 times the usual risk, and which is not reversed by orchidopexy. Surgery must be performed before the age of 2 years to preserve function.

Tortion of the testis

This presents with acute scrotal pain but lower abdominal pain may occasionally be present. Predisposing abnormalities include maldescended testes, transverse lying testes, and 'bell-clapper' testes with a long mesorchium. Torted testes are tender, and lie high in the scrotum. The differential diagnosis includes tortion of a pedunculated hydatid of Morgagni, acute epididymitis or orchitis, testicular trauma and idiopathic scrotal oedema. Acute infections will usually be secondary to urinary tract infections and this may be evident on urinalysis with traces of blood and protein, and leucocytes and bacteria on microscopy. Idiopathic scrotal oedema is painless and may be associated with signs of Henoch–Schoenlein purpura, though the appearance of the scrotum may be similar to a testicular torsion.

The only reliable method of ensuring the correct diagnosis is by surgical exploration of the testis. If this rule is followed, then no testicular tortion will be missed. The contralateral testis should also be fixed.

Gastrointestinal obstruction

1. Intussusception. Four out of 1000 children develop intussusception, which carries a 1% mortality. The intussusception is usually ileo-colic, but may be cob-colic or ileo-ileal, in which case it may occur at multiple sites. There is usually a lead point to intussusception in children, which may be a Meckel's diverticulum, a polyp, or a reactive Peyer's patch. Intussusception typically causes screaming episodes interspersed with periods of silence and pallor, and the passage of bloody mucus per rectum, which has been likened to redcurrant jelly. A sausage-shaped mass may be palpable in the abdomen. The diagnosis is confirmed by barium enema. Barium may enter the space between the intussusceptum and the intussuscepiens, giving rise to the 'coiled-spring' appearance of oedematous mucosal folds.

The instillation of barium frequently reduces the intussusception. The reduction should not be deemed to be complete until there is free passage of barium into the terminal ileum. Despite this, there is a 1–3% recurrence rate, which may be dealt with by repeated barium reduction (though this is less likely to succeed the second time) or surgery. Surgery is performed through a transverse incision, and the intussusceptum is gently pushed back through the investing intussuscepiens. Surgery must be undertaken if there are signs of peritonitis, and bowel must be resected if either a manual reduction is impossible, or if it is gangrenous.

2. Congenital causes of bowel obstruction. Malrotated bowel is prone to volvulus (volvulus neonatorum). Ladd's bands are congenital peritoneal adhesions that usually tether the right colon to the liver, and may result in obstruction. A Meckel's diverticulum often has a band at its apex which may tether it to the umbilicus, or to the mesentery of the distal ileum. The former acts as a fulcrum for volvulus of the ilium, and the latter can result in adhesion obstruction or internal herniation. Neonatal duodenal stenosis or atresia, common in Down's children, results in intractable vomiting. This is often identified in utero and gastrojejunostomy planned for the first few days of life. Strangulated inguinal hernia must never be overlooked as a cause of intestinal obstruction at any age.

Acute abdomen

The acute abdomen in children may not be due to a surgical condition. However, surgical problems can prove life-threatening if left to develop. Bowel ischaemia and perforation may occur over a very short period of time in children. It is important to review the child frequently and to have a low threshold for surgical exploration.

1.   Acute appendicitis.   Only 7% of all acute appendicitis occurs in the under-6-years age group, but this is responsible for up to one-third of deaths from appendicitis. The child is usually still, may have vomited and will not be hungry; facial flushing is prominent, there is a low-grade pyrexia (high fever if seen late), a tachycardia, and there is firm evidence of right-sided abdominal peritonism. A leucocytosis is common, but not requisite for the diagnosis. A child suspected of having acute appendicitis must undergo appendicectomy as soon after diagnosis as possible. If acute appendicitis is not apparent, a Meckel's diverticulum is sought.

2.   Constipation.   This may cause peritonism and can cause a leucocytosis, and often occurs without a history of prior episodes, unless the patient has megacolon or Hirschsprung's disease. The diagnosis may be very difficult to establish without a plain abdominal X-ray, which shows faecal loading throughout the colon. Underlying causes such as fissure-in-ano should be excluded. Faecal impaction is diagnosed by rectal examination, and requires manual evacuation of faeces under general anaesthesia.

3.   Mesenteric adenitis.   A generalized viral infection may result in mild enteritis with reactive enlarged mesenteric lymph nodes. This causes a diffuse, poorly localized, often peri-umbilical pain, which is not associated with vomiting. There is a history of a recent coryzal infection, and the child may have a high pyrexia and palpable cervical adenopathy. The abdomen may be tender but there will not be signs of peritonism. If there is doubt about the diagnosis, the child is admitted. Paracetamol will relieve the pyrexia and the pain.

4.   Gastro-enteritis.   Colicky abdominal pain with vomiting and diarrhoea, often a pyrexia and abdominal tenderness but no signs of peritonism should suggest a diagnosis of gastroenteritis. There may be others in the family with the same problem. Most causes are viral, but some prove to be bacterial, including *Salmonella* and *Campylobacter*. All are self-limiting, and the child may be admitted for assessment of hydration and correction with i.v. fluids if necessary.

5.   Other causes.   These include lower and upper urinary tract infections, renal and ureteric calculi, hydronephrosis, gallstones, pancreatitis, pneumonia, hepatitis, Henoch–Schoenlein purpura, diabetes, sickle-cell crisis, porphyria, and lead poisoning.

Further reading

Davenport M. Surgically correctable causes of vomiting in infancy. *British Medical Journal*, 1996; **312:** 236–239.

Davenport M. Acute abdominal pain in children. *British Medical Journal*, 1996; **312:** 498–501.

Drake DP. Neonatal surgery. In: Burnand KG, Young AE (eds) *The New Aird's Companion in Surgical Studies.* Edinburgh: Churchill Livingstone, 1992; 1373.

Related topics of interest

Intestinal obstruction (p. 190); Meckel's diverticulum (p. 218); Penile conditions and scrotal swellings (p. 251); Undescended testes (p. 335).

CRITICAL LEG ISCHAEMIA

Nick Wilson

The term 'critical leg ischaemia' implies the presence of limb-threatening impairment of arterial flow but attempts to define this condition objectively have met with difficulty.

Acute ischaemia

The ischaemia is dense because little or no collateral supply has developed. The clinical features are pain, pallor, pulselessness, paraesthesia, paralysis and coldness. The causes are as follows.

1. Acute on chronic ischaemia. Rupture or ulceration of an atheromatous plaque leads to thrombosis and occlusion.

2. Emboli. These may arise from the heart (mural thrombus on an area of recent infarction; left atrial thrombus in atrial fibrillation; thrombus on diseased or artificial valve), atherosclerotic plaques or aneurysms.

3. Aneurysm thrombosis. This is more likely to affect aneurysms of smaller vessels (e.g. popliteal aneurysm thrombosis).

4. External compression.

5. Ligation.

6. Traumatic arterial disruption. This may occur following closed injuries (e.g. supracondylar fracture of the humerus) or penetrating injuries (e.g. stab wound, gunshot injury).

Chronic ischaemia

The most widely accepted definition is that stated in the European consensus document: Chronic critical leg ischaemia, both in diabetic and non-diabetic patients is defined by either of the two following criteria:

1. Persistently recurring rest pain requiring regular adequate analgesia for ≥2 weeks, with an ankle systolic pressure ≤50 mmHg and/or a toe systolic pressure of ≤30 mmHg.
2. Ulceration or gangrene of the foot or toes, with an ankle systolic pressure ≤50 mmHg and/or a toe systolic pressure of ≤30 mmHg.

Approximately 15 to 20% of non-diabetic patients with intermittent claudication progress to critical leg ischaemia[c]. Diabetic claudicants are far more likely to progress to critical ischaemia. Approximately 60% of patients presenting with chronic critical leg ischaemia undergo early vascular reconstruction or percutaneous angioplasty and 20% undergo early primary amputation. One year after initial presentation 25% of patients have had a major amputation, 55% still have both legs and 20% have died[c]. Despite the fact that aggressive revascularization improves limb salvage the number of major amputations is set to double over the next 30 years as a result of the ageing population[b].

Pathophysiology

The changes that occur in the microcirculation during ischaemia are not well understood. When they become irreversible, gangrene or infarction occur. Platelets, white cells and their products, endothelial cells and the components of the coagulation and fibrinolytic systems are all implicated in the microcirculatory changes taking place in the face of severe ischaemia.

Assessment

Having assessed the leg clinically for pulses, ulceration, temperature capillary refilling, movement and sensory loss, the ankle/brachial Doppler pressure indices should be recorded. Either conventional or good quality intra-arterial digital subtraction arteriograms should be obtained to define the arterial anatomy. Even where embolus is the likely cause, an arteriogram should be undertaken to define co-existent atheroma. Evidence of coronary or cerebrovascular disease should be sought.

Treatment

Limb salvage is sought to avoid the mutilation, morbidity, mortality and expense associated with amputation.

1. General measures. Effective pain relief is essential. Positioning of the leg in a dependent position maximizes arterial inflow, but should be avoided if there is oedema. Co-existent infection should be treated with parenteral antibiotics or surgical drainage if indicated. Necrotic areas should be kept dry.

2. Medical conditions. It is important to treat any coexisting or causative medical conditions such as cardiac failure, which may impair perfusion pressure, diabetes mellitus or renal failure.

3. Thrombolysis/angioplasty. Intra-arterial catheter infusion of streptokinase, urokinase or tissue plasminogen activator is frequently successful at clearing arterial segments and is particularly useful in distal occlusions (e.g. following embolization from popliteal aneurysms). A stenosis or occlusion may then become apparent that can be dilated or recanalized using angioplasty. Thrombolysis can occasionally give rise to catastrophic limb ischaemia, probably through destabilization of thrombus and consequent embolization. Thrombolysis should be abandoned if this occurs and surgical reconstruction attempted.

4. Surgical reconstruction. The patient's general health, mobility, and social circumstances should be considered when planning reconstruction. Embolectomy may be performed via a groin approach under general or local anaesthesia, depending on the age and condition of the patient. An approach via the popliteal artery may be necessary less frequently. Intraoperative thrombolysis by injection down an irrigating embolectomy catheter is sometimes a useful adjunct if the embolectomy has failed to clear the distal circulation. Bypass of an occluded segment (aortofemoral, femoropopliteal, femorodistal) is frequently necessary. Arteriographic demonstration of a patent distal vessel is not always necessary if a patent vessel can be identified in the dependent foot on Doppler examinaton. Where multiple stenoses/occlusions are present, the proximal segments should be cleared or bypassed first. Femorodistal bypass procedures are time consuming and demand considerable dedication to achieving patency. For infra-inguinal distal reconstructions, autogenous vein should be used wherever feasible[b]. Various techniques (Miller cuff, Taylor patch, St Mary's boot) have been devised to enlarge the distal anastomosis and improve patency rates where prosthetic grafts are used. High reocclusion rates frequently mean that secondary procedures are frequently required. Unfortunately, graft patency does not always ensure limb salvage.

5. Fasciotomy. When ischaemia is prolonged and/or dense or there is paralysis or muscle tenderness, revascularization is likely to be followed by the development of a compartment syndrome. In these circumstances, full-length, three-compartment (anterior, posterior and peroneal) fasciotomy should be performed.

6. Primary amputation. In some patients amputation is inevitable, and should not be delayed by misplaced attempts at revascularization.

7. Pharmacological agents. A trial of pharmacological agents may be justified where a patient's ischaemia is not deteriorating rapidly. Prostanoids (PGI_2, PGE_1, iloprost) inhibit platelet activation, aggregation, adhesion and release actions, stabilize leucocytes and endothelial cells and cause vasodilatation. They have been used in end stage critical ischaemia and there is some evidence of ulcer healing, relief of rest pain and improved limb salvage[b]. These agents should be considered for patients in whom surgery or interventional radiology are inappropriate or in whom several weeks delay for a course of treatment is unlikely to be detrimental.

Trials have shown that long-term administration of low-dose aspirin reduces the frequency of fatal cardiovascular events in patients with peripheral vascular disease[b].

Further reading

Dormandy J, Heek L, Vig S. The fate of patients with critical leg ischemia. *Seminars in Vascular Surgery*, 1999; **12:** 142–147.

Luther M, Kantonen I, Lepantolo M, Salenius J, Group KY. Arterial intervention and reduction in amputation for chronic critical leg ischaemia. *British Journal of Surgery*, 2000; **87:** 454–458.

Related topics of interest

Amputations (p. 21); Intermittent claudication (p. 182); Vascular imaging and investigation (p. 350).

CROHN'S DISEASE

Nick Lagattolla

This is a chronic granulomatous inflammatory condition that can involve any part of the gastrointestinal tract. It may occur at any age, and the sex distribution is equal. The most common site affected is the terminal ileum. This is involved in 70% of patients, giving rise to the soubriquet of 'terminal ileitis' or 'regional ileitis'. The colon may also be involved, and Crohn's colitis is the only manifestation of disease in 20% of cases. Multiple sites are common: Crohn's disease occurs in a discontinuous pattern within the bowel such that affected areas may be separated by quite normal bowel. These affected areas are termed skip-lesions.

Pathology

Macroscopically the bowel wall becomes grossly thickened, and enveloped in mesenteric fat (fat wrapping). The histological hallmark is a non-caseating granuloma. This may not be found in up to 40% of specimens, however. There is transmural chronic inflammation of the affected bowel with local lymphadenopathy.

Various aetiological theories exist, including genetic, autoimmune, viral and mycobacterial infections, though a complex polygenic aetiology is most likely. There appears to be a strong relationship with smoking.

Presentation

Crohn's disease presents in a varied fashion. In children, failure to thrive and loss of weight may be the only features. In adults, the most common presentation is diarrhoea, which occurs in 80% of cases. Penianal lesions are present in 70%, and this may be the presenting feature of the disease. Abdominal pain is present in 60% of cases. Other features include abdominal distension, rectal bleeding, pyrexia, abdominal mass, or abdominal wall fistula.

Clinical manifestations and complications of chronic inflammatory bowel disease

There are many extra-intestinal manifestations of Crohn's disease, many of which also occur in ulcerative colitis.

- Oral and rectal aphthous ulceration.
- Clubbing of the nails.
- Pyoderma gangrenosum.
- Erythema nodosum.
- Large joint mono-arthritis and sacroileitis.
- Uveitis and episcleritis.
- Renal oxalate stones.

Hepatobiliary complications of both Crohn's disease and ulcerative colitis include:

- Cholelithiasis.
- Fatty change of the liver.

- Penicholangitis.
- Cirrhosis.
- Chronic active hepatitis.
- Cholangiocarcinoma.
- Sclerosing cholangitis.
- Amyloid deposition.

Investigations

A barium enema or small bowel enema may reveal characteristic features of Crohn's: rose thorn ulceration, deep fissures, skip lesions, fistulae, thickened bowel, string sign of Kantor (terminal ileal stricture) or a featureless (drain pipe) colon. The ESR and C-reactive protein are invariably raised in acute episodes, and the LFTs are often elevated. Anaemia is common.

Complications

1. *Acute inflammation.* This can result in peritonitis and any of its sequelae, particularly intra-abdominal abscess formation. Rarely, involved bowel may perforate. Crohn's colitis, as with any form of colitis, can become fulminant and develop into a toxic megacolon.

2. *Bleeding.* This may be a feature of a Crohn's colitis, but rarely occurs if small bowel is involved alone, and it rarely requires emergency surgery.

3. *Recurrence.* Up to 30% of patients having a bowel resection for Crohn's disease will require further procedures for recurrent disease. It has a predilection for recurring at anastomoses from previous resections.

4. *Bowel obstruction.* This results from a stricture, which is common in Crohn's, particularly in the small intestine. These are best treated by either a conservative bowel resection, or stricturoplasty if the strictures are multiple or there have been previous resections. It has been shown that bowel healing is not affected by the presence of Crohn's disease. Therefore wide resections of affected bowel are both unnecessary and counterproductive in the long term.

5. *Perianal disease.* Anal conditions such as perianal tags, penianal abscess, chronic fissures and fistula-in-ano are common. Acute perianal conditions need to be treated as they arise. Histologically the affected tissue may show changes of Crohn's disease. Fistulae may be very numerous and wide ranging, with openings throughout the perineum ('watering can perineum'). The chronically inflamed and infected perianal skin that results has been shown to be histologically indistinguishable from hydradenitis suppurativa. The end result of multiple procedures on the anus in the presence of Crohn's disease is a distorted, scarred and chronically inflamed anus that may be the source of great distress to the patient.

6. *Malignancy.* There is a risk of developing carcinoma in colon or small bowel affected with Crohn's disease. The prognosis is poor as the diagnosis is usually made late because the symptoms are put down to existent inflammation. The risk of malignancy in Crohn's disease is less than the risk of developing colonic carcinoma in ulcerative colitis.

7. Abdominal mass.   Persistent inflammation in affected bowel may result in a phlegmanous mass. This usually occurs in the right iliac fossa, representing terminal ileal disease, but may occur at any site. An inflammatory mass may resolve with continued anticolitic drugs and metronidazole, but persistence despite these measures is an indication for bowel resection.

8. Fistula.   Crohn's disease has a tendency to form fistulae. Entero-enteric, entero-colic, and entero-cutaneous fistulae are the most commonly encountered. These frequently follow surgery, however carefully undertaken.

Medical treatment

- 5-aminosalicylic acid-containing preparations may be of benefit. Colitis responds better than small bowel disease. However, there are no proven benefits in reducing recurrence following resection.
- Antibiotics, particularly metronidazole and ciprofloxacin are effective, though three months may need to be given.
- Steroids are used in acute episodes, though there is little to suggest that maintenance treatment with steroids prevents recurrence.
- Immunosuppression with azathioprine may be successful in severe disease, particularly in combination with steroids.

Surgical treatment

1. Small bowel.   The principle of surgery in small bowel Crohn's disease is to conserve as much bowel as possible. Stricturoplasty is preferred to resection, and if resection is necessary, then limited resection is performed. If a fistula becomes unmanageable, the affected segment may need to be removed. Intra-abdominal abscess must be drained.

2. Colonic.   Should symptoms persist in Crohn's colitis despite maximal medical therapy, the colon may be defunctioned by the formation of a split (loop) ileostomy. This has been shown to improve colonic inflammation. A subtotal colectomy with a permanent right iliac fossa end ileostomy may however become necessary. Crohn's disease is usually considered to be a contraindication to the formation of an ileoanal pouch.

Further reading

Alexander-Williams J. Small bowel Crohn's disease – surgical strategy. *Current Practice in Surgery*, 1991; **3:** 118–124.

Gobligher J. *Surgery of the Anus, Rectum and Colon*, 5th Edn. London: Baillière Tindall, 1984.

Rampton DS. Management of Crohn's disease. *British Medical Journal*, 1999; **319:** 1480–1485.

Schofield PF. Inflammatory disease of the barge bowel. *Surgery*, 1990; **85:** 2020–2026.

Related topics of interest

CUSHING'S SYNDROME

Christopher Lattimer

Cushing's syndrome was first described in 1932 by Harvey Cushing. He discovered eight patients with similar symptoms and signs. Six of these patients had basophil adenomas of the pituitary gland and they were later classified as having Cushing's disease. Women predominate with Cushing's disease (8:1) with a peak incidence in the second or third decade. The primary lesion is a basophil adenoma of the pituitary gland, which secretes excess levels of ACTH. This hormone acts upon the zona fasciculata of the adrenal cortex to stimulate an over-production of cortisol, which is responsible for the features of the disease.

Clinical features

These are all secondary to chronically elevated levels of circulating cortisol. Excess levels of cortisol can be produced in a number of ways but their effects on metabolism are similar. The clinical features can be divided into anatomical and metabolic. They comprise of truncal obesity, buffalo hump, plethoric moon face, proximal muscle wasting, skin atrophy, poor wound healing, osteoporosis, acne, excessive bruising, impotence, and growth retardation in children. Patients are usually hypertensive, accounting for 0.2% of newly diagnosed hypertensives with a 5-year survival, if untreated, of 50%. Diabetes, and psychiatric disturbances like depression, insomnia or overt psychosis can also be precipitated. Fatal complications include cerebral thrombosis and myocardial infarction, which are the commonest causes of death. Female patients may suffer from hirsutism, greasy skin, amenorrhoea and infertility. Cushingoid striae are purple. They can thus be distinguished from the white striae of simple obesity.

Aetiology

Cushing's syndrome is usually caused by excessive steroid administration. Primary Cushing's can be classified into ACTH dependent (pituitary or ectopic) or ACTH independent.

1. Ectopic ACTH (10%). This can be secreted by an oat cell carcinoma of the lung or a bronchial carcinoid (ectopic ACTH syndrome). It presents with a rapid onset of symptoms and is more common in men (2:1) and in the fourth to fifth decade.

2. Exogenous ACTH. This can be administered therapeutically in excess.

3. Adrenal cortisol (20%). Both benign and malignant tumours of the adrenal gland can secrete a variety of inappropriate glucocorticoids and corticosteroids. These occur more commonly in women (adenoma 3:1, carcinoma 2:1) in the third and fourth decades. The condition of nodular adrenal hyperplasia (NAH) occurs at around 18 years of age. It is characterized by the presence of multiple adrenal nodules up to 3 mm in diameter. In this condition, an excess of cortisol is produced with ACTH suppression.

4. **Exogenous cortisol.** The commonest cause of Cushing's syndrome is iatrogenic, the therapeutic administration of corticosteroids for conditions like rheumatoid arthritis, autoimmune diseases and chronic inflammatory disorders.

5. **Cushing's disease (70%).** Pituitary (ACTH)-dependent Cushing's is caused by a pituitary adenoma or microadenoma (<1 cm) which is nearly always benign.

Investigations

The aim of the investigations is firstly to establish the presence of hypercortisolism, secondly to determine its origin and finally to image the suspected organ involved.

1. **Diagnosis.** Hypercortisolism is determined by an elevated plasma cortisol and loss of the diurnal variation. Two tests are routinely used: the dexamethasone suppression test and the urinary-free cortisol. One mg of dexamethasone given at 11 pm suppresses the adrenal axis and in normal subjects cortisol levels the following morning will be low. No suppression will occur in those with Cushing's syndrome. A 24-hour urinary collection measuring cortisol gives an integrated measure of plasma-free cortisol. Cortisol is protein bound in normal individuals with a very low urinary excretion. If creatinine levels are concurrently measured the cortisol : creatinine ratio can be calculated and used instead of the long collection period required to estimate urinary excretion. False positive values can occur in alcohol abuse, obesity and depression. If diagnosis is still questioned midnight and morning cortisol levels are taken to assess if the normal cortisol diurnal ratio is intact (normally 1:4). A level of less than 1:2 is diagnostic. The level at 6:00 a.m. is normally higher than the 6:00 p.m. dip (a level less than 5 µg/dl is normal). All patients with non-pituitary Cushing's syndrome should exhibit resistance to suppression with a low-dose dexamethasone suppression test (0.5 mg is given every 6 hours for 2 days) by maintaining their hypercortisol state. Diurnal salivary cortisol estimations reflect plasma values and may also aid diagnosis.

2. **Origin.** It is often difficult to distinguish between pituitary-dependent Cushing's disease and ectopic ACTH production. The high-dose dexamethasone suppression test (2 mg is given every 6 hours for 2 days) may help to further localize the problem. Cushing's disease rarely produces the grossly elevated levels that are seen in ectopic ACTH syndrome. In pituitary Cushing's syndrome hypercortisolism is suppressed with this level of dexamethasone but hormone production continues with the hypercortisolism of adrenal or ectopic origin. Measurement of ACTH levels with a radioimmunoassay should distinguish an ectopic ACTH source from hypercortisolism of adrenal origin, because in the latter condition ACTH levels are low. Adrenal carcinomas secrete a variety of adrenal steroids (unlike adrenal adenomas) and a high level of DHEA-S (a specific adrenal androgen) is diagnostic. A chest radiograph or better still, a chest CT, should never be forgotten.

3. **Adrenal imaging.** A selenium-75-selenomethylcholesterol scintigram images the adrenal glands. Bilateral increased uptake is indicative of excess ACTH stimulation, whereas asymmetrical uptake is more indicative of nodular adrenal hyperplasia. Lateralized uptake is pathognomonic of an adrenal adenoma. Adrenal

carcinoma often shows poor uptake and the cortisol it produces suppresses the contralateral gland resulting in bilateral non-visualization. Furthermore, compared to that of benign disease, the hormone profiles of adrenal malignancy demonstrate increased levels of a large variety of steroid metabolic by-products. CT and MRI may be used in a complementary fashion to image the adrenal glands. Somatostatin analogue or PET scanning is occasionally of value. These investigations often allow a 'histological' diagnosis to be inferred in the majority of patients.

4. Pituitary imaging. In Cushing's disease, 10% of patients have tumours large enough to cause an enlarged sella on plain skull X-rays. Only half of the patients with pituitary microadenomas, however, have lesions visualized on a CT scan, which makes the confirmation of Cushing's disease difficult. MRI scanning is the preferable imaging modality, however, it may not identify tumours of less than 10 mm and 25% of the population have non-functioning micropituitary adenomas. If a chest radiograph or whole body CT fails to show evidence of an ectopic ACTH source in lung, pancreas or mediastinum, bilateral selective petrosal venous sampling for ACTH can confirm excess pituitary ACTH production. This is a difficult, but invaluable, technique only carried out at specialist centres.

Treatment

The treatment of Cushing's disease in patients where a pituitary microadenoma has been identified is carried out with a trans-sphenoidal microsurgical dissection and excision of the adenoma. Ninety per cent of patients are cured in this way, however long-term studies have demonstrated recurrence rates up to 50%. Surgical complications include corticotropin, thyroid-stimulating hormone or gonadotropin deficiencies as well as permanent or transient diabetes insipidus and anosmia. In patients demonstrating suprasellar tumour extension, direct excision together with hypophysectomy is associated with early recurrence of Cushing's disease of over 50%. In these patients, bilateral adrenalectomy is indicated with autotransplantation of 8 g of sliced adrenal into the rectus abdominis muscle. This prevents dependence on glucocorticoid and mineralocorticoid replacement, preserves reproductive function and prevents Nelson's syndrome. The major disadvantage to autotransplantation is that exogenous steroids may not be required and any residual pituitary lesion will be freed from steroid inhibition and encouraged to expand. External pituitary irradiation or interstitial radiotherapy can be administered as adjuvant therapy and primary therapy. The latter is especially indicated in children. Complete adrenal blockade can be achieved with Metyrapone which acts by inhibiting the conversion of 11-deoxycortisol to cortisol. It can be used as a poor alternative to surgery in Cushing's syndrome and has prophylactic value prior to surgery. Bilateral adrenalectomy is indicated:

- following unsuccessful pituitary surgery or if such surgery is impossible;
- in patients with rapidly progressive and severe hypercortisolism;
- in palliative treatment for ectopic corticotropin syndrome.

Replacement steroid therapy is required following adrenalectomy, and prophylactic antibiotics are helpful to prevent the wound infections cushingoid patients are prone to developing. Wound sutures should be left undisturbed for several more days than for normal patients. Adrenalectomy is now possible using endoscopic approaches.

Nelson's syndrome

In 1960, Nelson described a syndrome of hyperpigmentation, pituitary enlargement and ACTH elevation in patients following bilateral adrenalectomy for pituitary-dependent Cushing's disease. The hyper-pigmentation is due to the increased levels of ACTH and melanocyte-stimulating hormone (MSH). Treatment involves prophylactic pituitary irradiation at the time of adrenalectomy. If the syndrome becomes established (this occurs in 30% of patients), hypophysectomy or pituitary irradiation is indicated.

Further reading

Farndon JR, Dunn JM. Adrenal tumours. *Recent Advances in Surgery*, 1992; **15:** 55–68.
Lucarotti M, Farndon JR. Cushing's syndrome. *Current Practice in Surgery*, 1993; **5:** 172–177.
Wheeler MH. The adrenal glands. *The New Aird's Companion in Surgical Studies*, 1992; **44:** 1215–1232.

Related topics of interest

Adrenal tumours (p. 13); Renal tumours (p. 280).

DAY CASE SURGERY

Prakash Sinha

Day surgery is defined as a planned investigation or procedure on a patient who is admitted and discharged home the same day. In the UK the concept of complete hospital care for the surgical patient during the course of an 8 hour period arose primarily out of the lack of adequate inpatient resources as well as from the rapid developments of surgical technique and anaesthesia. The Royal College of Surgeons took the initiative and set standards and published guidelines in their *Guidelines for Day Case Surgery* in 1985 and again in 1992. Day case surgery currently accounts for 50% of elective surgery in the UK and 60% or more in the USA and Canada[b]. However in the USA day case surgery is termed 'Ambulatory Surgery' and includes patients who may spend up to 23 hours in hospital thus allowing a greater range of procedures to be included.

Benefits

The benefits of day case surgery are:

1. Early ambulation. This is preventive of the complications of venous thrombosis and pulmonary embolism.

2. Reduced waiting list. Seventy-five per cent of patients on the waiting list for greater than 3 months are suitable for treatment as a day case[b]. Offering them such a service decreases the waiting lists and reduces the cancellation rate because the competition with emergency admissions for beds is eliminated. There is also less time spent in hospital which is a positive benefit for many patients who fear hospitals, especially children.

3. Job satisfaction. This increases for nursing staff as they can rotate within the unit between theatre, anaesthesia, recovery and ward care as well as be guaranteed time off at weekends, Christmas and Easter.

4. Efficient management. Protocols are easier to establish and their implementation can be supervised because many patients require similar procedures which all require similar after care.

5. Reduced complications. If day case surgery is to be successful the complication rates must be reduced to an absolute minimum. Surgeons and anaesthetists recognize this need and should ensure the procedures are carried out by fully trained and experienced staff.

6. Financial. Day surgery operations cost less, saving expensive out of hour nursing and inpatient beds.

Unit management

The management and running of a day surgery unit should be consultant based. This requires an additional commitment to the already busy consultant programme and, consequently, this has not found universal favour. Whilst the principle of day surgery has many benefits, especially for the patients, it is an exception rather than the rule, that such a unit is correctly and optimally managed. There is considerable variation in consultant practice in the same hospital and between practices in neighbouring districts as to the type of surgery that should take place in a day surgery unit. For example some units have extended the day surgery facilities to incorporate laparoscopic cholecystectomy. Such inconsistencies between the classification of a day surgical operation has created audit problems and invalidated many of the statistical comparisons that are made to indicate performance and efficiency.

Cost

The cost of a day surgery unit must be balanced with its benefits to the working community and to improved patient care. Money is only saved in nursing salaries and hotel services if one ward patient bed is closed or substituted for every day surgical bed that is opened. This is not often the case and the resulting cost is usually in addition to the services that are already provided. Costs are further increased if consultant numbers increase to manage the service. More skilled nurses would be required to manage the greater proportion of severely dependent inpatients if comparatively more straightforward and self-caring patients were removed from the main wards. A well-run unit is also likely to attract boundary patients to the hospital who would otherwise go elsewhere for their treatment. This is not without even further cost.

Audit

Day case procedures should be frequently audited as they fulfil an increasing role in surgical practice. This includes patient satisfaction, availability of help after discharge, adequacy of post-operative instructions, suture removal and analgesia, the cost in time and resources on the GP and patient cancellation rates for medical reasons or inappropriateness in selection.

Essentials of a good day surgery unit

1. Selection of appropriate procedures and patients. The ideal day surgery patient should have a confined day surgical problem, good social circumstances for rehabilitation and domestic support, and be reasonably fit and healthy. The duration of procedure should be on an average 1 hour and certainly not exceeding 2 hours[c]. The procedure should not be associated with excessive blood loss or fluid shift. The decision of the suitability of the procedure should be made by the consulting doctor in the clinic and the patient sent for an assessment to the day unit. Very elderly and frail patients will not be suitable.

2. Pre-admission assessment and information regarding surgery. The patient should be booked in to the day surgery unit at the time of outpatient consultation where a nurse with the aid of a standard pro forma, will assess general fitness and the social support required. This will also confirm the appointment date for surgery, reduce patient anxiety on the day of surgery and dramatically decrease the patient cancellation rate. It is here that it is made sure that the patient will have a responsible adult to escort home and care for them for at least 24 hours. The domestic situation can be assessed as regards to easy access to toilet facilities. It is important that the residence is at a reasonable distance from the hospital (not more than 45 minutes drive) and there is access to telephone facility. Patients should be given an information leaflet at this stage explaining the surgery and postoperative expectations.

3. Anaesthesia and surgery with minimal morbidity and complications. Patients should be reasonably fit for anaesthetic. ASA 1, 2 and stable 3 patients are suitable for day surgery. At pre-assessment patients with major respiratory disease, cardiac disease, unstable hypertension and uncontrolled diabetes should be picked up. These patients will need to be assessed by an anaesthetist for fitness for day surgery[b]. Grossly obese patients are not suitable and as a guideline patients with BMI greater than 30 are not appropriate. Some units extend this limit to 35[b]. The procedures should have a very low risk of serious post-operative complications. All patients should be forewarned of any general complications if the risk is greater than 5%. The signs of postoperative haematoma and haemorrhage should be looked for before discharge.

4. Post-operative and post discharge analgesia/ discharge criteria and post-op instructions. Patients should be reasonably ambulant after surgery and before discharge. Pain must be controlled with oral analgesia after discharge. A supply of adequate prophylactic analgesia is given with general postoperative advice, an information leaflet and a phone number to call in case of emergency. In comparison to main ward patients, there is a small increase in readmission rate due to early post-operative complications. A phone call from the unit the following morning to make sure the patients are well is much valued by the patients.

5. Patient satisfaction. Simple questionnaires help to audit and improve the quality of service. Day patients themselves often have increased anxiety and frequently admit they would have preferred to stay in overnight; however, if recently discharged ward patients are asked the same question many would also have elected to remain a further night. Increased patient anxiety at being discharged too soon and being totally responsible for their own management has led to an increase in the use of the GP, the community nurse and readmission rates.

With increase in confidence of surgeons, nursing staff and patients in the concept of day surgery the criteria for suitability is being stretched to include older, less fit patients and more major surgery. This is possible due to better equipment and newer techniques in both surgery and anaesthesia. Equally important is quality service and patient satisfaction. Adequate pre- and postoperative information with the backup of community care and hospital accessibility in case of need will hold the key to the future success.

Further reading

Fleming WR, Michell I, Douglas M. Audit of outpatient laparoscopic cholecystectomy. Universities of Melbourne HPB Group. *Australian and New Zealand Journal of Surgery*, 2000 Jun; **70**(6): 423–427.
Royal College of Surgeons of England. *Guidelines for Day Case Surgery*, 1992; RCS, London.
White PF. *Ambulatory Anaesthesia and Surgery*, 1997, W.B. Saunders, London.

Related topic of interest

Clinical governance (p. 87).

DEEP VEIN THROMBOSIS

Nick Wilson

The significance of deep vein thrombosis (DVT) lies in its potential to cause pulmonary embolism and post-thrombotic calf pump failure. Virtually all venous thrombi arise in the deep veins of the legs or pelvis. The incidence of DVT in the general population is approximately 0.5%. Where no preventative measures are employed, the incidence of DVT in general surgical patients over 40 years undergoing major surgery is 30% and 60–80% in patients undergoing hip or knee replacement or surgery for hip fracture[b]. In patients recovering from myocardial infarction or cerebrovascular accident, the incidence is 20–60%[b].

Aetiology

1. Virchow's triad

- *Hypercoagulability:* Antithrombin III deficiency, protein C deficiency, protein S deficiency, factor V Leiden, antiphospholipid syndrome, heparin cofactor, alpha II macroglobulin, alpha I antitrypsin, fibrinolytic impairment, oral contraceptive.
- *Stasis:* Surgery, bed rest.
- *Vein wall damage:* Surgical injury, trauma, radiotherapy.

Risk factors include age, sex, race, operation, anaesthetic, pregnancy, trauma, immobilization, bed rest, malignancy, previous thrombosis, obesity, cardiac failure, myocardial infarction, contraceptive pill, congenital venous abnormalities.

Pathology

Thrombosis is frequently initiated in the vein valve sinuses of the soleal plexuses. Platelets adhere to the venous endothelium initially and fibrin and red cells are deposited between the layers of platelets giving rise to a laminated thrombus. This propagates to extend up the vein, being free or loosely attached to the wall initally. Thrombus then becomes firmly adherent to the endothelium, organizes, retracts and recanalizes, to varying degrees, destroying the endothelium and valves as it resolves.

Clinical features

Limb swelling, pain, tenderness, erythema and dilated superficial veins are the classic signs, but are frequently absent, even in a major thrombosis. A swollen white leg (phlegmasia alba dolens) or blue leg (phlegmasia cerulea dolens) may follow an extensive ileofemoral thrombosis. Clinical diagnosis is incorrect in 50% of patients when compared with venography[c]. The differential diagnosis includes ruptured Baker's cyst, cellulitis, lymphoedema, torn calf muscles and calf haematoma.

Investigations

Ascending venography remains the gold standard, although colour duplex ultrasound is non-invasive and is being used increasingly. It is, however, time consuming and relatively insensitive in the detection of below-knee thromboses. Plethysmography is used to detect reduced venous capacitance after a thrombosis, but has low accuracy in non-occlusive thrombi. It is used increasingly as a screening test.

Prevention

1. *General measures.* Early mobilization, hydration.

2. *Mechanical methods.* Graduated compression stockings, perioperative pneumatic compression, electrical calf stimulation, intermittent foot compression all reduce the incidence of perioperative DVT.

3. *Pharmacological.* Warfarin – postoperative bleeding can be troublesome. Low-dose heparin (5000 IU b.d.) is effective in preventing DVT and pulmonary embolism (PE), but at the risk of increased bleeding complications. Low-molecular-weight heparins have the advantage of once daily administration and are at least as effective as unfractionated heparin. A reduction in bleeding complications is most marked in patients undergoing hip or knee surgery. Dextran 70 has not been demonstrated to reduce the incidence of DVT, although it appears to reduce the incidence of PE. Problems with fluid overload and hypersensitivity have occurred.

Combinations of prophylactic techniques appear additive in their reduction of DVT risk, but even with careful prophylaxis, 5–20% of patients undergoing general surgical operations sustain a DVT and up to 0.2% have a fatal PE[b].

Treatment

Because clinical diagnosis is unreliable, objective venographic or duplex evidence of DVT should be obtained wherever possible before starting treatment. Both legs should be studied. A confirmed thrombosis should be treated with weight-adjusted bolus doses of low-molecular-weight heparin. APTT monitoring is not necessary. Warfarin should be started once the patient is stable and an international normalized ratio (INR) of 2.5–3.0 obtained. Warfarin should be continued for 3–6 months. Warfarin is not always given to patients who have suffered a minor calf thrombosis, since these rarely cause major PE. Most extensive DVTs start as calf thromboses, however, and the long-term effects on critical areas of the calf pump mechanism remain uncertain. Anticoagulation reduces the incidence of repeat thrombosis, but does little to prevent the post-thrombotic syndrome or protect from the complications of pulmonary embolus.

Thrombolysis may be used to resolve extensive, fresh thrombus. Surgical thrombectomy has no place in the treatment of distal thrombosis, but may prevent limb loss in the acutely ischaemic limb caused by extensive thrombosis.

Caval interruption by ligation, plication, clip, or filter may be required when there is fresh, non-adherent thrombus floating in the iliofemoral segment, especially where there are contraindications to anticoagulation or there has been an initial minor PE. The percutaneously inserted Greenfield filter is the technique of choice.

Pulmonary embolism

DVT is the source of 98% of PE, generally arising from the iliofemoral veins. Approximately 2–5% of DVT give rise to significant PE. Death occurs immediately or within the first hour in 10% of patients sustaining PE. A firm diagnosis of PE is made in a minority of the remaining 90%. Up to 70% of patients presenting with the features of PE have normal pulmonary angiograms.

Clinical features

Dyspnoea, haemoptysis, pleuritic chest pain and sudden death caused by interruption of venous return to the left heart are the cardinal features. A pleural rub may be detected.

Investigations

The chest radiograph may show oligaemia, consolidation and hilar enlargement. The electrocardiograph may show the S1 Q3 T3 pattern of right heart strain and the arterial blood gas analysis may show hypoxia and hypocarbia. Ventilation/perfusion isotope scanning shows varying probability of pulmonary embolism, but the gold standard is the pulmonary angiogram.

Treatment

Minor PE requires heparin anticoagulation once the source of the embolus has been confirmed. Acute massive PE requires emergency surgical embolectomy where there is marked pulmonary outflow obstruction. Fibrinolytic treatment may suffice where the haemodynamic effects are less severe. Once the PE has been confirmed, the legs should be studied with venography or duplex ultrasound to determine the extent of the DVT in case thrombectomy or venous interuption is required. Recurrent PE in the face of adequate anticoagulation is a strong indication for filter insertion.

Further reading

Browse NL, Burnand KG, Irvine AT, Wilson NM. *Diseases of the Veins, 2nd Edn.* London: Edward Arnold, 1998.

Related topics of interest

Calf pump failure and venous ulceration (p. 66); Postoperative care and complications (p. 265); Pre-operative assessment (p. 274).

DIVERTICULAR DISEASE

Nick Lagattolla

Diverticular disease or diverticulosis is an acquired condition of the colon, characterized by mucosal pouches herniating outward through the submucosa and muscularis externa. Congenital diverticula also occur, though these comprise all layers of the bowel wall, and are most common in the jejunum and duodenum.

Epidemiology

This is a common condition which affects upwards of 30% of individuals aged more than 60 years. The condition is rare in those aged less than 30. It is more common in females than males. The association of diverticulosis, cholelithiasis and hiatus hernia is known as Saint's triad. Diverticulosis is a disorder of modern civilization, probably reflecting dietary fibre content. Diverticular disease does not occur in rural African populations where the diet is rich in fibre and colonic transit time is greatly reduced compared with Westernized populations.

Pathology

Diverticula probably form because of disordered colonic peristalsis. The dysmotility may result from constipation. Peristalsis occurs in neighbouring segments of the colon causing high intraluminal pressure in between. This may cause the herniation of mucosa out through the bowel wall at anatomical points of weakness, often the site of entry of blood vessels. A constant finding is hypertrophy of the circular and longitudinal muscle resulting in a contracted, tortuous often gnarled colon with a narrowed lumen. Colonic diverticula often contain inspissated faecal matter.

Sixty per cent have involvement of the sigmoid colon. This is the part most commonly affected in isolation, and which results in most of the complications of diverticular disease. However, any part of the colon may be affected; 7% of cases have total colonic involvement. Diverticula may be giant, in which case the wall is particularly attenuated and prone to rupture. These often occur singly and are found in the sigmoid and the caecum equally. Colonic diverticula arise between the antimesenteric taenia and the omental and free taenia, at the site of entry of blood vessels. The appendix and rectum have a continuous longitudinal muscle layer rather than taenia, and thus do not have diverticula.

Complications and immediate management

1. *Pain.* Ninety per cent of patients with diverticulosis are symptomless. It may be associated with lower abdominal colic.

2. *Acute diverticulitis.* A diverticulum may become inflamed when an inspissated faecolith obstructs the neck of the diverticulum. Acute diverticulitis causes lower abdominal colic followed by constant left iliac fossa pain. Rebound tenderness and guarding result (this has been called 'left-sided appendicitis'). Most of the inflammatory and infective complications of diverticular disease affect the sigmoid colon, although the caecum is occasionally affected.

3. *Diverticular abscess.* Acute diverticulitis may result in purulent peritonitis or a localized diverticular abscess. There is severe pain, a high swinging pyrexia and a prominent leucocytosis. If an abscess becomes established, then diagnosis by ultrasound or CT scan may enable percutaneous drainage. Paracolic or subphrenic abscess may occur.

4. *Diverticular mass.* The local response to acute diverticulitis may be phlegmonous rather than purulent, resulting in a palpable and tender diverticular mass.

5. *Diverticular stricture.* Repeated episodes of inflammation in the sigmoid colon will eventually result in fibrosis, and thickening of the bowel wall. A stricture may result, often presenting with acute colonic obstruction.

6. *Faecal peritonitis.* Diverticula may perforate causing faecal peritonitis, which is a life-threatening complication, carrying a mortality of 50%. The patient may be endotoxic, requiring resuscitation with i.v. fluids and high doses of antibiotics.

7. *Haemorrhage.* This results from the neck of a diverticulum being sandwiched between a faecolith and colonic blood vessel. The vessels can erode, and bleeding is typically very brisk with the passage of bright red blood from the sigmoid (common), or dark red blood from the caecum (unusual).

8. *Fistula.* Inflamed segments of sigmoid colon may adhere to adjacent viscera via a diverticular abscess, which points and ruptures into it, establishing a fistula. The most common is a colovesical fistula. These result in recurrent lower urinary tract infections. Pneumaturia and faecaluria may occur. Colovaginal fistula is very debilitating and necessitates urgent correction. A paracolic abscess may rupture laterally through the parietes presenting as a left groin abscess (if on the right, consider an underlying appendicitis). If this discharges, a colocutaneous fistula arises. Coloenteric fistulae may cause diarrhoea.

Investigation

Diverticula can be seen on flexible sigmoidoscopy and colonoscopy. These examinations should not be carried out if acutely inflamed distal colon is suspected as perforation of the bowel may result. A CT scan will demonstrate diverticulosis and any associated acute complication. Diverticular disease is best diagnosed by barium enema 6 weeks following the resolution of symptoms.

Treatment

Acute diverticulitis or a diverticular mass requires a broad-spectrum cephalosporin combined with metronidazole. Should symptoms or a mass persist it is worth continuing metronidazole for some weeks. During resolution of the acute phase the patient is allowed a soft diet. A high-fibre diet is instigated when the inflammation has settled. If simple dietary measures do not prevent constipation, additional fibre supplements may be prescribed. Antispasmodics may relieve cramping pains, but may slow colonic transit time, and should be avoided.

Surgery

Diverticulitis is a common cause of an acute abdomen. If there is peritonitis, a laparotomy must be performed. The usual operation is a Hartmann's procedure, involving excision of the affected colon (usually the sigmoid), and fashioning of a left iliac fossa end colostomy. The distal end is either oversewn and fixed to the side of the pelvis, or brought to the abdominal skin as a mucous fistula, considerably facilitating the reversal of the end colostomy at a later date. This operation is applied to most acute conditions of the left colon presenting with either peritonitis or obstruction. It has been shown that excision of diseased sigmoid carries a better prognosis, compared with drainage and proximal loop colostomy, and left colonic anastomoses have high leak rates if performed in obstructed bowel or if there is peritonitis. Whilst Hartmann's procedure certainly retains an important role in emergency surgery, sigmoid resection with a primary colonic anastomosis can be safely performed following peroperative (on table) colonic lavage in experienced hands.

Elective resection may be performed for chronic symptoms resulting from diverticulosis, usually pain or recurrent bleeding. A sigmoid colectomy with primary anastomosis is usually sufficient.

Further reading

Elliott TB, Yego S. Five-year audit of the acute complications of diverticular disease. *British Journal of Surgery*, 1997; **84:** 535–539.

Golligher J. Diverticulosis and diverticulitis of the colon. In: *Surgery of the Anus, Rectum and Colon, 5th Edn.* London: Baillière Tindall, 1984.

Morgan PG, Hyland JMP. Management of diverticular disease. *Current Practice in Surgery,* 1994; **6:** 102–107.

Rotherberger DA, Wiltz O. Surgery for complicated diverticulitis. *Surgical Clinics of North America,* 1993; **73:** 975–992.

Schoetz DJ. Changing concepts in diverticular disease. *Diseases of the Colon and Rectum,* 1983; **26:** 12–18.

Related topics of interest

Intestinal obstruction (p. 190); Lower gastrointestinal haemorrhage (p. 207).

ENDOSCOPY

Nick Lagattolla

Endoscopy is the visualization of the luminal surface of hollow viscera. A large number of organs can be inspected. The need for exploratory operations has thus diminished and diagnostic potential is greatly enhanced. Techniques have become widely available to visualize coelomic cavities and even fascial compartments, and these will be mentioned.

Gastroscopy

Gastroscopy (oesophagogastroduodenoscopy) allows visualization of the oesophagus, stomach and duodenum under light sedation. The patient is placed in the left lateral position, head on a pillow, and the neck slightly flexed. The throat is sprayed with lignocaine, and either diazemuls or midazolam may be used for sedation, though often none is required. The gastroscope is manoeuvred into the pharynx, and the patient is asked to swallow, while the endoscope is gently inserted into the oesophagus. The endoscope has channels that allow for biopsies, suction, flushing. Air is blown through the endoscope to distend the gastrointestinal lumen in order to pass the endoscope under a clear field of view.

Gastroscopy is used for diagnostic purposes, for example, to localize the source of upper gastrointestinal bleeding or in the investigation of dyspepsia. It may also be therapeutic. Bleeding gastric or duodenal ulcers may be injected with a solution of adrenaline which may reduce the incidence of rebleeding. Oesophageal strictures may be dilated after introduction of a guidewire past the stricture. Similarly, pyloric stenosis may be dilated. Malignant strictures of the oesophagus may be palliatively treated by laser via the endoscope.

Colonoscopy

This allows the full length of the colon to be examined under sedation. The bowel must be prepared prior to colonoscopy. It may be used for a great number of purposes: to confirm and assess the extent of colitis; to biopsy lesions identified on barium enema; to snare polyps and retrieve them for histology; regularly to follow-up colitics to check for malignant or dysplastic changes; to differentiate acute colonic pseudo-obstruction from organic causes of obstruction and to deflate the colon; to identify angiodysplasias in the colonic mucosa (a source of bleeding) and to treat them.

Proctosigmoidoscopy

In the general surgical outpatient department, proctoscopy and rigid sigmoidoscopy are invaluable. Proctoscopy examines the anus and the distal folds of rectal mucosa, and sigmoidoscopy is used to visualize the rectum. In the presence of an acute anal condition such as thrombosed haemorrhoids, fissure-in-ano or anorectal abscess, proctoscopy and sigmoidoscopy should not be performed. The anal canal will almost certainly be in spasm, and the procedure will be exceptionally painful, if not impossible.

On proctoscopy, first-degree (bleeding) haemorrhoids can be injected with 3% phenol to good effect, and second-degree (prolapsing) haemorrhoids can be banded. Sigmoidoscopy will identify proctitis and biopsies can be taken. Polyps and rectal carcinomas may be seen and biopsied. Flexible sigmoidoscopy enables a view through to the sigmoid colon, and this can be performed in the outpatient setting.

Endoscopic retrograde cholangiopancreatography (ERCP)

ERCP is performed using a side-viewing gastroduodenoscope. The ampulla of Vater is identified and cannulated. Contrast is injected and radiographs outlining both the biliary tree and pancreatic duct are obtained. Biliary strictures and bile duct calculi can be identified. Chronic pancreatitis results in characteristic pancreatic duct strictures with intervening dilated segments. Brushings and biopsies of neoplastic obstructions of the common bile duct or ampulla may be obtained for diagnostic purposes. ERCP also has important therapeutic roles. The sphincter of Oddi can be incised (sphincterotomy) to extract biliary calculi thus relieving obstructive jaundice. Stents can be inserted to bypass structures or obstructing calculi. The combination of ERCP followed by laparoscopic cholecystectomy has almost replaced the operation of open cholecystectomy, intraoperative cholangiography and exploration of the common bile duct. ERCP may be complicated by acute pancreatitis or (rarely) haemorrhage following a sphincterotomy.

Intraoperative endoscopy

1. Enteroscopy. This is intraoperative visualization of the interior of the small bowel and this has been of use in the surgery of Crohn's disease to identify co-existing skip lesions and to dilatate stenoses.

2. Choledochoscopy. The extrahepatic biliary tree and its larger intrahepatic branches are visualized. The choledochoscope is inserted through a longitudinal choledochotomy during exploration of the common bile duct. Choledochoscopy can determine whether an obstruction is calculous or neoplastic.

3. Colonoscopy. This may be of use in the identification of sites of colonic bleeding during surgery when no source can easily be identified.

Chest

Bronchoscopy is performed under local anaesthesia. Thoracoscopy requires a general anaesthetic. It provides a view of the pleural cavity enabling biopsy of pleural masses, aspiration of effusions, and insufflation pleurodesis. Mediastinoscopy requires general anaesthesia, and enables a view of the superior and anterior mediastinal structures through a small suprasternal incision. Masses, particularly enlarged lymph nodes, can be biopsied.

Urinary tract

Cystoscopy with a rigid cystoscope is performed under general or spinal anaesthesia, and enables transurethral resection of the prostate, bladder neck or bladder tumours, extraction of calculi, or insertion of ureteric stents. The bladder is best viewed using a 60° angled cystoscope and the bladder base and ureteric orifices using a 30° cystoscope. The ureters may be entered with a ureteroscope enabling laser or contact lithotripsy of ureteric calculi. The urethra is viewed using a 0° urethroscope prior to cystoscopy, and strictures may be incised with a urethrotome. Nephroscopy is performed under general anaesthesia after percutaneous nephrostomy followed by dilatation of the tract. Renal calculi may be extracted.

Laparoscopy

The peritoneal cavity is insufflated with carbon dioxide using a Veres needle inserted immediately below the umbilicus. A 10 mm diameter port is inserted and the peritoneal cavity is visualized directly. This may be used for diagnostic purposes but, increasingly, laparoscopy is used to achieve an operative procedure, such as cholecystectomy, gastric fundoplication, biopsy of intraperitoneal or hepatic lesions, rectopexy, herniorrhaphy, tubal ligation, or colonic mobilization prior to colectomy. Surgery is performed following insertion of 10 mm or 5 mm operating ports, through which a variety of laparoscopic equipment can be inserted.

The complications of laparoscopic procedures include haemorrhage from the anterior abdominal wall port sites or retroperitoneal vessels, port site incisional hernia, and it may predispose to lower limb venous thromboembolism because of raised intra-abdominal pressure.

Other

There are many applications of 'endoscopy'.

- Angioscopy using fine flexible angioscopes has been applied to peripheral arteries and veins. Arterial occlusions can be located and recanalized. Carotid arteries may be angioscoped following endarterectomy to check for suture line thrombus or intimal flaps. Veins have been screened in situ by angioscopy prior to use as arterial bypass grafts.
- Angioscopy has been used to identify incompetent deep vein valves to allow accurate positioning of plicating sutures to restore valvular competence.
- Cruroscopy allows inspection and interruption of incompetent perforating veins passing through the deep fascia of the lower leg (SEPS: subfascial endoscopic perforator ligation).
- The interior of the cerebral ventricles may be visualized during a craniotomy by ventriculoscopy.

Related topics of interest

Gallstones and their complications (p. 130); Lower gastrointestinal haemorrhage (p. 207); Minimal access surgery (p. 224); Upper gastrointestinal haemorrhage (p. 338).

ENDOVASCULAR TECHNIQUES

Nick Wilson

Rapid advances in coronary angioplasty have led to the development of peripheral arterial angioplasty and subsequently arterial stenting. These techniques are used mainly in the management of occlusive disease, but aneurysm stenting is being evolved and assessed. Advances in catheter and stent technology are extending the application of these procedures, but many major problems persist precluding their universal application in the management of arterial disease. In the UK most of the techniques are undertaken by interventional radiologists, but the younger generation of vascular surgeons is gradually acquiring the necessary skills.

1. **Carotid angioplasty/stenting.**   The place of endarterectomy in the treatment of high-grade symptomatic carotid stenosis is well established. Angioplasty has the potential to avoid cranial nerve injuries and a neck incision with its attendant risk of haematoma formation. The technique also has advantages for the treatment of surgically inaccessible lesions and recurrent stenoses. A stent may be placed following angioplasty to stabilize an ulcerated plaque and avoid restenosis. Embolization during guidewire placement and balloon inflation is a potential complication and devices are being introduced to improve cerebral protection. A high degree of operator skill is required and few centres offer the technique currently. The benefits and risks remain uncertain, but angioplasty/stenting carries a similar 30-day major stroke/mortality rate to surgery although the restenosis rate appears higher [b].

2. **Thoracic aortic aneurysm stenting.**   Surgical correction of thoracic aortic aneurysms carries a high mortality (10–20%) and morbidity with a major risk of a spinal cord ischaemia resulting in paraplegia. Endovascular stent placement has a mortality of 1–4% and paraplegia occurs in 1–2%. The technique awaits full assessment in prospective trials.

3. **Abdominal aortic aneurysm stenting.**   This has the benefit of avoiding the respiratory, cardiac and metabolic insults associated with the long incision and aortic cross clamping inherent in open surgery. Patients still require a general anaesthetic for introduction of the device through the femoral artery, but can return home the next day. Anatomically, only 30% of potential patients are suitable as at least 1.5 cm of normal aorta below the renal arteries is necessary for graft fixation. Tortuous iliac arteries can preclude introduction of the stent and relatively normal calibre distal iliac arteries are required to anchor the bottom of the stent. Stent grafts are available in straight or bifurcated configurations, the later having more widespread application. The devices are evolving rapidly but stent failure, graft migration, arterial dissection, distal embolization/thrombosis and endoleaks are still major problems precluding their general use and resulting in revision or removal of 30% of grafts [c]. Endoleaks are classified as follows.

Type 1.   Leakage of aortic blood into the aneurysm sac through a defect between the top or the bottom of the stent and the aorta.

Type 2. Backbleeding into the sac from patent lumbar or inferior mesenteric arteries.

Type 3. Bleeding into the sac from the stent lumen caused by a tear in the graft fabric.

The place of aortic stenting has been assessed in various registries (RETA, EUROSTAR) and currently a randomized prospective trial (EVAR) is underway comparing a variety of endovascular techniques with open surgery.

4. Renal artery angioplasty/stenting. Renal artery stenosis can cause refractory hypertension and impairment of renal function. The place of open renal artery reconstruction and angioplasty/stenting has been unclear, but recent randomized trials have indicated that angioplasty has no advantage over antihypertensive medication in the treatment of hypertension[b].

5. Aortoiliac angioplasty/stenting. Angioplasty can be used to dilate aortic and iliac artery stenoses and occlusions. Patency rates are high (80% at 5 years)[c]. Bilateral iliac occlusions/stenoses can be dilated simultaneously using the 'kissing balloon' technique or where only one iliac artery can be recanalized, a unilateral procedure may be used in conjunction with femoro-femoral bypass grafting. The place of stents remains unclear with most interventionalists reserving them for the treatment of recurrent disease. These techniques are suitable for patients with critical limb ischaemia or intermittent claudication where appropriate.

6. Femoropopliteal angioplasty. This is a less durable procedure than iliac angioplasty and the overall patency rate is 50% at 1 year for occlusions up to 10 cm in length. Critically ischaemic legs can be treated this way as can claudicants in appropriate circumstances although the disappointing patency rate makes a supervised exercise programme preferable in many patients. Where transluminal passage of a guidewire cannot be achieved or for occlusions greater than 10 cm length in patients with critical ischaemia, the subintimal approach can be attempted. The arterial wall is intentionally dissected with the guidewire and the lumen re-entered distal to the occlusion. Not all centres can reproduce favourable results[c]. Complications of angioplasty include inadvertent wall dissection, embolization, vessel rupture, thrombosis, groin haematoma and false aneurysm formation. Devices are available to seal the puncture site and false aneurysm formation is increasingly treated using ultrasound-guided thrombin injection (which thromboses the sac) rather than open surgical repair.

7. Tibial artery angioplasty. For patients with critical limb ischaemia, tibial artery angioplasty may result in limb salvage. The subintimal approach is usually required and a high degree of operator experience and skill is required.

Adjunctive treatment

Most patients undergoing angioplasty are given antiplatelet treatment. This protects them against myocardial infarct and stroke, but the effect on patency rates, claudication distance and limb salvage is unclear [a]. Aspirin is the standard agent, but dipyridamole, clopidogrel, ticlopidine and abciximab are being investigated individually or in combination with aspirin or each other.

Brachytherapy (intraluminal radiotherapy) is being investigated for the prevention of restenosis caused by fibrointimal hyperplasia. Early results are promising but access to radiotherapy facilities is limited.

Embolization

Vascular malformations and tumours can be embolized using catheter-delivered coils and/or foam to reduce their vascularity and prominence or to cause infarction in the case of tumours. Upper and lower gastrointestinal tract bleeding can also be treated in this way, but the bleeding must be active at the time of the procedure or the damaged vessel will not be apparent at angiography. A high degree of radiological skill is required.

Further reading

CAVATAS. Endovascular versus surgical treatment in patients with carotid stenosis in the Carotid and Vertebral Artery Transluminal Angioplasty Study (CAVATAS): a randomised trial. *Lancet*, 2001; **357:** 1722–1723.

Van Jaarsveld BC, Krijnen P, Pieterman H *et al.* The effect of balloon angioplasty on hypertension in atherosclerotic renal-artery stenosis. Dutch Renal Artery Stenosis Intervention Cooperative Study Group. *New England Journal of Medicine*, 2000; **342:** 1007–1014.

Thomas SM, Gaines PA, Beard JD. Vascular Surgical Society of Great Britain and Ireland: RETA: the registry of endovascular treatment of abdominal aortic aneurysms. *British Journal of Surgery*, 1999; **86.**

Related topics of interest

Aneurysms (p. 24); Cerebrovascular disease (p. 76); Critical leg ischaemia (p. 100); Intermittent claudication (p. 187); Renovascular surgery (p. 284); Vascular imaging and investigation (p. 350); Vascular malformations and tumours (p. 353).

FEMORAL HERNIA

Nick Wilson

Epidemiology and aetiology

Femoral hernias are more common in women than in men in the UK (M : F = 2.5 : 1). In women, indirect inguinal hernias and femoral hernias are equally common. Femoral hernias account for 11% of all groin hernias, but account for between 35% and 50% of all strangulated groin hernias. Approximately 50% of femoral hernias present with strangulation. The cumulative probabilities of strangulation at 1 month and 21 months after diagnosis are 22% and 45%, respectively. Bowel resection is twice as likely during operations for strangulated femoral hernia as for strangulated inguinal hernia and the mortality for such surgery lies between 3% and 15%.

Femoral hernias are always acquired and usually occur from middle age onwards. They are commonest in multiparous women and may follow a period of weight loss. Ten per cent of femoral hernias follow a previous operation for inguinal hernia. Femoral hernias are usually irreducible and frequently exhibit no cough impulse. Omentum is the usual content of a femoral hernia, but if bowel is contained it is frequently in the form of a Richter's hernia, this phenomenon occurring most frequently on the right.

Femoral hernias share the same basic pathology as all other lower abdominal hernias. A defect in the transversalis fascia and overlying muscles occurs, allowing a peritoneal protrusion to occur.

Differential diagnosis

- Inguinal hernia
- Saphena varix
- Enlarged lymph node
- Psoas bursa or abscess
- Obturator hernia
- Lipoma
- Femoral aneurysm
- Sarcoma
- Ectopic testis

Management

Because of the high risk of strangulation, femoral hernia should always be repaired promptly after diagnosis. The principles of repair include isolation and removal of the peritoneal sac, repair of the transversalis fascia, and reinforcement of this repair. Three approaches are described:

1. Abdominal, suprapubic, preperitoneal or extraperitoneal (Henry, McEvedy). This approach utilizes a vertical midline or Pfannenstiel incision to repair bilateral hernias or an oblique, muscle-splitting incision over the lateral border of rectus abdominis (linea semilunaris) for unilateral hernias. The hernias are reduced and the femoral canal closed without breaching the peritoneum, unless there is a suspicion of strangulated bowel. This is a good approach for a strangulated hernia.

2. *Inguinal or high (Lothiessen).* The posterior wall of the inguinal canal is opened to give access to the femoral canal from above. Femoral and inguinal hernias may be repaired simultaneously by this method which is therefore useful if the exact nature of the hernia is unclear. The inguinal canal must be repaired carefully to avoid a subsequent inguinal hernia.

3. *Crural or low (Lockwood).* An incision is made directly over the hernia, just below and parallel to the medial half of the inguinal ligament. The sac is identified, opened and ligated. The femoral canal is closed using either non-absorbable sutures or a polypropylene cylindrical plug taking care not to damage or narrow the femoral vein. An upturned flap of pectineal fascia may be used to reinforce the repair. This approach should be reserved for elective operations, but if compromised bowel is discovered, a separate paramedian incision should be performed.

The chance of recurrence following the extraperitoneal high approach or the low crural approach is 5–10%. A higher recurrence rate accompanies the inguinal approach, although this can be substantially reduced if the inguinal canal is carefully repaired using the Shouldice or Lichtenstein technique.

Further reading

Sanchez–Bustos F, Ramia JM, Fernandez Ferrero F. Prosthetic repair of femoral hernia: audit of long term follow-up. *European Journal of Surgery*, 1998; **164**: 191–193.

Related topics of interest

FLUID REPLACEMENT

Chris Perera

The ultimate goal of fluid therapy is to ensure that tissue perfusion is not compromised and that both oxygen delivery and CO_2 removal are adequate. The Confidential Enquiry into Perioperative Deaths (CEPOD) has recognized that inadequate rehydration and oliguria prior to surgery carries with it a high mortality. Total body water is distributed into the intracellular compartment (two-thirds) and the extracellular compartment (one-third). A quarter of the extracellular fluid exists as plasma. These ratios are maintained together with electrolyte balance and acid-base balance by various homeostatic mechanisms.

Simplified theoretical effective volumes of distribution of infused isotonic solutions of an ideal colloid, saline and glucose

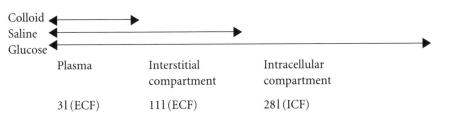

Total body water = 14l (ECF 33%) + 28l(ICF 66%) = 42l

Renin-angiotensin-aldosterone

This mechanism is activated by sympathetic stimulation, falls in blood pressure and alterations in Na^+ flux across the renal tubules. Renin is secreted by the juxta-glomerular apparatus, and activates circulating angiotensinogen to form angiotensin I. This is then converted to angiotensin II by converting enzyme, found in high concentrations in the lungs. Angiotensin II is itself a powerful vasoconstrictor and stimulates the release of aldosterone from the zona glomerulosa of the renal cortex. Aldosterone acts mainly on the distal convoluted tubule to encourage the preferential resorption of sodium at the expense of potassium and hydrogen ions. This system is the most powerful single mechanism for the control of plasma volume, electrolyte and acid-base balance.

Antidiuretic hormone (arginine vasopressin)

This hormone is released from the posterior pituitary in response to anxiety, operative trauma, falls in blood pressure and changes in plasma osmolality. It acts upon the collecting ducts to reduce the excretion of water.

Atrial naturetic peptides

These have been identified in cardiac tissue and are released in response to increases in plasma volume. They act on the kidney to provide an increased diuresis independent of the renin-angiotensin-aldosterone mechanism.

Sodium

Sodium is considered the skeleton upon which the extracellular fluid hangs. The normal plasma concentration is maintained between 135 and 145 mmol/l. The normal daily requirement is 1–2 mmol/kg/day. Excess loss of sodium and therefore water occurs in vomiting, diarrhoea, high output fistulae, profuse sweating, Addison's disease and third space sequestration like intestinal obstruction or peritonitis. Assuming that the total body water is three-fifths of the body weight the saline deficit can be estimated:

Saline deficit (mmol) = 3/5 Body weight (kg)   (140 Plasma Na conc.)

Potassium

Potassium is 97% intracellular. Normal plasma values are between 3.5 and 4.5 mmol/l. The normal daily requirements vary from 05–1.0 mmol/kg/day.

1. Hypokalaemia. Deficiency from gastrointestinal fluid loss or a metabolic alkalosis (pyloric stenosis) results in weakness, confusion and ileus, or even cardiac arrest in systole. Diagnostic ECG changes include a prolonged PR interval, depressed ST segments and inverted T waves.

2. Hyperkalaemia. This is often secondary to renal failure and can be treated with 10% dextrose (1 l) with 10 units of added Actrapid as a single infusion. Ten per cent calcium gluconate 10 ml or salbutamol 5 mg nebulized or 400 µg s/c promotes entry of K^+ ions into cells. Ionic exchange resins can be administered rectally. Severe cases require dialysis. Characteristic ECG changes include peaked T waves, absent P waves, a widened QRS complex, slurring of the ST segment into T wave. Eventually, cardiac arrest occurs in diastole.

Metabolic response to trauma

The duration and extent of the metabolic response to trauma (release of cortisol, ADH, aldosterone) depends upon the severity of the insult. Burns and crush injuries are particularly strong stimuli whereas day case procedures hardly elicit any response. Awareness of this has important implications in postoperative fluid balance.

Postoperative management

During the first postoperative day it is essential to establish a urinary output of greater than 0.5 ml/kg/hour. This should be effected primarily by ensuring the patient is adequately hydrated without precipitating cardiac failure. Intensive monitoring of the CVP and if necessary, the pulmonary artery wedge pressure should be performed if problems in maintaining normal blood pressure and adequate urine output (in the presence of presumed adequate filling) still arise. A 200 ml colloid/crystalloid fluid challenge is a useful way of establishing this. The fluid bolusing should be continued until a sustained rise in CVP occurs, for example >3 mmHg after 15 minutes, rather than be limited by a predetermined CVP value. If a hydrated patient continues to produce only small volumes of urine, frusemide should be administered to challenge the metabolic response to trauma and provide a diuresis. Occasionally, some hypertensive patients or patients in poor cardiovascular health fail to establish a good urinary output despite adequate filling and frusemide. Restoration of blood pressure to 'normal' levels (i.e. in a hypertensive patient) or the commencement of a renal (low-dose) dopexamine infusion can often encourage the kidneys to perform again. Maintenance of an adequate diuresis is a requisite for renal health and the prevention of renal failure. A rising potassium, urea or creatinine indicates renal failure. Potassium supplements should not be given in the first post-operative day because tissue damage and blood transfusions provide a rich source of plasma potassium.

Fluid and electrolyte maintenance

The normal fluid requirement is 3 l/day. Pyrexia, nasogastric aspirate, ileus, peritonitis, fistula, diarrhoea and unhumidified ventilation increase these requirements, and adjustments should be made in the replacement regime. Up to 1 l of fluid can be lost each hour during a laparotomy, excluding major blood loss. Serial haematocrit, electrolyte, urea and creatinine estimations give an indication as to the state of hydration. A typical short-term fluid maintenance regime involves 3 l of dextrose saline/24 hours with 60–80 mmol of KCl added in divided doses. This will provide the required daily amount of sodium and potassium. This regime will have to be supplemented according to the fluid and electrolyte losses of the individual patient. Alternatively, 3 l of dextrose saline can be administered, but this only provides 90 mmol of sodium. Patients on long-term dextrose saline infusions may consequently become sodium deficient. Gastrointestinal losses should be replaced with saline, volume for volume, with added potassium supplements.

Pyloric stenosis

The repetitive vomiting of pyloric stenosis results in a metabolic alkalosis. It also provides a situation where acid is lost from the stomach and a paradoxical acid urine may be excreted. This happens because the distal convoluted tubule preferentially conserves potassium rather than hydrogen ions when sodium is resorbed.

Further reading

Grocott MPW *et al.* Fluid therapy. *Baillière's Clinical Anaesthesiology*, 1999; **13**: 363–381.
Knighton J *et al.* Postoperative fluid therapy. *Anaesthesia and Intensive Care Medicine*, 2000; **1**: 16–19.
Salmon JB, Mythen MG. Pharmacology and physiology of colloids. *Blood reviews*, 1993; **14**: 114–120.
Schierhout G, Roberts I. Fluid resuscitation with colloid or crystalloid solutions in critically ill patients: a systematic review of randomised trials. *British Medical Journal*, 1998; **316**: 961–964.
Webb AR. Fluid management in intensive care – the avoidance of hypovolaemia. *British Journal of Intensive Care*, 1997; **7**: 59–64.

Related topics of interest

Blood transfusion (p. 53); Burns (p. 62); Nutrition in the surgical patient (p. 233).

GALLSTONES AND THEIR COMPLICATIONS

Nick Lagattolla

Gallstones are common, affecting about 20% of the population. Although the typical patient is said to be 'fat, fertile, fair, female and over forty', men and women are probably equally affected, and gallstones may even occur in childhood. They frequently co-exist with diverticular disease and hiatus hernia (Saint's triad). Most gallstones are symptomless, but a wide variety of clinical entities may result. Cholecystectomy, the removal of the gallbladder, is the most common elective operation performed.

Formation and composition

Eighty per cent of gallstones have alternate laminae of cholesterol and calcium salts (mixed). Such stones are invariably multiple, numbering from a few to many hundreds, and are faceted. Twelve per cent of stones are small, multiple and dark, containing bilirubin salts (pigment stones). They may be separate or concreted together (mulberry stones). These may complicate haemolytic anaemias. Eight per cent of gallstones are composed primarily of cholesterol. These stones are usually single (solitaires) and tend to be soft and large.

The formation of gallstones revolves around three factors:

- Bile is rendered 'lithogenic' by an increase in cholesterol relative to bile salts which render it soluble. A reduction in bile salts, as may follow ileal resection or Crohn's disease of the terminal ileum, may effectively precipitate cholesterol in the bile.
- A nidus may be necessary for the stones to form, and this may be provided by bacteria or foreign bodies.
- Some degree of stasis is also required.

Diagnosis

1. Clinical. Gallstones may cause flatulence, dyspeptic symptoms, nausea, and postprandial discomfort. This overlaps with other foregut pathologies, particularly peptic ulceration and hiatus hernia, and a clinical diagnosis may be difficult. Murphy's sign, the arrest of inspiration (due to pain) while pressure is being applied to the right hypochondrium, is indicative of cholecystitis.

2. Ultrasound scan. Ultrasound scanning is a rapid non-invasive test demonstrating stones in the gallbladder with acoustic shadows behind them. The gallbladder wall may be thickened in acute cholecystitis. The gallbladder is usually small and shrunken. The scan will also identify bile duct dilatation if there are stones within the extrahepatic bile ducts, though stones in the distal common bile duct are rarely visualized due to overlying intraduodenal gas.

3. Plain radiology. Plain abdominal X-rays will detect only 10% of gallstones. Rarely, a thin rim of calcification is seen within the wall of the gallbladder (porcelain gallbladder). Limey bile may be visible rarely.

4. *Special radiology.* ERCP and magnetic resonance cholangiopancreatography (MRCP) can show gallstones in the gallbladder though this structure is not always opacified. They are ideal for confirming bile duct disorders and calculi. Oral cholangiography concentrates an oral bolus of contrast in the gallbladder. Radiolucent stones become obvious filling defects on X-rays.

Complications: stones within the gallbladder

1. *Biliary colic.* Intermittent epigastric pain may radiate to the right and may be induced by fatty food. The patient may need to be admitted and opiate analgesia may be required. The pain usually subsides within 24 hours. The pain is not caused by gallbladder contraction as in cholelithiasis the gallbladder is non-contractile.

2. *Acute cholecystitis.* Stasis in a hollow viscus allows infection to supervene. In the gallbladder this results in severe pain in the right upper quadrant which is constant. The patient has a pyrexia and a tachycardia, and a leucocytosis will be present. The signs include rebound tenderness or guarding. This requires antibiotics covering Gram-negative organisms. Approximately 10% of patients with acute cholecystitis may be transiently jaundiced. This may arise from compression of the common bile duct from oedematous tissue in the region of the neck of the gallbladder where a calculus has impacted.

3. *Empyema of the gallbladder.* Very severe acute cholecystitis with a high swinging pyrexia suggests an empyema of the gallbladder. This may result from infection within a mucocele or from a severe cholecystitis. An air-fluid level is seen on a plain abdominal X-ray.

4. *Acute acalculous cholecystitis.* Rarely, the gallbladder may become inflamed in the absence of gallstones. This may occur in those who are already severely debilitated, particularly patients in intensive care. This commonly results in a necrotic gallbladder.

5. *Emphysematous cholecystitis.* Severe infections with anaerobic gas-forming organisms may occur in diabetics. Gas is seen in the wall of the gallbladder on a plain radiograph. This may occur in the absence of stones.

6. *Mirizzi syndrome.* A gallstone impacted in Hartmann's pouch, usually a single large solitaire, may result in obstructive jaundice by impinging on the common bile duct. This is Mirizzi type 1 syndrome, and should be diagnosed preoperatively, as there is a risk of damage to the common bile duct. Pressure on the common bile duct from the large calculus may result in necrosis of the intervening tissue, with a resultant cholecystocholedochal (or cholecystohepatodochal) fistula. This is Mirizzi type 2 syndrome. ERCP should demonstrate these conditions.

7. *Mucocele.* Impaction of a calculus in the neck of the gallbladder resulting in stasis and continued formation of mucus results in a mucocele.

8. *Carcinoma.* There is a small risk of malignancy in the gallbladder mucosa in association with gallstones. It is five times more common in females than males. Up to 0.5% will have carcinoma-in-situ if closely examined histologically. Rarely, advanced gallbladder carcinoma presents as a hard right upper quadrant mass and jaundice through lymph node involvement at the porta hepatis. This is usually unresectable, and the prognosis is poor.

Complications: stones outside the gallbladder

1. Pancreatitis. Acute and chronic pancreatitis may result from the passage of gallstones through the common bile duct. Approximately 50% of pancreatitis is gallstone-related.

2. Biliary stricture. Chronic calculous inflammation may result in a benign bile duct stricture. This may cause obstructive jaundice and predispose to ascending cholangitis, with further inflammation and further tendency for stricture formation. This requires careful evaluation by ERCP before cholecystectomy and a biliary drainage procedure.

3. Obstructive jaundice. This results from impaction of a calculus in the distal common bile duct. Multiple calculi may be present. ERCP will identify the problem, and a sphincterotomy can be performed through which stones can be retrieved. Any residual stones fall through the sphincterotomy. If ERCP is unsuccessful or unavailable, surgery to remove stones from the bile ducts is required. This procedure entails cholecystectomy with exploration of the common bile duct.

4. Ascending cholangitis. This is a severe infection, usually complicating benign obstruction of the biliary tree. The infecting organisms are usually Gram-negative bacilli. Endotoxic shock may result. A diagnosis may be made clinically in the presence of Charcot's triad: fever with rigors, jaundice, and an enlarged tender liver. It requires prompt diagnosis, i.v. fluids, antibiotics directed toward coliforms, and urgent relief from the obstruction. ERCP and sphincterotomy with stone extraction or temporary stenting is urgently undertaken. Open surgery is hazardous in acute cholangitis.

5. Gallstone ileus. A large solitaire may erode into the duodenum and impact at the narrowest point of the small bowel, typically two feet proximal to the ileocaecal valve or at an existent pathological stricture. This presents as a small bowel obstruction. A plain abdominal X-ray may show obstructed small bowel, a large calcified gallstone in the right iliac fossa, and air outlining the biliary tree, although the whole triad is rarely seen.

Management of gallstones

1. Gallbladder calculi. Elective cholecystectomy is required if symptomatic. Surgery should be urgent in severe acute cholecystitis, empyema, or emphysematous or necrotizing cholecystitis.

2. Common bile duct calculi. Following acute pancreatitis or obstructive jaundice, or if the LFTs are abnormal or the common bile duct is dilated on ultrasound, the bile ducts should be screened prior to cholecystectomy by ERCP. This is essential in established jaundice or ascending cholangitis. Alternatively, intra-operative cholangiography is performed.

Surgery

1. *Cholecystectomy.* Right subcostal (Kocher's) or transverse incisions are ideal for open surgery. Tiny incisions may be used (mini-cholecystectomy), however laparoscopic cholecystectomy has become the preferred procedure, with a conversion rate to an open cholecystectomy of 5%, and a low complication rate once the technique has been mastered.

2. *Intra-operative cholangiography.* Cholangiography may be performed during open or laparoscopic surgery. The X-rays obtained or the views on the image intensifier are scrutinized for filling defects (calculi), biliary dilatation and flow of contrast into the duodenum. If common bile duct calculi are suspected, the duct is explored.

3. *Exploration of the common bile duct.* The duodenum is mobilized (Kocher's manoeuvre). The opened common bile duct is irrigated to flush out loose calculi. Choledochoscopy locates impacted calculi which are extracted with Desjardin's forceps or a Fogarty catheter. Transduodenal sphincteroplasty plus stone extraction is rarely required. The common bile duct is closed over an extemal biliary drain (T-tube), through which a cholangiogram is performed at 10 days. The T-tube is removed if there are no stones and there is free flow into the duodenum.

Treatment of retained common bile duct calculi

T-tubes may be repeatedly flushed with saline if cholangiography confirms small retained calculi. Alternatively, methyl terbutyl ether instilled through a T-tube will dissolve residual stones. Larger calculi may be extracted using forceps introduced along a dilated T-tube tract (Burhenne technique). Extracorporeal lithotripsy has been used successfully. The results of these techniques may be improved by endoscopic sphincterotomy.

Postcholecystectomy syndrome and recurrent symptoms

Early recurrence of the often vague epigastric or dyspeptic symptoms for which the patient was relieved of their gallbladder is frequently referred to as the postcholecystectomy syndrome. In some of these patients, the true cause of their symptoms may be discovered, but often the problem persists, and proves very difficult to treat.

Medical treatment

Gallstones may dissolve with oral ursodeoxycholate and chenodeoxycholate (bile acids). Treatment takes many months to complete, and has been shown to dissolve only small uncalcified stones successfully. A functioning gallbladder is necessary for bile acids to work. There is a high recurrence rate, as the root cause of the problem, the gallbladder, remains in situ. Their use is thus limited.

Further reading

National Institutes of Health consensus development conference statement on gallstones and laparoscopic cholecystectomy. *American Journal of Surgery*, 1993; **165:** 390–398.

O'Leary DP, Johnson AG. Future directions for conservative treatment of gallbladder calculi. *British Journal of Surgery*, 1993; **80:** 143–147.

Perissat J, Huibregtse K, Keane FBV *et al*. Management of bile duct stones in the era of laparoscopic cholecystectomy. *British Journal of Surgery*, 1994; **81:** 799–810.

Cuschieri A, Lezoche E, Morino M *et al*. EAES multicentre prospective randomized trial comparing two-stage vs single-stage management of patients with gallstone disease and ductal calculi. *Surgery and Endoscopy*, 1999; **13:** 952–957.

Related topics of interest

Acute pancreatitis (p. 8); Jaundice – investigation (p. 203); Minimal access surgery (p. 224).

GASTRIC CANCER

Christopher Lattimer, Simon Gibbs

Nearly all gastric cancers detected in the UK are advanced adenocarcinomas with an appalling overall 5-year survival rate of 5–10%. In comparison, in Japan, where the disease is commonest, over 30% of all gastric cancers are detected early and the overall 5-year survival rates exceed 50%. Japanese experience in mass screening, appreciation of the more radical D2 gastrectomy and different disease behaviour patterns all contribute to improved survival.

Demography

The incidence of gastric cancer has fallen dramatically in the Western world over the past 30 years. Gastric cancer is twice as common in males, peaks in incidence between 55 and 65 years, is associated with blood group A and *Helicobacter pylori* and occurs more frequently amongst the lower social classes. There is a genetic link as stomach cancer can run in families, but environmental factors such as diet and methods of food preservation are also important.

Types

Gastric cancer can be divided into intestinal and diffuse types. The intestinal type matches geographical areas of increased incidence and is usually accompanied by an area of chronic gastritis. The diffuse type bears no such relationship.

Risk factors

Chronic gastritis, gastric ulcers and gastric polyps are lesions often considered pre-cancerous. The gastric remnant following a partial gastrectomy for benign disease has an increased risk of developing a gastric carcinoma. Autoimmune gastritis (pernicious anaemia) is subject to dysplastic change which may then become neoplastic. Populations where gastric cancer is common have a high incidence of chronic gastritis, mucosal atrophy and subsequent intestinal metaplasia, all of which are associated with *H. pylori*. Over 90% of carcinomas are found in areas of gastritis and 10% of patients with chronic gastritis develop a carcinoma. Gastric adenomatous polyps are considered premalignant, and the larger the polyp the higher the incidence of malignancy. There is no convincing evidence that chronic gastric ulcers undergo malignant change, but any gastric ulcer should be biopsied.

Presentation

Clinical presentation depends upon lesion site and disease advancement. The commoner antral lesions may cause outlet obstruction with vomiting and a succussion splash or fistulate into the colon. Cardiac lesions may cause dysphagia or regurgitation. Fundal lesions are often silent, with anorexia and increasing satiety after meal times. Irrespective of site, many first present with indigestion pains and dyspepsia. Carcinomas may perforate, ulcerate causing anaemia and lead to ill health with weakness and weight loss. A knobbly liver or the carcinoma itself may be palpable. A left supraclavicular node mass (Virchow's node) (Troisier's sign) or ascites indicates advanced disease. Jaundice may be caused by nodal compression at the porta hepatis, direct ductal involvement or by progressive liver replacement.

Diagnosis

The mainstay of diagnosis for early lesions is to perform an upper GI endoscopy on all patients with a recent onset of dyspepsia or indigestion-like pains. All suspicious lesions and unusual areas of gastritis should be biopsied or undergo brush cytology. Linitis plastica (leather bottle stomach) is suggested if the stomach fails to distend on insufflation. Repeat biopsies at the same site (trench biopsy) may be required to reach the areas of submucosal infiltration that are typical for these carcinomas. Double contrast barium radiology is complementary to diagnosis. A filling defect, mucosal irregularity or stricture may be visualized.

Staging

Ultrasound and CT scan allow visualization of distant metastases in the liver and lungs, which normally precludes surgery. Endoscopic ultrasound should be performed for all patients in whom surgery is considered. The ultrasound probe is located in the end of an 'end viewing' endoscope, and is passed like a normal gastroscope to the level of the tumour. It generates a radial ultrasonic image thus allowing T and N staging, permitting a much more accurate assessment of local operability. Laparoscopy allows exclusion of small peritoneal deposits or small metastases and allows cytology and biopsy of any suspicious lesions. Enlarged lymph nodes can also be seen. The lesser sac can sometimes be entered safely and any posterior extension into the pancreas can be visualized. Accurate staging of the disease helps prevent unnecessary laparotomy, although the presence of involved nodes does not always preclude surgery.

Preoperative nutrition

Many patients who present with a gastric carcinoma are malnourished. If oral feeds can be tolerated and there is no obstruction then high calorie and protein supplemented liquid feeds can be given under the guidance of an experienced dietitian, prior to surgery. If oral feeding is not possible, then a radiologically placed nasojejunal tube may be useful. In obstructed lesions TPN can be used prior to surgery but this should be replaced by a jejunal feeding route created at surgery. In severely cachectic patients, operation may need to be delayed to allow correction of profound nutritional disability.

The D2 gastrectomy

The D2 gastrectomy has been shown to increase survival in gastric cancer patients in Japanese series. All the lymph node groups which drain the stomach are classified according to their site (supra/infra pyloric, right/left cardiac, greater/lesser curve and those groups along and at the origins of the arterial supply to the stomach). The primary tumour is documented in the upper, middle or lower third of the stomach. N1 nodes are situated within 3 cm of the primary. N2 nodes are all those mentioned above greater than 3 cm from the primary. N2 nodes could all become N1 nodes if the tumour was sited in a different region. A D2 resection involves removing all the

N1 and N2 nodes with a 5 cm clearance of the tumour. The operative mortality for a D2 gastrectomy should not exceed 5%. Although there are undoubtedly some patients who would benefit from having a D2 resection rather than a D1 (those with disease that has just started to spread to the N2 nodes), there is as yet no convincing European data that this type of resection increases overall 5 year survival if performed routinely for all patients undergoing surgery for gastric cancer. It is hoped that with more accurate staging, patients who would benefit from D2 type resection will be identified pre-operatively and their operation tailored accordingly.

Anastomosis

Gastrointestinal continuity is restored after a radical lower partial gastrectomy with a Roux-en-Y anastomosis. Bilroth 1 gastrectomy is considered ill advised because the anastomosis will be sited on the original tumour bed. Continuity after total gastrectomy is established by Roux-en-Y loop. A naso-jejunal tube is placed allowing aspiration of the gastric remnant or oesophagus, and enteral feeding via the jejunum. Once a contrast swallow shows integrity at 7 days, oral feeding can be started.

Palliative surgery

With better preoperative staging less palliative resections are now performed. Most patients, particularly the elderly, will not benefit from surgery if there is no chance of complete resection. In younger patients with longer life expectancy, resection may still be appropriate to debulk the disease prior to other palliative treatments. If patients have gastric obstruction however (such as in pyloric stenosis), a gastrojejunostomy is indicated to divert the gastric contents directly into the jejunum.

Post-gastrectomy symptoms

Gastrectomy is associated with post-gastrectomy symptoms in 20% of cases. These include diarrhoea, osmotic (early) and hypoglycaemic (late) dumping, anaemia and malnutrition. Mild dumping usually responds to simple dietary manipulation and an experienced dietitian should be consulted. If dumping is severe and fails to settle, it can be treated with anti-peristaltic segments which can be fashioned surgically to hold up emptying into the jejunum. Roux-en-Y construction with an anastomosis at least 50 cm distal to the upper resection limit eliminates biliary reflux, which dogged patients who had Polya or Bilroth I gastrectomies. Vitamin B_{12} injections may be needed in total gastrectomy patients, who fail to secrete intrinsic factor.

Prognosis

Disease stage is the best prognostic indicator. Well-differentiated lesions carry a better prognosis than the poorly differentiated or signet cell types. Vascular invasion is associated with future liver metastasis. Serosal invasion, perforation and poor differentiation are associated with peritoneal dissemination. Lymph node metastases are associated with both. Upper gastric lesions are often advanced with a poor prognosis. There is no convincing evidence that chemotherapy or radiotherapy prolongs survival.

Lymphoma

Gastric lymphoma is the commonest extranodal primary site for non-Hodgkin's lymphoma, and is strongly associated with *H. pylori*. Most are B-cell lymphomas arising from mucosa-associated lymphoid tissue (MALT). They present similarly to gastric carcinomas. Therapy depends on stage and involves resection and adjuvant chemotherapy for early stage lesions (Ann Arbor stage I, II), chemotherapy and/or radiotherapy for advanced stages (III, IV). Some early low-grade MALT lymphomas respond to *Helicobacter* eradication therapy alone. Careful observation is required if chemotherapy or radiotherapy is initiated in advanced lesions, as perforation may occur.

Carcinoid tumour

Carcinoid tumours usually form a polypoidal mass in the body or fundus. The carcinoid syndrome of flushing, diarrhoea and bronchospasm occurs when liver metastases secrete large amounts of 5-hydroxytryptamine (serotonin, 5-HT), but in many cases of gastric carcinoid 5-hydroxytryptophan and histamine are released rather than 5-HT, leading to atypical skin blotches rather than whole body flushes. Resection is the mainstay of treatment and offers 5-year survival rates of over 75%. Chemotherapy has also been employed in those not fit or too advanced for surgery.

GI stromal tumours (GIST)

Gastric leiomyomas and leiomyosarcomas most often present with bleeding due to ulceration. Malignant diagnosis depends on the number of mitoses present and whether the lesion recurs! Resection offers 5-year survival rates approaching 50%.

Further reading

McCulloch P. Description of the Japanese method of radical gastrectomy. *Annals of the Royal College of Surgery of England*, 1994; **76**: 110–114.

Raines SA. Surgery for cancer of the stomach. In: Griffin SM, Raines SA (eds) *Upper Gastrointestinal Surgery – A Companion to Specialist Surgical Practice*. W.B. Saunders, London, 1999; 145–190.

Siewert JR *et al.* Benefits of D2 lymph node dissection for patients with gastric cancer and pN0 pN1 lymph node metastases. *British Journal of Surgery*, 1996; **83**: 1144–1147.

Related topics of interest

Nutrition in the surgical patient (p. 233); Oesophageal cancer (p. 237).

GASTROINTESTINAL FISTULAE

Nick Lagattolla

A fistula is an abnormal connection existing between two epithelial linings. The gastrointestinal tract provides much scope for the formation of a diverse variety of fistulae.

Pathology

Fistulae can arise between two different parts of the gastrointestinal tract, or between the bowel and a separate structure. An enterocutaneous fistula is an abnormal connection between the gastrointestinal tract and the skin. An end fistula arises from a segment of discontinuous gastrointestinal tract (e.g. a duodenal stump), while in a lateral fistula, the connection is with the side of an intact viscus and intestinal continuity is maintained. A simple fistula has a single tract from involved bowel to the abdominal wall, whereas a complex fistula will have multiple tracts often is associated with abscess cavities.

Fistula types

The varieties most encountered are:

- Vesicocolic.
- Colovaginal.
- Enterocutaneous.
- Gastrocolic.
- Ileocolic.
- Colocutaneous.
- Enteroenteric.

Aetiology

There are five main causes of gastrointestinal fistulae. The aetiology is important when establishing a plan of treatment.

1. Iatrogenic. Anastomotic leakage is a common cause of enterocutaneous fistula. This principally arises from bowel end ischaemia, suture line tension, or construction of an anastomosis in a high-risk situation such as intraperitoneal sepsis or distal obstruction with subsequent anastomotic breakdown. Most enterocutaneous fistulae are ultimately iatrogenic in origin.

2. Gastrointestinal disease. Fistulae frequently arise secondary to sigmoid diverticular disease, particularly colovaginal, vesicocolic and left groin colo-cutaneous fistulae. Other inflammatory causes include appendicitis presenting with chronic discharge through the right groin, Crohn's disease (entero-enteric, entero-colic) and intestinal tuberculosis.

3. Malignancy. Colonic carcinoma causes colo-cutaneous fistulae by direct invasion of the abdominal wall or after spontaneous perforation, abscess formation with discharge through the abdominal wall. Radical local surgical resection can be therapeutic, though this is inappropriate in patients with disseminated malignancy. Gastrocolic fistula is rare, arising as a complication of gastric carcinoma more commonly than colonic carcinoma. As a cause of fistula, malignancy is less frequently encountered than inflammatory bowel and diverticular disease.

4. Radiotherapy. Pelvic irradiation especially may lead to damage and inflammation of small or large bowel with fistula formation.

5. Trauma. Penetrating wounds to the abdomen can cause fistulas, particularly when the trauma results in multiple intestinal perforations with subsequent sepsis and abscess formation.

General treatment principles

Cutaneous fistulae close spontaneously in most circumstances. Approximately 60% should close within 1 month on conservative treatment. Closure will not occur if there is distal obstruction, a complex or chronic abscess cavity or direct mucocutaneous epithelial continuity. These features suggest a surgical solution is likely. Closure less readily occurs if the involved bowel is diseased or if the patient is malnourished. Internal fistulae may be asymptomatic (e.g. entero-enteric) and are unlikely to close. Colovaginal and vesicocolic fistulae require resection of the involved segment of bowel; many would advocate a stoma as opposed to primary anastomosis, though if the latter is chosen, there must be interposition of omentum between the anastomosis and the secondarily involved viscus. Other indications for surgery are failure to improve, continued metabolic or nutritional complications, or generally if the patient is not thriving.

Management of enterocutaneous fistula

These are chronic by nature, and are very debilitating for the patient. They require a team approach from medical and nutritional teams, and pharmacist, physiotherapist and stoma nurses. Initial resuscitation needs to be followed by longer-term nutritional support and detailed assessment of the pathophysiology of the fistula:

1. Fluid and electrolyte loss. A high output fistula (>500 ml/day) can lead to large fluid and electrolyte losses with insiduous circulatory collapse from isotonic dehydration. Appropriate resuscitation needs to be guided by accurate measurement of all fluid losses. Serum levels of electrolytes need to be tested frequently until fluid balance is achieved. Thereafter twice-weekly estimations of haematological and biochemical indices should be sufficient.

2. Skin protection. Proteolytic enzymes in upper gastrointestinal secretions cause skin excoriation and damage. Skin protection is essential around the site of a fistula. Reducing the volume of a high output fistula helps skin management and reduces fluid and electrolyte losses. This can be achieved by restricting oral intake, though somatostatin analogues are commonly used. Other pharmacological agents (H_2 antagonists, omeprazole) have been used with varying degrees of success.

3. Nutritional support. Correction of nutritional deficiencies and long-term parenteral nutrition are often necessary for patients with proximal gastrointestinal high-output fistulae. Oral intake should be stopped, which reduces intestinal secretion and fistula output. Intravenous feeding should be commenced in any patient with an enterocutaneous fistula other than a low output terminal ileal or colonic fistula. This rests the bowel and restores nutritional status, providing optimal conditions for spontaneous fistula closure.

4. *Control of sepsis.* An abscess cavity may complicate an enterocutaneous fistula and should be suspected in the presence of persisting pain, pyrexia, tachycardia, leucocytosis and a falling serum albumin. Confirmation and delineation of an abscess cavity is best achieved by a sinogram using gastrograffin or dilute barium. Ultrasound and CT scanning are also useful and may allow percutaneous drainage. Abscess cavities need to be drained to eliminate sepsis and convert a complex cavity into a simple tract, which can close spontaneously. Antibiotics should not be used unless there is septicaemia or surrounding cellulitis.

5 *Haemorrhage.* This can be life-threatening from eroded vessels within the fistula tract or abscess cavity. Erosion of arteries occurs as a result of sepsis or the action of digestive enzymes (especially in the stomach). Treatment may require urgent resection of the fistula but arterial embolization can be considered.

Further reading

Coutsoftides T, Fazio VW. Small intestine cutaneous fistulas. *Surgery and Gynecological Obstetrics*, 1979; **149:** 333–336.

Williams JG, Wong WD, Rothenberger DA, Goldberg SM. Recurrence of Crohn's disease after resection. *British Journal of Surgery*, 1991; **78:** 10–19.

Related topics of interest

Crohn's disease (p. 103); Diverticular disease (p. 116); Nutrition in the surgical patient (p. 233).

GASTROINTESTINAL POLYPS

Nick Lagattolla

Polyps are swellings arising from the gastrointestinal epithelium. Occasionally, through the action of peristalsis, they may develop a stalk, which can become very long. Polyps with a stalk are called pedunculated, and those with a flat or broad base are termed sessile. Polyps may be single or multiple and can occur at any age, peaking between 55–65 years. The majority of gastrointestinal polyps occur in the colon, however, the stomach and small intestine are other sites.

Pathology

Polyps may be classified as malignant or benign, however, this can be confusing as many benign polyps have malignant potential. A practical classification includes adenomatous (or neoplastic), hamartomatous, inflammatory and miscellaneous polyps.

1. Adenomatous. Adenomatous polyps are benign neoplasms arising from the gastrointestinal epithelium, occurring in up to 20% of the population. They are almost always found in the colon, but may occur in the stomach, duodenum or small bowel. There are different types based on morphology. All adenomatous polyps comprise glandular tissue, but this may be arranged differently giving rise to a pathological classification. Eighty per cent of adenomatous polyps are found in the rectosigmoid. They are an important cause of rectal bleeding, although they may be discovered incidentally. Large rectal polyps may present as a prolapsing mass at the anus. Any polyp may act as the lead point of an intussusception.

(a) *Tubular adenoma.* These are polyps that are macroscopically solid and consist of many curled acini. They comprise about 65% of all colonic polyps and may occur anywhere in the gastrointestinal tract, but are most common in the colon. They often develop a stalk, and thus become pedunculated.

(b) *Villous adenoma.* These are usually sessile, and appear fronded, soft and velvety macroscopically. Microscopically they consist of multiple villi. These are more common in females, and comprise about 15% of all polyps. They are most frequently found in the rectum or the caecum, are usually solitary, and may be large at presentation, possibly involving the full circumference of the colon. Large rectal villous adenomas produce inordinately large amounts of mucus. Copious amounts of mucus and slime are passed per rectum, best described as a clear and somewhat lumpy jelly. This is a potassium-rich alkaline mucus. If this is lost in excess over a long period, patients will become hypokalaemic and may even develop a metabolic acidosis.

(c) *Tubulovillous adenoma.* If there are tubular and villous histological features, the polyp is a tubulovillous adenoma. These are more common in males than females, and account for about 20% of gastrointestinal polyps. In 20% of cases these are multiple.

2. Hamartomatous

(a) *True hamartoma.* These occur sporadically or as part of the Peutz–Jehger's syndrome. They vary greatly in size, and have well-defined fibrous and smooth muscle layers interspersed with epithelial structures histologically. They may carry a small increased risk of malignancy.

(b) *Juvenile polyps.* These are large, fleshy, hamartomatous polyps that usually occur in childhood. They are more common in boys, and there may be a family history. They cause rectal bleeding and may intussuscept. They have a typical histological appearance of a well-defined fibrous stroma interspersed by large cystic epithelial lined spaces. They are usually solitary, but may be multiple in the juvenile polyposis syndrome. Juvenile polyposis is associated with an increased risk of malignancy, although solitary juvenile polyps are not.

3. Inflammatory. These arise in inflamed colonic mucosa, typically in ulcerative colitis. They represent islands of regenerating epithelium, are usually multiple, and are often called pseudopolyps.

4. Miscellaneous

(a) *Metaplastic polyps.* These are usually small and are of no clinical significance. They are commonly encountered in the colon, and are differentiated from neoplastic polyps by their fronded or serrated microscopic appearance. They are usually sessile, but may, rarely, be pedunculated. They are common in the rectum and at stomas.

(b) *Lymphoid.* These are sessile accumulations of benign lymphoid cells, and have little clinical significance.

(c) *Other benign tumours.* Any submucosal tumour may become pedunculated and appear polypoid. In the colon, this is usually a submucosal lipoma or leiomyoma. They may be the cause of intussusception.

The polyp cancer sequence

All adenomatous polyps carry the potential to become malignant. Features most likely to be associated with malignancy in a polyp are size (greater than 1.5 cm diameter), greater number, the presence of cytological atypia in the epithelium, sessile or villous morphology, and polyposis syndromes. The epithelium of an excised or biopsied polyp must be scrutinized carefully for the presence of signs of developing malignancy. Hyperplasia, atypia or mitotic figures all suggest epithelial dysplasia, and if this is ignored, then invasion and frank malignancy will result. If a pedunculated polyp is excised, the stalk must be examined for invasion in view of the above. Excluding the colonic carcinomas developing in ulcerative colitis and hereditary non-polyposis colonic cancer, 80% of all carcinomas probably arise as a consequence of the polyp–cancer sequence. Villous adenomas have a higher risk than tubular adenomas of developing malignant change.

Polyposis syndromes

1. Familial adenomatous polyposis (FAP). This comprises multiple colonic adenomatous polyps, otherwise known as adenomatous polyposis coli (APC). This is inherited as an autosomal dominant gene on chomosome 5 with near-complete penetrance. The APC gene normally functions as a tumour suppressor. The sheer quantity of colonic polyps combined with their early onset, give rise to the very high risk of gastrointestinal carcinoma, usually occurring by the age of 30. The treatment for this condition is total colectomy with formation of an ileo-anal pouch, or sub-total colectomy and ileorectal anastomosis with frequent endoscopic screening of the rectal mucosa. Polyps may also occur at other sites in the gastrointestinal tract, particularly in the duodenum. Extra-intestinal tumours may also occur. The patient's family must be screened for the disorder.

2. Gardner's syndrome. This overlaps heavily with familial adenomatous poly-posis, though differentiation is useful as this syndrome represents the association of multiple colonic adenomatous polyps with multiple extracolonic tumours, often hamartomatous. These include dental and epidermoid cysts, bone exostoses, abdominal wall desmoid, cerebral and thyroid tumours.

3. Hereditary flat adenoma syndrome. Also termed attenuated familial adeno-matous polyposis, the genetic origin being very close to the APC gene. The adenomas are typically in the right side of the colon, and are flat or sessile. Duodenal adenomas also occur.

4. Peutz–Jegher's syndrome. This is the association of multiple, variably sized small bowel hamartomatous polyps with perioral pigmentation. The polyps may cause multiple episodes of entero-enteric intussusception. The polyps may, rarely, occur in the colon or stomach. There is a potential for malignant change.

5. Juvenile polyposis syndrome. This comprises hamartomatous polyps throughout the small intestine and colon, and carries a risk of malignant change in the colon.

6. Others. Canada–Cronkite syndrome is the association of total gastrointes-tinal polyposis, with ectodermal abnormalities including alopecia, nail dystrophies and hyperpigmentation. Turcot's syndrome may be part of the spectrum of FAP, though the polyps are fewer in number, with a reduced risk of carcinoma; however there is an association with cerebral malignancies.

Treatment

Polyps should be removed by diathermy snare polypectomy during colonoscopy. These must be retrieved for histological examination. Should a polyp be found to harbour non-invasive carcinoma or dysplasia, or if there are multiple polyps or recurrent polyps, then colonoscopic follow-up is mandatory. If a pedunculated polyp is frankly malignant, but with no evidence of invasion into the stalk, then the patient may be similarly followed-up. However, if there is evidence of an incomplete excision, then the patient should undergo colonic resection.

Pedunculated rectal polyps may be snared through an operating sigmoidoscope under general anaesthesia. Alternatively, if they are sessile, they may be excised locally after infiltration of saline to separate the lesion from the muscularis. The mucosal defect is often left open.

Large benign polyps may be removed colonoscopically or using the operating sigmoidoscope in a piecemeal fashion, but if this is not possible, a laparotomy, colotomy and open polypectomy or a limited colectomy may be better. If a polyp is seen to be histologically malignant after initial biopsy, then there is no option other than a colectomy.

Further reading

Campbell WJ, Spencer RAJ, Parks TG. Familial adenomatous polyposis. *British Journal of Surgery*, 1994; **81:** 1722–1733.

Desai DC, Neale KF, Talbot IC *et al.* Juvenile polyposis. *British Journal of Surgery*, 1995; **82:** 14–17.

Talbot IC. Colonic polyps. *Surgery*, 1992; **10:** 182–186.

Related topics of interest

Colorectal carcinoma (p. 91); Lower gastrointestinal haemorrhage (p. 207).

GASTRO-OESOPHAGEAL REFLUX

Simon Gibbs, Christopher Lattimer

Minor gastro-oesophageal reflux is a normal physiological process. However excessive reflux, known as gastro-oesophageal reflux disease (GORD), can result in symptoms of heartburn, regurgitation, chest pain, acid brash, asthma and even dysphagia. Hiatus herniae are often associated with GORD, although not all patients with hiatus herniae have reflux symptoms. Oesophagitis is usually associated with GORD, although symptoms have poor correlation with endoscopic findings. Treatment of GORD depends on severity of both symptoms and endoscopic findings, and ranges from simple conservative lifestyle changes through anti-acid medical therapies to anti-reflux surgery.

Hiatus hernia

This is a disease of all ages but is commoner in the elderly. It is defined by the protrusion of part of the stomach through the oesophageal hiatus of the diaphragm into the chest cavity. There are two types: sliding and rolling. Sliding is by far the commonest type and is characterized by the herniation of the gastro-oesophageal junction (GOJ) through into the chest. In rolling type a portion of the fundus herniates and the GOJ remains in the abdomen. As both of these types of hernia enlarge then they come to form a common type; the large incarcerated hernia which has elements of both with up to three quarters of the stomach in the chest. These large hernias can develop complications such as haemorrhagic gastritis due to reduced ability to empty, and acute torsion leading to obstruction, ischaemia and perforation. Over a period of 10 years, 30% of patients with large hiatus herniae will develop life-threatening complications[b].

Lower oesophageal sphincter

The non-anatomical lower oesophageal sphincter is 1–4 cm long and can be identified physiologically. It has a resting pressure of 20–40 mmHg, relaxing with coffee, fatty foods, chocolate, secretin, glucagon and cholecystokinin, and contracts after the administration of cholinergic and alpha-adrenergic drugs. Reflux is encouraged with a hypotensive sphincter, increases in abdominal pressure, gastric distension, and episodes of inappropriate sphincter relaxation from vagal overactivity.

Gastric content

Duodeno-gastric reflux, gastric outlet obstruction, gastric distension and the acid nature of the gastric content all promote gastro-oesophageal reflux. The hyperacidity of duodenal ulcer disease and the Zollinger–Ellison syndrome both encourage oesophagitis. Reflux of duodenal contents into the lower oesophagus is now thought to promote adenocarcinoma[b].

Anatomy

A length of intra-abdominal oesophagus helps prevent reflux and is an important feature of some surgical treatments[b]; the loss of an intra-abdominal segment contributes to reflux, such as in a sliding hiatus hernia. However reflux can still occur with a normal intra-abdominal length. The acute angle (angle of His) of the gastro-oesophageal junction was believed to act as a valve, and some surgical repairs attempt to refashion this angle. Reduced lower oesophageal sphincter pressure is considered the most important factor in the genesis of GORD[b].

Presentation

Heartburn and regurgitation are the commonest symptoms. They are often relieved by milk and antacids and are often precipitated by rich, fatty or spicy meals, and exacerbated by recumbent posture. Chest pain mimicking angina can also occur. Dysphagia can be due to stricture, oesophagitis or a reflux-induced motility disorder. Rarer symptoms include odynophagia (painful swallowing), aspiration pneumonitis, bronchospasm and upper gastrointestinal haemorrhage with anaemia.

Investigations

1. Endoscopy. Endoscopy is the investigation of choice allowing direct mucosal visualization and tissue sampling. Oesophagitis can be graded by endoscopic appearance (erythema, ulceration, stricture) according to various classifications.

The indentation of the right crus identifies the diaphragm, the landmark for diagnosis of a hiatus hernia. A Barrett's oesophagus is identified when the squamo-columnar junction (Z-line) is at least 3 cm higher than the gastro-oesophageal junction. Biopsies should be taken to prove the diagnosis and exclude dysplasia.

2. pH and manometry. Twenty-four hour ambulatory oesophageal pH recording and static manometry are essential for diagnosis of significant GORD, especially in symptomatic patients with no oesophagitis at endoscopy. A pH electrode is placed 5 cm above the gastro-oesophageal junction and a 24-hour recording of pH is taken. The area above trace and below the line of pH 7 is derived by a computer and a De Meester score is calculated. The normal range is 5–14, but in severe reflux can go up to at least 150. Surgery is considered if the De Meester score is elevated and the patient is symptomatic. Asymptomatic patients with elevated scores are offered surgery if there is evidence of oesophagitis, or if the patient is young and PPI dependent. Static manometry is also performed to detect motility disorder, which may be the cause of symptoms in the absence of GORD, and to measure LOS pressure. A Bernstein acid perfusion test is also usually performed. (Symptom reproduction following lower oesophageal instillation of 0.1 M HCl indicates a positive test.)

3. Barium swallow. This may demonstrate reflux directly and is also useful for demonstrating strictures, hiatus herniae, and disorders such as achalasia. Bread soaked in barium can be a useful medium to demonstrate peristaltic abnormalities.

4. Indications for surgery. All patients with symptomatic reflux and elevated De Meester scores who are not controlled by PPIs are offered fundoplication surgery if they are fit enough. Young asymptomatic patients are offered surgery to avoid them having to take PPIs for the rest of their life. Patients with Barrett's oesophagus are also offered fundoplication in this author's practice, as there is some evidence that this may halt malignant transformation[c].

Treatment

1. General. General treatment includes weight reduction, elevation of the head of the bead for nocturnal symptoms, avoiding fatty foods, coffee, meals just before bed-time, and stopping smoking. Drinking milk which is alkaline can give temporary relief, but milk fats also promote more acid secretion.

2. Medical. Anti-acids such as Gaviscon may be all that is required. If failure of control persists an H_2-receptor antagonist may be used, particularly if there is oesophagitis. Endoscopic evidence of healing may then permit reducing the dose or switching to more simple therapy. Metoclopromide and Domperidone are sometimes useful to enhance oesophageal and gastric clearance of acid. Proton pump inhibitors (PPIs) are used in more resistant cases and are also indicated for the treatment of benign strictures in conjunction with balloon dilatation or bougienage. The frequency of dilatation usually decreases with time. An anti-reflux operation is indicated in young people with resistant strictures. The mode of action of all medical therapies is to reduce acid exposure by decreasing production of acid, or moving acid downstream more rapidly.

3. Surgery. Fundoplication is now the mainstay of anti-reflux surgery, and can be performed as an open procedure or laparoscopically. Laparoscopic operation allows a quicker recovery and discharge from hospital, but requires advanced laparoscopic instrumentation and operator skills. Open operation allows more accurate assessment of tension of the wrap and crural repair. The operative procedures are essentially the same for both modes of surgery and give very similar results[b].

Nissen fundoplication, the most commonly performed procedure, involves mobilization of the distal oesophagus, crural approximation and wrapping the mobilized fundus posteriorly around the oesophagus through 360°, and thus is a total fundoplication. Gas bloat and dysphagia can be diminished by making the wrap 'floppy', i.e. not too tight. More recently partial fundoplications (< 360°) have been developed which have now been shown to reduce gas bloat and dysphagia without compromising anti-reflux effect[a]. Fundoplications can be performed through either abdominal or thoracic approaches. A shortened oesophagus can be lengthened by a Collis gastroplasty with fundoplication around the neo-oesophagus. In this author's practice, there is now no place for the Angelchick prosthesis.

4. Barrett's oesophagus. The acquired condition of Barrett's oesophagus predisposes the patient to a 50-fold increase in incidence of adenocarcinoma[a]. Endoscopic surveillance and biopsy is per-formed every 18 months, or more frequently if dysplasia is found. Severe dysplasia or carcinoma-in-situ are indications for oesophagectomy if fit for surgery[b]. If unfit, patients may be entered into trials of photodynamic therapy. Anti-reflux procedures seem to prevent progression of Barrett's, unlike PPIs[c], although reversal of Barrett's change is not common.

Further reading

Griffiths Pearson F *et al. Hiatal Hernia, Gastroesophageal Reflux, and Other Complications – Esophageal Surgery,* 1995; Part IV.

Mughal M, Bancewicz J. Gastro-oesophageal reflux – pathophysiology and treatment. *Recent Advances in Surgery,* 1991; **14:** 17–35.

Watson DI *et al.* Prospective randomisation double-blind trial between laparoscopic Nissen fundoplication and anterior partial fundoplication. *British Journal of Surgery,* 1999; **86:** 123–130.

Related topic of interest

Oesophageal dysmotility (p. 242).

GOITRE

Nick Wilson

The term goitre is used to describe any form of enlargement of the thyroid gland. Morphologically, three varieties of goitre are recognized:

- Diffuse goiter.
- Multinodular goiter.
- Solitary nodule (50% are actually dominant nodules in a multinodular goitre).

Pathologically, thyroid abnormalities causing goitre are as follows:

- Simple goitre.
- Multinodular colloid goitre.
- Graves' disease.
- Thyroid 'cyst'.
- Thyroiditis.
- Thyroid adenoma.
- Malignant thyroid neoplasms.

Simple goitre

May be diffuse or nodular. Result from increased TSH drive in the face of relative T_4 and T_3 deficiency. Physiological goitres occur to meet increased demand for thyroxine (puberty, pregnancy, lactation).

Iodine-deficiency goitres occur endemically in regions (usually mountainous – Alps, Andes) of iodine deficiency or sporadically. They can also be caused by antithyroid drugs (iodides, propyl-thiouracil, carbimazole, thiocyanate, lithium) and foodstuffs (halogens, cassava, soya beans). Dyshormogenesis (absence of an enzyme) is familial and rare. Iodine transport, oxidation, coupling or thyroglobulin synthesis may be affected. Radiation to the head and neck may cause nodular goitre and thyroid cancer.

Multinodular colloid goitre

Usually euthyroid. Symptoms include visible swelling, discomfort, cough, dyspnoea, dysphagia, hoarseness and anxiety about malignancy. Mild hyperthyroidism sometimes occurs (Plummer's syndrome).

Graves' disease

This is an autoimmune disorder caused by polyclonal immunoglobulins stimulating thyroid cell membrane TSH receptors. Female : male = 10 : 1. The peak incidence occurs at 20–40 years. The goitre is usually diffuse, often with a bruit. Exophthalmos, pretibial myxoedema, thyroid acropachy are other classic signs. Patients are hyperthyroid and describe weight loss, fatigue, heat intolerance, palpitations, tremor, diarrhoea and menstrual disorders. Treatment is by antithyroid drugs, radioiodine or thyroidectomy. Mild disease may resolve spontaneously but the majority of patients will require treatment.

Thyroid 'cyst'

True cysts (a space-containing fluid lined by epithelium) are rare. Nodules containing colloid degeneration, necrosis or haemorrhage are however quite common. Aspiration of clear fluid with negative cytology does not exclude malignancy. If aspiration does not provide complete and lasting resolution, surgical excision is required.

Thyroiditis

The aetiology of these conditions is largely unknown. Some varieties have an autoimmune basis in which reduced suppressor T-cell function probably allows sensitization to thyroid antigens of helper T-cells which stimulate B-cells to produce autoantibodies. These are common conditions, usually affecting women.

1. **Acute suppurative thyroiditis.** Now rare. Results from the spread of haematogenous infection (*Staphylococcus aureus*, β-haemolytic streptococcus, *Streptococcus pneumoniae*) usually to a goitrous gland. The signs are of acute infection and treatment is by antibiotics or, occasionally, surgical drainage.

2. **Sub-acute thyroiditis.**
- de Quervain's thyroiditis. Self-limiting and probably caused by viral infection. The gland enlarges diffusely and flu-like symptoms are prominent. Mild hyperthyroidism occurs initially, followed by slight hypothyroidism. Isotope scanning reveals low uptake. Treatment is symptomatic.
- Postpartum thyroiditis. Affects 5% of women. An autoimmune condition causing thyroid dyfunction within a year of delivery, there is a modest, firm goitre and hyperthyroidism or hypothyroidism may occur. Antithyroid drugs, radioiodine and surgery are contraindicated and the condition resolves spontaneously.
- Silent thyroiditis. A painless, diffuse goitre with mild hyperthyroidism, but none of the features of Graves' disease. It occurs at any age and affects males more frequently than other varieties. Usually self-limiting, but may recur.

3. **Chronic thyroiditis.**
- Riedel's thyroiditis. Dense fibrosis of the gland occurs which is of normal or reduced size. The thyroid remains non-tender but becomes very hard ('woody'). Patients are usually middle-aged and euthyroid. Malignancy must be excluded.
- Hashimoto's thyroiditis is characterized by a large, rubbery goitre with hyperthyroidism progressing to hypothyroidism as the immune process destroys the gland. Antithyroid drugs or thyroxine may be necessary, but steroids are unhelpful. Surgery may be required if the gland is unresponsive to thyroxine and if malignancy is suspected.
- Atrophic thyroiditis. The end result of autoimmune thyroiditis, leaving a fibrotic, shrunken gland, usually with hypothyroisism. Thyroxine is the only treatment required.

Thyroid adenoma

See Thyroid neoplasms (p. 324).

Malignant thyroid neoplasms

See Thyroid neoplasms (p. 324).

Investigation of goitre

Morphological and functional aspects are important. Ultrasound scanning demonstrates single or multiple solid or 'cystic' lesions. Standard CXR views will indicate retrosternal extension and tracheal deviation. CT scanning shows tumour transgression of the thyroid capsule or retrosternal extension. Scintiscanning using ^{123}iodine or technetium^{99m} is rarely justified. FNAC is very accurate (in experienced hands) in the diagnosis of goitres and is easily performed in the clinic. The technique will not distinguish between follicular adenoma and follicular carcinoma.

Thyroid function is assessed by TSH, T_3 and T_4. Total T_4 may be misleading because hyperthyroidism may be caused by raised T_3; TBG may be increased during pregnancy or oestrogen therapy – e.g. oral contraceptives (low T_4); TBG may fall during liver disease or nephrotic syndrome (high T_4). Thyroid autoantibody titres should be measured if thyroiditis is suspected.

Treatment for goitre

Endemic goitre can be treated with thyroxine, but older patients with established goitre rarely benefit from thyroxine. Thyroxine is commonly given to suppress multinodular goitre and may be effective in the early stages, but frequently does not reduce the size of an established, nodular goitre[c]. It is usually effective in suppressing dyshormogenetic goitres.

Propylthiouracil and carbimazole are used to treat hyperthyroidism. These drugs are usually given for 14–24 months and more than 50% of patients relapse after cessation of treatment. Agranulocytosis may occur on treatment and regular FBC is necessary. Beta-blockers are used to control tachycardia, sweating and tremor.

Radioiodine as ^{133}I can be offered to patients beyond reproductive age. The choice between radioiodine and surgery should rest with the patient when the pros and cons of each treatment have been explained.

Surgery is appropriate in the following circumstances:

- Discomfort;
- Unacceptable appearance of goiter;
- Dyspnoea, dysphagia or retrosternal extension;
- Failure of thyroxine to suppress goiter;
- Possible malignancy – solitary cold nodule (p. 326);
- Thyrotoxicosis (p. 173).

Further reading

Young AE. The thyroid gland. In: Burnand KG, Young AE (eds) *The New Aird's Companion in Surgical Studies (2nd Edn)*. London: Churchill Livingstone, 1998; 459–483.

Related topics of interest

Hyperparathyroidism (p. 170); Hyperthyroidism – treatment (p. 173); Thyroglossal tract anomalies (p. 322); Thyroid neoplasms (p. 324).

HAEMORRHOIDS

Deya Marzouk

Aetiology and pathogenesis

The anal canal submucosa forms a series of 'cushions'. The three main cushions are found in the left lateral, right posterior and right anterior positions (3, 7 and 11 o'clock). They consist of venous dilatations surrounded by a network of smooth muscle, elastic and fibrous tissue, as well as the overlying mucosa. The submucosal smooth muscles are anchored to the internal sphincter and the longitudinal muscle passing through the internal sphincter fasciculi. This network of muscle supports the anal canal lining during defecation. It returns the anal canal lining to its initial position after the temporary downward displacement in defecation.

Haemorrhoids are prolapsed anal cushions. They are caused primarily by deterioration and disruption of the fibromuscular supporting framework of the cushions from the 3rd decade onwards, allowing them to slide downwards and allowing the submucosal vessels to engorge as they prolapse. This is especially liable to occur as a result of constipation and straining. In some patients this is aggravated by a tight internal anal sphincter. Heredity may play a role either environmentally (same family having similar dietary or bowel habits) or through inheritance of weakened fibrocollagenous supporting tissue.

Increased intra-abdominal pressure as a result of pregnancy or pelvic tumours may increase venous engorgement leading to development of secondary haemorrhoids.

Clinical features and diagnosis

Haemorrhoids are commoner in males. They are rare below 20. Common symptoms include:

- Bleeding per rectum, during or after defecation, which is bright red in colour and separate from stools (on surface, not mixed within). It is often slight and noted on the toilet paper. Sometimes it is more pronounced and drips into the pan, but is rarely massive.
- Prolapsed haemorrhoids
- Slight mucus discharge which may lead to pruritis ani may occur in patients with prolapsed haemorrhoids.
- Mild anal discomfort. Acute or severe pain is not a symptom of haemorrhoids unless there is complication such as thrombosis or the patient is suffering from another condition (e.g. anal fissure or abscess).
- Mild obstructive defecatory symptoms occur in patients with bulky prolapsed haemorrhoids.

Digital rectal examination and proctoscopy confirms the diagnosis. Haemorrhoids are classified according to their location in the anal canal into:

- **Internal:** above the dentate line (their vessels arise from the superior haemorrhoidal plexus), they are covered with pink rectal mucosa.

- **External:** below the dentate line (their vessels arise from the inferior haemorrhoidal plexus), they are covered with violet anal mucosa or skin.
- **Internal-external:** mixture of the above two types, usually with a groove between them.

Haemorrhoids are further classified by the degree of prolapse and for purposes of treatment into:

First degree:	Project into the lumen during straining, but don't prolapse
Second degree:	Prolapse during defecation, then is reduced spontaneously into the anal canal
Third degree:	Prolapse during defecation, require manual reduction
Fourth degree:	Prolapsed irreducible haemorrhoids

All patients should have at least rigid sigmoidoscopy to exclude colorectal cancer (flexible sigmoidoscopy is desirable in most patients above 40 years). Barium enemas and/or colonoscopy are needed if bleeding is mixed with stools or there is change in bowel habits.

Bleeding haemorrhoids needs differentiation from colorectal cancer and proctocolitis. Prolapsing haemorrhoids needs differentiation from mucosal rectal prolapse, anal warts, anal carcinomas, prolapsed rectal polyps or skin tags associated with anal fissures. Finally, they should be distinguished from rectal varices in patients with portal hypertension.

Treatment

1.   Conservative medical treatment.   Indicated in first- and early second-degree as well as in long-term management after treatment of other degrees. This relies mainly on avoiding constipation and straining as well as increasing dietary fibre intake. Astringent creams, e.g. Xyloproct or Proctosedyl, give moderate symptomatic relief to symptoms.

2.   Injection sclerotherapy.   Indicated for uncomplicated first-degree bleeding **internal** haemorrhoids. Five per cent phenol in almond oil or 5% ethanolamine oleate solution is used for injection. Three ml are injected submucosally into the root of each major haemorrhoid, well above the dentate line. Two or three sites can be injected per session. Injection can be repeated after 4 weeks, but it is not recommended to repeat it more than 2 or 3 times. It usually gives good short-term results. Rarely injections may cause ulceration (when done very superficially), pain, abscess and oleogranuloma.

3.   Rubber band ligation.   This is indicated in bleeding and prolapsing 2nd-degree and early 3rd-degree **internal** haemorrhoids. It is contraindicated in patients on anticoagulants, bleeding disorders or immune deficiency. It may be also wise to stop aspirin and non-steroidal anti-inflammatory drugs 1 week before the procedure. Up to 3 sites can be treated in the same session and it can be repeated after 4–6 weeks.

Banding is applied using Barron's applicator inserted via a proctoscope (or similar applicators). The applicator is loaded first with one or two rubber rings (bands), and a toothed grasper (or suction) is used to grasp the haemorrhoid (1 cm above the dentate line) and pull it inside the applicator, which is then fired to strangulate the haemorrhoidal pedicles. After 7–10 days the banded tissue sloughs, which may result in a minor bleeding episode. Other complications include pain, if rings are applied near the dentate line. Very rarely sepsis may follow; this is evidenced by a triad of symptoms: late worsening pain, fever and late urinary retention. This calls for re-examination, drainage of any abscesses, excision of any necrotic tissues and administration of triple antibiotics. Good results occur in about 70% of patients. Post-treatment analgesia, stool softener and Sitz baths are recommended.

4. Infrared photocoagulation. Indicated for first- and second-degree haemorrhoids. The probe is inserted via an anoscope and is applied to haemorrhoids above the dentate line for 1–2 seconds. It is applied to 3 or 4 sites over the apex and sides of each major haemorrhoid. This produces a circular burn about 2–5 mm in depth. Results are comparable to sclerotherapy and banding. Pain and complications are very rare.

Operative treatment of haemorrhoids

Haemorrhoidectomy is associated with less need for further future therapy[b]. Surgery is usually indicated in 3rd- and 4th-degree haemorrhoids. There are now two main competing techniques: traditional excisional haemorrhoidectomy and stapled haemorrhoidectomy (the latter is only suitable for 3rd-degree haemorrhoids).

Excisional haemorrhoidectomy often calls for sound judgement to tailor it to the needs of the patient.

1. Open haemorrhoidectomy (Milligan–Morgan, St. Marks haemorrhoidectomy). This is the traditional method of excisional haemorrhoidectomy, in which prolapsed haemorrhoidal tissues are excised using scissors or diathermy usually at the three main sites (leaving three mucocutaneous bridges, at least 1 cm in width each) and leaving the resultant wounds open. This is still the most widely practiced haemorrhoidectomy.

2. Closed haemorrhoidectomy (Ferguson). This is a similar technique, but it ends with closure of the wounds. It is more popular in the United States.

3. Laser haemorroidectomy. Laser may be used either for vaporization of the tissues overlying the haemorrhoids, resulting in an ulcer and fixation (non-contact laser) usually in 2nd-degree haemorrhoids, or used as knife for performing a Milligan–Morgan haemorrhoidectomy. Either the CO_2 or Nd-YAG is used. There have been claims that it results in less pain[c], but these claims are not yet substantiated.

4. Stapled haemorrhoidectomy (Longo procedure, PPH (procedure for prolapse and haemorrhoids). This new procedure aims at pulling the prolapsed cushions back into place rather than resecting them. This is done by excising a cylinder of the lower rectal mucosa and submucosa and reanastomosing them using a specially designed circular stapling instrument. It is indicated in 3rd-degree haemorrhoids (but not in 4th-degree) and seems to be associated with less post-operative pain and faster return to normal activity[a]. However, long-term results are not known yet.

5. Choice of operation. Each method has advantages and disadvantages, for example closed haemorrhoidectomy may result in more residual skin tags (if wounds become disrupted and they often do). Stapled haemorrhoidectomy deals well with circumferential haemorrhoids, but is often unable to deal with 4th-degree haemorrhoids or unequally bulging circumferential haemorrhoids, resulting in residual haemorrhoids.

6. Postoperative management. This should include adequate analgesia, stool softeners and frequent Sitz baths. Metronidazole treatment for 7 days postoperatively is recommended to decrease potential for septic complications after stapled haemorrhoidectomy. It also seems to decrease postoperative pain following open haemorrhoidectomy[a].

Haemorrhoidectomy may be done as a day case surgery, although larger haemorrhoids probably need to be done as an in-patient procedure. In-patients should stay in the hospital until the first bowel motion after haemorrhoidectomy, as the degree of pain in individual patients is unpredictable.

7. Complications of haemorrhoidectomy. While postoperative pain is not strictly a complication, it may be considerable in some patients, even when local anaesthetic has been injected into the wounds of excisional haemorrhoidectomy. Other complications include reactionary or secondary haemorrhage. Very rarely anal stenosis (if too much skin is excised) or defects in continence (sphincters damaged by an inexperienced operator).

8. Other techniques no longer used. Parks submucosal haemorrhoidectomy (high recurrence rates). Whitehead haemorrhoidectomy (risk of continuous mucus leak and wet anus). Lord's maximal anal dilatation, using four fingers of both hands (risk of incontinence).

Cryodestruction (profuse mucoid discharge associated with foul smell for few weeks and very long healing times).

9. Thrombosed interno-external haemorrhoids. Prolapse and consequent thrombosis of internal haemorrhoids is exceedingly painful. Treatment consists of hospital admission, ice packs, elevation of the foot of the bed and analgesia. Alternatively the condition may be treated by an emergency haemorrhoidectomy, which must be done carefully with preservation of sufficient mucocutaneous bridges.

10. Thrombosed external haemorrhoids. Thrombosis of the subcutaneous plexus of veins at the anal margin is also very painful. This is treated adequately by incision and expression of the clot under local anaesthetic, but may be prone to recurrent future episodes. Formal excision probably results in far less incidence of recurrence. Untreated the acute episode often resolves spontaneously after few days, leaving a skin tag.

Further reading

Carapeti EA, Kamm MA, McDonald PJ, Philips RKS. Double-blind randomised controlled trial of effect of metranidazole on pain after day-case haemorrhoidectomy. *Lancet*, 1998; **351**: 169–172.

Fazio VW. Early promise of stapling technique for haemorrhoidectomy. *Lancet*, 2000; **355**: 768–769.

MacRae HM, McLeod RS. Comparison of haemorrhoidal treatment: a meta-analysis. *Canadian Journal of Surgery*, 1977; **40**: 14–17.

Mehigan BJ, Monson JRT, Hartley JE. Stapling procedure for haemorrhoids versus Milligan–Morgan haemorrhoidectomy: randomised controlled trial. *Lancet*, 2000; **355**: 782–785.

HEAD INJURY

Nick Lagattolla

Pathology of head injury

The Monroe–Kelly doctrine confirms that the skull cannot easily accommodate an increase in volume of its contents without a significant rise in intracranial pressure (ICP). Cerebral perfusion pressure (CPP) equals the systemic arterial pressure (SAP) minus the ICP. This relationship is fundamental and explains the pathophysiology of brain injury.

Brain injury causes swelling. This volume increase causes a rise in ICP and thus a fall in CPP, resulting in brain ischaemia. Deterioration in cerebral function causes respiratory failure resulting in reduced PaO_2 and a rise in $PaCO_2$, which both cause cerebral vasoconstriction, further aggravating ischaemia. This leads to infarction which causes more brain swelling. If this vicious cycle is not interrupted, the inevitable outcome is death, as total brain failure occurs when ICP = SAP, and the CPP is zero.

A rise in the ICP results in displacement of parts of the brain. In earlier phases this is seen as midline shift. Later stages result in herniation of the cingulate lobe under the adjacent falx (subfacial herniation), the uncus through the tentorial hiatus to compress the oculomotor nerve and midbrain, and the cerebellar tonsil through the foramen magnum compressing the medulla oblongata. These are terminal events.

Mechanism of brain injury

Trauma may either injure the brain, or the extracerebral vessels. Rupture of extra-cerebral vessels results in intracranial bleeding, indirectly causing further brain injury. Trauma severe enough to cause brain injury usually also results in skull fracture. However, skull fracture is not requisite for either direct brain injury or intracranial bleeding.

Brain injury may occur at the site of the trauma ('coup' injury). Acceleration of the brain away from the source of injury with an abrupt stop at the opposite side also results in injury ('contre-coup' injury).

1. Intracranial bleeding. Extracerebral bleeding occurs in the extradural or subdural spaces. Intracerebral bleeding results from coup or contre-coup injury. All result in haematomas that raise the ICP.

- *Cerebral contusion.* Injuries range from mild contusion to large intracerebral haematoma. Mild contusions resolve. Large haematomas are acute space-occupying lesions, and need to be evacuated.
- *Extradural haematoma.* The thin pteryon anterior to the ear fractures easily, and rupture of the underlying middle meningeal artery may result. A compact

haematoma lying between the periosteal layer of the dura mater and the inner table of the skull results. The classical sequence of events is loss of consciousness as a result of the blow, followed by some recovery (the so-called 'lucid-phase'), before consciousness is lost again. CT scan shows characteristic convex haematoma. Treatment is by craniotomy, evacuation of the haematoma, and clipping of the bleeding artery. Small extradural haematomas may result from blood oozing from skull fractures.

- *Acute subdural haematoma.* This is far more common than extradural haematoma. It results from bleeding communicating veins in the less restricted subdural space, and thus develops rapidly. Prompt evacuation is required.
- *Chronic subdural haematoma.* The elderly are prone to develop subdural haematomas. Cerebral atrophy places the communicating veins under tension, and these rupture easily. Because of cerebral atrophy, there is a greater space for blood to accumulate. The haematoma may remain undiscovered for a long time. As the content alters, it becomes osmotically active, slowly expanding, and presenting as a chronic confusional state.

2.   Direct parenchymal injury.   The brain has a layered structure. A force applied to the parenchyma causes shearing stresses and the layers may move over each other. This direct parenchymal disruption is impossible to visualize by any means, and may occur without any appreciable intracranial bleeding. The prognosis is poor.

Evolution of clinical signs

With cortical disruption, convulsions may occur, the level of consciousness reduces, and there may be Cheyne–Stokes respiration. As corticospinal tracts are disrupted, contralateral weakness occurs. With involvement of the midbrain, hyperventilation may occur. The ipsilateral pupil becomes fixed and dilated. With involvement of the upper pontine respiratory centre, the respiratory pattern develops with episodes of hyperventilation separated by periods of apnoea. If the lower pons is involved, there may be prolonged inspirations and expirations. Blood pressure elevation and bradycardia signify involvement of the medullary cardiovascular regulatory centre.

Evaluation of clinical signs

Conscious level may be rapidly evaluated using the Glasgow Coma Scale (GCS). The highest score possible is 15, and the lowest is three. This serves to assess neurological state in standard terms, and second, to monitor the progress of a patient following a head injury and to identify quickly any deterioration in condition.

External examination may reveal signs of a brain skull fracture: blood or CSF issuing from the ear, Battle's sign (bruising around the mastoid area), bilateral periorbital haematomata ('panda eyes') or haemotympanum.

The Glasgow Coma Scale

Motor response	Obeying commands	6
	Localizing to pain	5
	Withdrawal to pain	4
	Flexion to pain	3
	Extension to pain	2
	No movement	1
Verbal response	Orientated	5
	Confused	4
	Inappropriate speech	3
	Incomprehensible sounds	2
	No verbal response	1
Eye opening	Spontaneous eye opening	4
	Eyes open to request	3
	Eyes open to pain	2
	No eye opening	1

Management of head injury in casualty

Indications for skull X-ray include loss of consciousness, convulsions, amnesia, severe trauma, global or focal neurological signs, GCS less than 15, and the presence of large scalp haematoma or tenderness. Evidence of facial injuries requires facial X-rays and nasal views. If the skull is fractured, if there is any neurological abnormality or if there is any difficulty in assessing neurological state (e.g. due to intoxication) the patient must be admitted and hourly neurological observations undertaken. There should be low thresholds for admission for children and the elderly. CT scan must be considered if there is a skull fracture or if there is any neurological abnormality. Patients with depressed skull fractures must be referred to a neurosurgical unit, as these need to be elevated.

Management of severe head injuries

1. *Initial*

- The patient's neck must be stabilized until either a CT scan or X-rays have shown no fracture of the cervical spine.
- Early assessment must be made of the GCS, arterial blood gases, pupillary response, respiratory pattern, and cardiovascular state. If there is evidence of respiratory dysfunction, or if the blood gases show respiratory failure, the patient must be ventilated immediately.
- The brain swelling is treated by infusing 1 g/kg mannitol intravenously, and a urinary catheter is inserted.
- In the presence of gross neurological changes, a CT scan of the head and neck is performed to exclude a surgically correctable focal lesion.

2. Surgical

- The presence of an intra- or extracerebral haematoma necessitates referral to a neurosurgical unit for evacuation.
- Depressed skull fractures must be referred for debridement and elevation. There is a high risk of epilepsy if bone fragments are in contact with the brain.
- Multiple burr holes in the parietal, frontal and occipital bones may achieve decompression in diffuse cerebral oedema.
- If there is any doubt about the potential for surgery in a patient with a severe head injury, the case and CT scans must be discussed early with neurosurgeons.

3. Supportive

- Continued management should be undertaken in an intensive care unit.
- The ICP may be monitored by the insertion of an ICP bolt through which the ICP can be transduced.
- Bolus doses of intravenous mannitol are given, titrated against the ICP, and continued for 4 days.
- Ventilation is continued, and if there is evidence that this is likely to be required for more than 1 week, a tracheostomy (open or percutaneous) is performed.
- Two litres of fluid are given intravenously per day and U&E are monitored daily.
- If prolonged unconsciousness is likely, a nasogastric tube is passed for enteral feeding.
- Care is taken to avoid pressure sores, and physiotherapy is given to chest and limbs.
- Continuous cerebral monitoring by EEG may be useful.
- Phenytoin is given intravenously if there have been seizures, a penetrating head injury, a depressed skull fracture, or if the patient requires longer than 48 hours of ventilation.

Further reading

Jennett B, Teasdale G. *Management of Head Injuries*. Philadelphia: Davis, 1981.
Molloy C. Head injuries. Part 1: management of the unconscious patient. *Surgery*, 1993; **11:** 545–549.

Related topic of interest

Trauma management (p. 328).

HEPATIC TUMOURS AND BILIARY CANCER

Deya Marzouk

Hepatic tumours

Malignant tumours are commoner than benign ones. Metastases are commoner than primary liver cancer in North America and Western Europe. Primary liver cancer is more common in the east and Africa.

Evaluation of patients with liver masses should take into account patient's history (e.g. oral contraceptive usage, cirrhosis, hepatitis B infection or previous malignancy), tumour markers (CEA, α-fetoprotein) and radiological investigations.

Ultrasonography distinguishes solid from cystic lesions. In some patients it is more sensitive than CT in detection of metastases. Spiral CT, biphasic CT and MRI are useful in delineating hepatic masses and its relation to major vascular and biliary structures as well as determining resectability of malignant masses. They are gradually replacing hepatic arteriography and CT portography. Intraoperative ultrasonography is the most sensitive technique in detecting hidden metastases, assessing resectability and planning surgery[b].

Symptomatic masses deemed potentially resectable should not be biopsied. Biopsies risk tumour seeding and infiltration of diaphragm. It may induce massive bleeding in hepatic adenomas and other vascular lesions. Biopsy should only be considered in unresectable tumours to guide further therapy or if a solitary lesion can be excised by a wedge resection[b].

Benign hepatic tumours

Haemangiomas

The commonest benign hepatic neoplasm. The majority are cavernous haemangiomas and are more common in women. Most are asymptomatic and are found incidentally. Rarely large haemangiomas may cause right upper quadrant pain or consumptive coagulopathy. Diagnosis is made by dynamic CT scan with iv contrast that shows a characteristic peripheral enhancement with centripetal filling.

Observation is indicated for asymptomatic patients especially with lesions less than 4 cm in diameter. Symptomatic lesions are resected.

Hepatic adenomas

The majority of hepatic adenomas occur in women who have used oral contraceptive pills[c]. Most patients have symptoms; 50% have abdominal pain, 20–30% may present with acute intraperitoneal bleeding from sudden rupture. Patients may have hepatomegaly or present with upper abdominal mass. Pregnancy is associated with tumour growth and increased incidence of acute bleeding.

Adenomas are difficult to differentiate radiologically with certainty from hepatocellular carcinoma. They show as a cold defect on radionuclide imaging. CT and MRI scans show areas of haemorrhage and necrosis. Angiography shows a hypervascular lesion with peripheral blood supply.

Patients should stop oral contraceptive pills and alternative contraception be used. Pregnancy should be avoided until the adenoma is removed. Surgical treatment is advised because of the tendency to bleed and to exclude malignancy.

Focal nodular hyperplasia (FNH)

FNH is found predominantly in young women (not related to oral contraceptives). Most are asymptomatic. Large lesions rarely present with hepatic enlargement or pain. At least half may decrease in size or appear to resolve during follow-up.

FNH are usually isodense on CT scan. It may show early filling with contrast in biphasic CT and contrast-enhanced MRI. It disappears in the venous phase and may show a central scar. It does not show as a defect on radionuclide imaging. Angiography shows a hypervascular lesion which may be stellate in appearance.

Asymptomatic patients are observed. Symptomatic patients (or lesions that can not be confidently diagnosed radiologically) need resection.

Bile duct adenomas

These lesions are usually small and found incidentally during laparotomy. They may be confused with metastatic liver lesions.

Primary hepatocellular carcinoma (HCC)

Hepatocellular carcinoma (HCC) accounts for 75% of primary hepatic malignancies. Other types include cholangiocarcinoma of the intrahepatic ducts (20%), angiosarcoma, hepatoblastoma, mixed hepatocellular and cholangiocarcinoma as well as other sarcomas. AIDS patients may develop primary hepatic lymphomas and Kaposi sarcoma.

Aetiology

HCC is associated with hepatitis B and C infection, cirrhosis and aflatoxin B1. It is also rarely associated with use of synthetic androgens, haemochromatosis, tyrosinaemia, alpha 1 antitrypsin deceficiency and type 1 glycogen storage disease.

Clinical features

Most patients present with right upper quadrant pain and hepatomegaly. Loss of weight, anorexia, fever or jaundice may also occur. Severe sudden abdominal pain may occur with intralesional bleeding. Shock may follow intraperitoneal bleeding which may occur in up to 10% of patients. Sudden deterioration in cirrhotic patients or development of ascites may indicate a hepatoma.

Diagnosis

The diagnosis may be suggested by elevated alpha fetoprotein (AFP), which occurs in 75–90% of cases, elevation of liver alkaline phosphatase and GGT or by US, CT and MRI scans. CT angiography, CT portography or biphasic CT is used to evaluate resectability.

Screening for high-risk patients, e.g. those with long-standing hepatitis B infection, should be done using AFP and liver US every 4 months to detect these tumours whilst small and operable.

Treatment

1. Surgical resection. Resection is possible in 20% of all patients. Only 50–70% of patients undergoing exploration will have resection with curative intent. Recurrence rates following resection range from 30–70% of patients. Cirrhosis limits surgical resection options because of inability of cirrhotic liver to regenerate and the consequent risk of postoperative hepatic failure. Anatomic segmentectomies or lobectomies are usually needed. Liver transplantation has been tried for unresectable tumours but has a high recurrence rate.

2. Chemotherapy. Systemic chemotherapy using doxorubicin has a response rate less than 20%. Combination chemotherapy has similar disappointing results. Hepatic artery ligation alone or in combination with hepatic arterial chemotherapy as well as hepatic artery embolization has been tried with limited success.

3. Radiotherapy. External beam radiotherapy may be used for palliation of symptomatic unresectable HCC, but dose must be limited to 25–30 Gy to avoid radiation hepatitis.

4. Percutaneous ethanol injection (PEI). Percutaneous injection of 95% ethanol under US control (10 ml once a week) has been used with some success in treatment of HCC in patients with cirrhosis or who are poor surgical risk. This has also been tried as a primary treatment for small HCC less than 3 cm in diameter [b].

Prognosis

Prognosis following hepatic resection averages 15–30% after 5 years.

Fibrolamellar hepatocellular carcinoma

This is a special histological variant, which is characterized by slower growth and consequently better prognosis. Five-year survival after resection is 50–60% versus 25% in classic HCC It occurs primarily in younger patients (90% are younger than 25 years). It is not associated with hepatitis B or cirrhosis and AFP is usually normal.

Liver metastases

Liver metastases are common in colorectal, gastric, oesophageal, pancreatic, breast, lung cancers, carcinoid tumours and melanomas. Lymphomas and leukaemia also involve the liver.

Diagnosis

Asymptomatic liver metastases may be suspected during follow-up from elevation of CEA (especially in colorectal cancer), elevation of alkaline phosphatase, GGT & 5'-nucleotidase or are detected by ultrasound or CT scans done every 6–12 months. Symptomatic disease presents with weight loss, right upper quadrant pain or hepatomegaly.

Treatment

Treatment depends on whether liver metastases are likely to be the only site of metastastic disease. Abdominal tumours draining into the portal circulation (e.g. colorectal, carcinoid etc.) may have metastases limited to the liver and may be suitable for resection. Nonportal tumours (e.g. breast, lung cancers or melanomas) are usually widely disseminated and are not normally considered for liver resection.

1. Surgical resection. Occult liver metastases in the remaining liver must be excluded first. Intraoperative ultrasound seems to be the best modality for doing so. Resection may be a nonanatomic wedge resection for peripherally located metastases, anatomic segmentectomies for more centrally located lesions or classic lobectomies or trisegmentectomy depending on location, number and extent of metastases.

Liver resection for metastatic disease is only established in colorectal cancer. Twenty per cent of patients with recurrent colorectal cancer have metastases limited to the liver. Of these, one quarter have limited hepatic involvement suitable for resection (5% of all patients with colorectal cancer). Five-year survival after potentially curative resection average 25%[b].

2. Palliative treatment. Non-resectable metastases may be treated by combination chemotherapy, cryosurgery or percutaneous injection of alcohol.

Current chemotherapy regimes for metastatic colorectal cancer include 5-fluorouracil and folinic acid. Second line chemotherapy includes oxaliplatin and irinotecan. Chemotherapy may be delivery systemically or via hepatic arterial infusion, using an implantable subcutaneous port.

Biliary cancer

Extrahepatic bile duct cancer

Extrahepatic bile duct cancer (cholangiocarcinoma) is extremely rare (0.2–0.3% of cancers). Unlike gallbladder cancer, it is slightly more common in men and generally occurs between 50 and 70 years. 15–20% may occur below 45 years.

1. Aetiology. Unknown. Increased incidence occurs in sclerosing cholangitis, ulcerative colitis, cystic dilatation of the biliary tree including choledochal cyst and Caroli's disease, infestation with *Clonorchis sinensis* as well as the radio-contrast Thorotrast. Cystic dilatation of the biliary tree may be related to anomalous pancreaticobiliary ductal junction that may induce mucosal hyperplasia, metaplasia, dysplasia and subsequent carcinoma.

2. Pathology. They are usually slow-growing small lesions. Local invasion results in infiltration of portal vein, hepatic artery and liver parenchyma. They metastasize to regional and paraortic nodes as well as by bloodstream in late stages. Most are adenocarcinomas and may be papillary, nodular and sclerosing. The papillary subtype has better prognosis, while the sclerosing type tends to be poorly differentiated and has the worst prognosis.

They are classified by location into hilar (50%), mid-duct, distal and diffuse. Bismuth classified hilar tumours according to their location relative to the confluence of hepatic ducts and proximal extension into 5 types. Type I: the common hepatic duct, Type II common hepatic duct and confluence, Type IIIa confluence and right hepatic duct, Type IIIb confluence and left hepatic duct, Type IV, confluence and proximal extension into both hepatic ducts. Hilar cholangiocarcinomas arising at the confluence of right and left hepatic ducts are called Klatskin's tumour.

3.   Clinical features.   Cholangiocarcinoma usually presents with obstructive jaundice, pruritis, vague abdominal pain, nausea and weight loss. Patients may also present with cholangitis and septicaemia. Prolonged biliary obstruction results in liver and renal dyfunction, coagulopathy, pruritis, progressive malnutrition and recurrent cholangitis. If biliary obstruction is not relieved then death from liver failure occurs soon. Mid and distal cholangiocarcinomas may lead to a distended palpable gallbladder.

4.   Investigations and diagnosis.   Initial investigations are usually carried out for obstructive jaundice and include liver function tests, abdominal US and CT scans. These may reveal a dilated biliary tree or a mass. CT scan is better in delineating masses. ERCP is even more definitive in diagnosing small masses and delineating the exact extension of these tumours within the biliary tree. It also allows brush cytology to obtain histological proof of the diagnosis and may be employed in placing stents. Klatskin tumours normally display a Mercedes sign with 3 strands radiating from the centre. ERCP needs to be carried under broad-spectrum antibiotic cover and vitamin K to normalize coagulation. CT angiography and MRI may be used to determine invasion of surrounding structures and resectability.

5.   Treatment.   Resection is the best hope for cure and also offers the best palliation and longer survival, compared with other treatments.

6.   Surgical resection.   Hilar tumours frequently invade major hepatic vascular structures and are only resectable in 20–30% of patients explored. This involves resection of the hepatic duct bifurcation and Roux-en-Y hepaticojejunostomy. Resection may need to include segmental hepatic resection as well to achieve tumour free margins.

   The resectability rate is higher in mid and distal bile duct tumours, 40% and 50% respectively. Tumours of the middle third are treated by local resection of bile duct and reconstruction by choledocho- or hepatico-jejunostomy. Tumours of the lower third require a Whipple's pancreaticoduodenectomy and reconstruction by choledocho- or hepaticojejunostomy.

7.   Liver transplantation.   Liver transplantation is no longer recommended for unresectable hilar tumours, because of high rate of recurrence.

8.   Palliative treatment.   In unresectable hilar tumours, palliative surgical bypass using left (round ligament approach) or right hepaticojejunostomy (through gallbladder bed) may be used. This may be accompanied by transhepatic U tube stent placement. Distal and mid bile duct tumours requiring bypass need a choledocho-, cholecysto- or hepaticojejunostomy.

The gallbladder may be removed to prevent acute cholecystitis from blockage of cystic duct by tumour or stents. Coeliac ganglion blockade (using 95% alcohol) to control pain may also be carried out.

Alternatively the tumour may be stented endoscopically (ERCP) or radiologically (PTC). Endoscopic stenting using self-expanding metallic stents is gaining popularity as the preferred method of stenting nowadays[b].

9. Chemotherapy. Chemotherapy using 5-fluorouracil alone or in combination with mitomycin C, adriamycin (FAM) or cisplatin produce response rates less than 15%[b].

10. Radiotherapy. Radiotherapy (following stenting), using external beam irradiation, intraoperative radiotherapy or irradiation with 192 Ir wires have all been tried, but efficacy is not established, although some reports suggest that it may improve survival compared with stents only.

11. Prognosis. Prognosis is poor. Five-year survival is 30% for patients with distal tumours and 15% for patients with hilar tumours.

Gallbladder cancer

Gallbladder cancer is rare, affecting 2.5 per 100 000 population annually. Incidental gallbladder cancer is found in 0–5–1% of all cholecystectomy specimens. Many of these cancers remain asymptomatic in elderly people until death.

1. Epidemiology and aetiology. Gallbladder cancer is commoner in Southwestern USA, Israel, Chile, Japan and Northeastern Europe. It is also very common in American Indians, where it represents 8.5–25% of all their cancers.

Gallbladder cancer is strongly associated with gallstone disease, which is present in 75–95% of patients. It appears that the risk is greater with larger stones and with the duration of gallstone disease. Calcified gallbladders (porcelain gallbladder) carries a 12–60% risk of malignancy. Other factors include: adenomatous gallbladder polyps (esp. >12 mm) and adenomyomatosis. Anomalous pancreaticobiliary ductal junction may induce mucosal hyperplasia, metaplasia and dysplasia and predispose to gallbladder and other biliary cancers. Chemical carcinogens in certain industries such as rubber, automobile, wood-finishing, and metal-fabricating industries may also contribute.

2. Pathology. Carcinoma of gallbladder usually arises in the fundus or neck of gallbladder and invades surrounding organs, especially the liver (50% of cases), duodenum and colon. Lymph node metastases occur in 50–75%. Cystic and porta hepatis nodes are involved first, lesser omentum and coeliac nodes are affected later. Distant spread may be seen in terminal disease.

Adenocarcinoma represents 90–95% of these tumours. Other tumours include anaplastic carcinoma and squamous cell carcinoma. The papillary subtype of adenocarcinoma has less tendency to invade locally or send lymph node metastases and carries a better prognosis.

3. Clinical features. Gallbladder cancer usually affects patients in their 7th and 8th decades of life and is 3–4 times more common in women. It usually remains asymptomatic until advanced. Symptoms fall into one of three groups:

1. Symptoms of gallbladder disease (biliary pain, nausea) occur in up to 50%. A recent increase in symptoms in patients who had cholelithiasis for 10–25 years may also signify development of carcinoma.
2. Symptoms of malignant biliary obstruction occur in up to 35% of patients with jaundice, weight loss, anorexia and persistent aching upper quadrant pain.
3. Acute cholecystitis may occur in 10–15% of patients.

Physical examination may reveal nothing. Alternatively a palpable gallbladder mass or hepatomegaly may be felt. In advanced cases, patients may have jaundice, cachexia and ascites.

4. Diagnosis. More than 90% of gallbladder cancers are diagnosed intra-operatively. Preoperative diagnosis may be suggested by calcification of the gallbladder wall on plain abdominal X-ray, presence of a gallbladder mass, or localized thickness that do not move with change in position on abdominal US or CT scans as well as liver or other organ invasion or nodal spread on CT. The diagnosis may also be made during investigations for obstructive jaundice using ERCP or PTC. When diagnosis is suspected preoperatively CT angiography may be used to assess resectability.

5. Treatment. Surgery is the mainstay of treatment. Resectability rate is approximately 30%. Curative resections are only possible in 3%[b].

6. Surgical resection.. Cholecystectomy may be sufficient for incidental carcinomas discovered on pathological examination, which are limited to the mucosa. More invasive tumours usually need extended cholecystectomy including wedge hepatic resection (3 cm macroscopic margin), en-bloc resection with adjacent organs and hepatoduodenal lymphadenectomy.

7. Palliative treatment. Relief of jaundice may be achieved by placement of stents endoscopically (during ERCP), under radiological guidance (during PTC) or during surgery. Alternatively internal bypass by hepaticojejunostomy to segment III duct via ligamentum teres approach may be used. Cholecystectomy may be also performed (if at all feasible) to prevent development of acute cholecystitis. Finally, coeliac ganglion block for pain relief may be done using 95% alcohol either intra-operatively or by percutaneous injection.

8. Chemotherapy and radiotherapy. The role of adjuvant and palliative chemotherapy and radiation therapy is not well defined, because of the poor response rates. Chemotherapy using FAM (5-fluorouracil, adriamycin and mitomycin C) has a response rate of 20%[c]. External beam radiotherapy may be used to reduce abdominal pain.

Further reading

Colorectal Cancer Collaborative Group. Palliative chemotherapy for advanced colorectal cancer: systemic review and meta-analysis. *British Medical Journal*, 2000; **321:** 531–535.

Giorgio A, Tarantino L, de Stefano G, Perrotta A, Aloisio V, del Viscovo L, Alaia A, Lettieri G. Ultrasound-guided percutaneous ethanol injection under general anesthesia for the treatment of hepatocellular carcinoma on cirrhosis: long-term results in 268 patients. *European Journal of Ultrasound*, 2000; **12:** 145–154.

Launois B, Reding R, Lebeau G, Buard JL. Surgery for hilar cholangiocarcinoma: French experience in a collective survey of 552 extrahepatic bile duct cancers. *Journal of Hepatobiliary Pancreatic Surgery*, 2000; **7:** 128–134.

Nevin JE, Moran TJ, Kay S, King R. Carcinoma of the gallbladder: staging, treatment and prognosis. *Cancer*, 1976; **37:** 141–148.

HYPERPARATHYROIDISM

Christopher Lattimer, Nitin Gureja

Parathyroid glands are small, oval-shaped tan glands, lying posterior to the thyroid, and often numbering 4 (90.6%), but 5 (5.1%), and 3 (0.6%) can occur.

The superior parathyroid glands arise from the 4th pharyngeal pouch, whilst the inferior arise from the 3rd pharyngeal pouch; and they progress caudally with the thymus. The inferior glands are much more variable in position then the superior.

The blood supply is often from the inferior thyroid artery; and venous drainage by the superior, middle and inferior thyroid veins.

Parathyroid glands are composed of 3 main cells:

- chief cells.
- oxyphil cells.
- water clear cells.

Parathormone

Parathormone is an 84-amino-acid peptide precursor, which is excreted as a precursor (pre-pro-parathormone), and which is cleaved prior to secretion. It is metabolized in the liver to the *N*-active metabolite. Its secretion is in response to low ionized Ca levels, detected by two receptors: a 120-kDa protein similar to G-protein receptors, and a 500-kDa protein similar to LDL receptors.

Secretion of PTH causes:

- An increase in bone resorption
- An increase in steoclastic activity
- An increase in 1,25-hydroxylation of vitamin D3
- A decrease in calcium excretion
- An increase in phosphate excretion

Hyperparathyroidism

Can be classified into 3 types:

- **Primary:** where the normal feedback of Ca is disturbed and hence have increased PTH secretion.
- **Secondary:** have disturbance of Ca homeostasis and hence have increase in gland size; e.g. chronic renal failure patients.
- **Tertiary:** when in 2° hyperparathyroidism, the parathyroid glands become autonomous.

Primary hyperparathyroidism

The incidence is approximately 30 per 100 000, with a female to male preponderance of 2:1. It is more common in the over 60s age group. In 85% of cases it seems to be caused by an adenoma; 12% of cases by hyperplasia, and 1–2% of cases due to carcinoma.

The exact pathogenesis is unknown, but seems to be related to resetting of the Ca set point. It may also occur due to genetic abnormality at chromosome 11; and is associated with MEN 1 and MEN 2A syndromes.

1. **Symptoms and signs.** Clinical presentation can be summarized by the tetrad of 'Stones, bones, moans and abdominal groans'. More commonly with the use of multichannel biochemistry tests, an increasing number are asymptomatic.

Skeletal complaints are mainly of arthralgia and myalgia. Patients rarely have osteitis fibrosa cystica. Excessive PTH secretion can result in distinctive radiographic appearances of subperiosteal bone resorption around the phalanges and clavicles; and in severe cases of 'brown tumours'. Renal abnormalities include nephrocalcinosis, calculi, and renal failure. Hypertension is an association with 1° hyperparathyroidism, which is not always reversed after parathyroidectomy. Commonest abdominal manifestation is colicky abdominal pain, but pancreatitis and peptic ulcer disease are also associated.

Psychiatric manifestations include depression, anxiety and confusional states.

2. **Laboratory diagnosis.** Elevated serum calcium (especially ionized Ca), and PTH levels are suggestive of hyperparathyroidism. In 50% of patients the serum phosphate level is also decreased. An elevated 24-hour urine excretion for calcium differentiates this from familial hypercalcaemic hypocalciuric syndrome.

The alkaline phosphatase may also be elevated especially if there is bony involvement. Malignant causes of hypercalcaemia are excluded by calculating the chloride-phosphate ratio {(chloride-84) × (albumin-15)/phosphate}. A value over 500 is suggestive of primary hyperparathyroidism, whilst a value of under 400 suggests another cause. Plain radiographs of the hand and skull ('pepperpot skull') may aid in making the diagnosis.

The 1991 American National Institutes of Health (NIH) consensus statement regarding best practise for patients presenting for the first time with asymptomatic primary hyperparathyroidism concluded that preoperative imaging was not indicated.

The use of Tc-99m sestamibi scanning in localization of ectopic parathyroid tissue, yields a sensitivity of 97% in adenomatous disease, and a sensitivity of 76% in multiple gland disease. CT, MRI and US scans give similar sensitivities in locating ectopic parathyroid tissue (~63%).

3. **Differential diagnosis.** Other causes of hypercalcaemia should be excluded (malignancy, sarcoidosis, multiple myeloma, milk alkali syndrome, etc.).

4. **Management.** All symptomatic patients should undergo parathyroidectomy if fit enough for the procedure. Asymptomatic patients should be followed up 6 monthly. Patients who are likely to be lost to follow up or who are under the age of 50 years should be offered surgery. Medical management of hyperparathyroidism is subsatisfactory.

5. **Surgery.** Consent is obtained prior to the procedure, and risks of a failed neck exploration, recurrent laryngeal nerve injury, and postoperative hypocalcaemia are obtained. A surgeon experienced in parathyroid surgery, under general anaesthetic

undertakes the surgery. In the presence of adenomatous disease, the diseased gland is excised and careful search made for the presence of any further adenomas.

In the case of hyperplasia, a $3\frac{1}{2}$ parathyroidectomy is undertaken. Alternatively a total parathyroidectomy is undertaken, with transplantation of slivers of the gland of the most normal appearance in the non-dominant forearm.

Secondary hyperparathyroidism

Most often seen in renal patients, due to a disturbance of calcium homeostais. This is best managed medically, only indications for surgery being:

- Persistent hypercalcaemia despite medical management, and dietary restriction.
- Bone pain and pathological fractures.
- Ectopic calcification.
- Persistent itching.

At surgery a total parathyroidectomy is performed with auto-transplantation, or a three quarter gland excision.

Parathyroid carcinoma

Parathyroid carcinoma is a rare cause of hyperparathyroidism (~1–2%). Often the biochemistry in cases of parathyroid carcinoma is severely deranged with very high serum calcium and alkaline phosphatase.

At operation, the gland is often found to be firm and may show evidence of invasion into surrounding tissues. If suspected, an en-bloc dissection of the surrounding tissues including a thyroid lobectomy should ensue.

Overall the prognosis is poor.

Further reading

Consensus Development Panel. Diagnosis and management of asymptomatic primary hyperparathyroidism: Consensus Development Conference Statement. *Ann Int Med*, 1991; **114:** 593–597.

Nussbaum SR. Pathophysiology and management of severe hypercalcaemia. *Endocrinol Metab. Clin. North Am*, 1993; **22:** 343.

Serpel JW, Campbell PR, Young AE. Preoperative localisation of parathyroid tumours does not reduce operating time. *British Journal of Surgery*, 1991; **78:** 589–590.

Uden P, Chan A, Duh Q-Y, Siperstein A, Clark OH. Primary hyperparathyroidism in younger and older patients: Symptoms and outcome of surgery. *World Journal of Surgery*, 1992; **16:** 791.

HYPERTHYROIDISM – TREATMENT

Nick Wilson

Causes of hyperthyroidism

- Diffuse toxic goitre (Graves disease).
- Toxic multinodular goiter.
- Toxic solitary nodule.
- Thyroiditis.
- Metastatic thyroid carcinoma.
- Factitious thyroxine ingestion.
- Pituitary tumours secreting TSH.
- Choriocarcinoma/hydatidiform mole.
- Neonatal thyrotoxicosis.

Treatment

Normal thyroid function should be restored as quickly and safely as possible.

*1. **Antithyroid drugs.*** Thionamides (propyluracil, carbimazole) prevent the binding of iodine with tyrosine residues and the coupling of iodotyrosines to form iodothyronine. Carbimazole also suppresses thyroid stimulating antibody production. These drugs act quickly and are usually given for 6 months initially. Relapse occurs within 1 year of stopping treatment in 65% of patients. A small dose of thyroxine given with the drug will prevent iotrogenic hypothyroidism. They are particularly suitable for rendering patients euthyroid prior to surgery. Adverse effects include nausea, pruritis, rashes, arthritis, agranulocytosis and aplastic anaemia.

Iodide (Lugol's iodine) inhibits T_4 and T_3 release and may be given for 10 days pre-operatively in patients who are unable to take thionamides or are poorly controlled. The vascularity of the thyroid may be reduced marginally.

β-blockers (propranolol) control the manifestations of thyrotoxicosis and can be used in combination with thionamides to prepare patients for surgery. If used, propranolol should be continued for 1 week postoperatively as thyroxine has a long half-life.

*2. **Radioiodine.*** ^{131}I effectively destroys thyroid tissue and is cheap, easy to use and safe. It should not be used in children or pregnant women and is best avoided in patients in their reproductive years, although there is no evidence that radioiodine causes leukaemia, thyroid cancer, fetal or genetic damage. Radioiodine takes 2 months to control hyperthyroidism and antithyroid drugs are required to cover this period. More than one dose may be required if the initial response is inadequate. Hypothyroidism occurs at 3% per year after treatment and prolonged follow-up is therefore required and treatment with thyroxine may be necessary.

*3. **Surgery.*** Preoperative control of hyperthyroidism is essential, using carbimazole in most patients, with the addition of β-blockers in the severely thyrotoxic patient. The vocal cords should be checked for a pre-existing paresis, particularly if there has been previous thyroid surgery.

Where surgery is indicated (see below), bilateral subtotal thyroidectomy is performed for diffuse conditions such as Graves' disease or multinodular goitre, leaving 3–4 grams (the area of a thumbnail) of thyroid on each side. This reduces the likelihood of postoperative hypothyroidism, and parathyroid or recurrent laryngeal nerve damage. Patients with a toxic solitary nodule should be treated by unilateral subtotal lobectomy.

Possible postoperative complications are:

- Bleeding causing airway obstruction. Equipment to open the wound must be available.
- Recurrent laryngeal nerve damage.
- Parathyroid damage causing hypocalcaemia. Serum calcium should be monitored.
- Hypothyroidism. May affect up to 40%. Give thyroxine replacement.
- Recurrent hyperthyroidism. Antithyroid drugs or radioiodine should be used.

Treatment strategies

1. *Graves' disease (diffuse toxic goitre).* Patients over 45 years are best treated with radioiodine. Antithyroid drugs should be given for several weeks until the isotope has been effective. Younger patients should be treated with antithyroid drugs (carbimazole) initially. Propranolol should be added in severe cases or where tachycardia and tremor are prominent. Treatment should be stopped after 6 months and patients reviewed regularly. Relapse will affect 65% and these patients should then undergo subtotal thyroidectomy. Patients with large, toxic goitres may benefit from early surgery.

2. *Toxic multinodular goitre.* Surgery is the treatment of choice as radioiodine and antithyroid drugs do not substantially reduce the size of the gland or resolve the local symptoms.

3. *Toxic adenoma.* Subtotal lobectomy is required.

4. *Recurrent hyperthyroidism after surgery.* Repeat surgery is hazardous and in young patients, antithyroid drugs are used. Radioiodine is preferable for patients over 45 years.

5. *Children.* Antithyroid drugs should be given for 2 years and repeated in the 50% who relapse. If surgery is required, a radical resection is necessary, as the gland has a great tendency to grow back. Parathyroids and recurrent laryngeal nerves must be preserved. Prolonged follow-up is necessary, to detect abnormal thyroid function. Radioiodine is contraindicated.

6. *Thyrotoxicosis occurring in pregnancy.* Antithyroid drugs should be given, but hypothyroidism must be avoided. Fetal hypothyroidism may be induced. Free, unbound hormones must be measured during pregnancy, since TBG levels are abnormal. Surgery during the second trimester may be preferable in patients who are difficult to control. Radioiodine is contraindicated.

7. *Thyroid crisis.* Rare. A life-threatening condition occurring in patients inadequately controlled before surgery or hyperthyroid patients enduring stress (infection, other surgery). Dyspnoea, tachycardia, hyperpyrexia, restlessness, confusion, delerium, vomiting and diarrhoea occur. Carbimazole, Lugol's iodine, and propranolol should be given. Cooling, rehydration and oxygen therapy should be given, and other respiratory, cardiovascular and psychiatric measures should be employed as necessary.

Further reading

Young AE. The thyroid gland. In: Burnand KG, Young AE (eds) *The New Aird's Companion in Surgical Studies (2nd Edn)*. London: Churchill Livingstone, 1998; 459–483.

Related topics of interest

Goitre (p. 150); Hyperparathyroidism (p. 170); Thyroglossal tract anomalies (p. 322); Thyroid neoplasms (p. 324).

INCISIONAL AND OTHER ABDOMINAL HERNIAS

Nick Wilson

Incisional hernia

Incisional hernias occur when a weak surgical or traumatic wound allows the protrusion of a peritoneal sac. A swelling appears which gradually enlarges. The hernia may affect the whole wound or just one portion, frequently the lower end. The contents may become irreducible and episodic subacute intestinal obstruction, incarceration and strangulation may follow. The overlying skin may become thin, atrophic and ulcerated. Occasionally, spontaneous rupture may occur, caesarean and gynaecological wounds being particularly prone to this complication.

Incisional hernia complicates 6% of abdominal wounds at 5 years and 12% at 10 years. The incidence in males and females is approximately equal. Predisposing factors include:

- Postoperative haematoma and necrosis.
- Wound infection.
- Poor technique.
- The presence of drains and stomas in wounds.
- Age.
- Obesity.
- Diabetes, jaundice, renal failure, immunosuppression.
- Malignant disease.

Incisions particularly liable to hernia formation are lower midline, lateral muscle splitting incisions and sucostal incisions.

Incisional hernias may be left untreated where symptoms and deformity are minor, they may be controlled by the use of a corset or surgical belt or they may be repaired surgically. Prior to surgical repair, patients with large hernias may undergo induction of pneumoperitoneum to enlarge the peritoneal cavity, facilitating hernial reduction at operation without impairing respiratory function. Surgical repair may be performed using:

- Layer-to-layer anatomical repair where the defect is of moderate size with no tissue loss.
- The Keel repair (Maingot). The old scar is excised but the underlying peritoneum is left intact and reduced by invagination into the abdomen and sutured in this position. Successive layers of peritoneum and aponeurosis are further invaginated and sutured using non-absorbable material.
- Synthetic mesh. This technique is widely used and results in a lower recurrence rate than the older techniques described above. Recurrence rates using mesh are approximately 10–20% [b].

Paraumbilical and umbilical hernia

In adults the hernial defect occurs through the linea alba, usually just above the umbilicus, resulting from obesity or raised intra-abdominal pressure. They rarely occur before the age of 40. Males and females are affected equally. Untreated, they may reach very large dimensions with excoriation and ulceration of the overlying skin. Abdominal pain and a lump are the commonest symptoms. Intestinal obstruction and strangulation are common complications. Surgical repair using Mayo's technique should be undertaken although patients are frequently obese and in poor health.

Epigastric hernia

Epigastric hernias occur in the midline, through a small defect in the linea alba, usually halfway between the xiphoid process and the umbilicus. They usually comprise a pea-sized protrusion of fat which may draw a small peritoneal sac into the defect. They are frequently acutely painful, paricularly during exercise. Patients are often manual workers and 30% have co-existing upper abdominal complaints including gastric and duodenal ulcer.

Repair involves closure of the linea alba defect after reduction of the fat and/or sac.

Spigelian hernia

Spigelian hernias represent less than 1% of abdominal hernias. The male to female ratio is 1 : 1.5. They occur in the linea semilunaris on the lateral border of rectus abdominis. The sac usually lies intraparietally between internal and external oblique just medial to the iliac crest at the level of the arcuate line. Patients present with a painful, reducible lump. The diagnosis can be confirmed by ultrasound scanning. Repair is by excision of the sac and closure of the defect using a Mayo-type repair.

Obturator hernia

These are rare and the male to female ratio is 6 : 1. They are commoner in middle and old age and the incidence on the right side is twice that on the left. The peritoneal sac passes through the obturator canal into the thigh, lying deep to pectineus, and emerging in the femoral triangle between pectineus and adductor longus as it enlarges. Strangulation is frequently the initial presentation, and the diagnosis is usually made at laparotomy. The hernia may compress the geniculate branch of the obturator nerve causing pain in the medial aspect of the knee (Howship–Romberg sign). There is usually tenderness medial to the femoral vessels. Vaginal examination allows palpation of the hernia. CT scanning is helpful where the diagnosis is suspected but does not seem to affect the outcome.

Repair is performed via an abdominal incision. The obturator membrane is stretched or divided from within and the sac reduced. Closure of the canal is not usually required.

Lumbar hernia

Lumbar hernia may be primary (occurring usually through the inferior lumbar triangle of Petit, or less frequently through the superior lumbar triangle), or secondary following a renal operation, perinephric abscess or local muscular paralysis following poliomyelitis, spina bifida or a seat belt injury.

A primary hernia is easily repaired by direct suture of the defect or by using an extraperitoneal prosthetic mesh. Secondary incisional hernias usually require prosthetic mesh.

Gluteal and sciatic hernia

Both are very rare. A gluteal hernia passes through the greater sciatic notch, above or below piriformis. A sciatic hernia passes through the lesser sciatic notch. Intestinal obstruction is the usual presentation and the diagnosis is rarely made before laparotomy. Pain may be referred through the sciatic nerve. Repair is performed via an abdominal incision, reducing the hernia from within and closing the defect with sutures or prosthetic mesh.

Perineal hernia

An anterolateral perineal hernia occurs in multiparous women, occurring spontaneously or after childbirth or trauma. The hernia protrudes into the posterior vaginal wall or labium majus.

A posterolateral perineal hernia passes through levator ani into the ischiorectal fossa.

The commonest perineal hernia occurs postoperatively following vaginal hysterectomy or abdominoperineal excision of rectum. The other varieties are all rare.

Further reading

Devlin HB, Kingsnorth AN. The abdominal wall and hernias. In: *The New Aird's Companion in Surgical Studies (2nd edn)*. Edinburgh: Churchill Livingstone, 1998; 665–691.
Luiendijk RW, Hop WC, van den Tol MP *et al.* A comparison of suture repair with mesh repair for incisional hernia. *New England Journal of Medicine*, 2000; **343:** 392–398.

Related topics of interest

Femoral hernia (p. 125); Inguinal hernia (p. 179).

INGUINAL HERNIA

Nick Wilson

Epidemiology and aetiology

A hernia is a protrusion of an organ through an abnormal defect in its surrounding structures and in the abdomen, this invariably means the protrusion of a viscus through a muscle or fascial defect. Abdominal hernias comprise a defect, sac (peritoneum) and sac contents.

Inguinal hernias are the commonest type of groin hernia and are present in 2% of live born babies (4% of male babies), the incidence rising in premature and low-birth-weight babies. The development of inguinal hernia is commonest in the first 3 months of life and is caused by failure of the processus vaginalis to close. The neck of the hernia is at the internal inguinal ring, lateral to the inferior epigastric vessels, and such hernias are indirect by definition. All indirect hernias arise as a consequence of the failure of the processus vaginalis to close. Direct inguinal hernias (defect and neck of the hernial sac medial to the inferior epigastric vessels) virtually never occur in infants. The ratio of males to females affected is 9 : 1. A female infant developing an inguinal hernia may have the testicular feminization syndrome and chromosome studies should be performed to exclude this. At all ages inguinal hernias are commoner on the right than the left (5 : 4). Appoximately 60% of children with an inguinal hernia present with incarceration but this rarely progresses to strangulation, 95% resolving with sedation and elevation in gallows traction.

The incidence of inguinal hernia in adult males is 6–12% and one tenth this in adult females. In males, 60% are direct, 35% direct and 5% combined ('saddlebag' or 'pantaloon'). Inguinal hernia patients account for 6% of all general surgical admissions and currently occupy 5% of all general surgical beds. Approximately 80 000 inguinal hernia repairs are performed annually in England and Wales, 10% of these for recurrence.

Clinical features and differential diagnosis

Pain, a dragging sensation and swelling in the groin are the commonest symptoms. The onset of severe pain suggests strangulation. Examination of the patient lying supine may reveal a swelling in the inguinal canal, or, if the hernia has reduced, a defect at the internal ring. A cough impulse may be felt at the external ring. Invagination of the scrotal skin into the inguinal canal is painful and should be avoided. Control of the hernia by pressure applied directly over the internal ring suggests indirect herniation, although it is often difficult to differentiate. The patient should also be examined standing when the hernia is more likely to be apparent. The opposite groin should always be checked for undetected hernias and, in men, the testes should be examined for hydrocele or epididymal cyst, in particular.

Other conditions that may mimic inguinal hernia include:

- Femoral hernia.
- Saphena varix.
- Hydrocele of the cord or of the canal of Nuck.

- Lipoma of the cord.
- Ectopic testis.
- Inguinal lymph nodes.
- Psoas abscess.
- Ilofemoral aneurysm.

Complications

- Incarceration (irreducibility).
- Intestinal obstruction.
- Strangulation.
- Reductio en masse.
- Testicular oedema, ischaemia or infarction.
- Maydl's hernia.
- Richter's hernia.
- Littre's hernia.
- Sliding hernia.
- Herniation of overies/uterus.

The annual probability of strangulation in an inguinal hernia is 0.3–3.0% with the risk weighted towards the first 3 months after the hernia is first noticed. Indirect hernias are 10 times more likely to undergo strangulation than direct hernias. The mortality of strangulated inguinal hernia in adults is 7–14%.

Management

Indirect and symptomatic direct inguinal hernias should be repaired to relieve symptoms and to eliminate the small long-term risk of strangulation. Easily reducible direct inguinal hernias which are not at significant risk of strangulation need not necessarily be repaired, especially in the elderly. Such patients should be reviewed within 1 year. Irreducible inguinal hernias and those presenting with a history of less than 4 weeks should be repaired promptly to avoid strangulation.

The most widespread technique used currently is the tension-free Lichtenstein repair where a prosthetic mesh is sutured over the posterior inguinal wall. Recurrence rates are 2–4% and the technique is easy to learn. The plug-and-patch technique involves inserting a polypropylene plug shaped like a shuttlecock into the hernial defect with an overlying loose patch. This is marginally quicker to perform and allows a quicker recovery than the standard Lichtenstein repair but is more expensive. Multiple or complex recurrent defects are repaired using a prosthetic mesh introduced preperitoneally. The use of local anaesthesia for the repair of inguinal hernias is safer in high-risk patients and allows prolonged analgesia with consequent early mobilization and reduced risk of urinary retention. Deep vein thrombosis and pulmonary embolism rates are reduced and recurrence rates are not affected. In appropriate patients, day case hernia repair is desirable and the majority of uncomplicated inguinal hernias should now be treated this way.

Laparoscopic repair has been assessed in various trials and the transabdominal preperitoneal (TAPP) hernia repair is the most widely used technique[b]. Recurrence rates are low at around 2%[b]. Patients recover more quickly than following open repair, but the potential for serious complications is greater and the technique is more expensive[b]. A general anaesthetic is necessary. The National Institute for Clinical Excellence (NICE) has recommended that laparoscopic repair be used only for recurrent and bilateral hernias.

Further reading

Chung RS, Rowland DY. Meta-analysis of randomized controlled trials of laparoscopic vs conventional inguinal hernia repairs. *Surgery Endoscopy*, 1999; **13:** 689–694.

Devlin HB. *Management of Abdominal Hernias.* London, Butterworth, 1988.

The MRC Laparoscopic Groin Hernia Trial Group. Laparoscopic versus open repair of groin hernia: a randomised comparison. *Lancet*, 1999; **354:** 185–190.

Related topics of interest

Femoral hernia (p. 125); Incisional and other abdominal hernias (p. 176).

INTENSIVE CARE

Nick Lagattolla

Vital functions are monitored in the intensive care unit (ICU) to assess progress, identify impending organ failure and, as a consequence, to sustain organ function. The main systems monitored are the cardiac, pulmonary, renal and cerebral. Arterial and venous blood tests are performed regularly and the results are charted to demonstrate trends. Renal, pulmonary and cardiac organ support is readily delivered as necessary.

Indications

The indications are many and varied, and the local criteria for ICU admission do vary; however, on many ICUs where surgical patients are dealt with, indications will typically include:

- existing single or multiple organ failure.
- need for intensive monitoring for impending organ failure.
- systemic sepsis.
- post-operative care for major surgery.
- requirement for ventilatory support.
- major head injury.
- severe chest injury.
- multiple trauma.

Some specific conditions requiring ICU (not elsewhere discussed) merit further consideration:

Endotoxic shock and the sepsis syndrome

Generalized infection with Gram-negative bacilli may result in endotoxic shock. The bacterial walls of these organisms consist of lipopolysaccharide endotoxin, which is a potent stimulus to the humeral and cellular inflammatory response. There is an early rise in circulating levels of inflammatory cytokines, such as tumour necrosis factor-α and interleukin-1β and these initiate a cascade of events that ultimately comprise septic shock. This may be clinically diagnosed by the association of hypotension with peripheral vasodilatation (warm peripheries), which is readily distinguished from cardiogenic or haemorrhagic shock, which result in peripheral vasoconstriction ('cold and clammy' peripheries). Multi-organ failure may supervene. Endotoxaemia most commonly complicates biliary, urological or gastro-intestinal tract-related infections, as these are most likely to be due to Gram-negative bacilli. Prompt diagnosis, correction of the relative hypovolaemia, and treatment with high-dose broad-spectrum antibiotics active against the Gram-negative organisms may be life-saving.

Adult respiratory distress syndrome (ARDS)

This is one of the commonest clinical problems in the ICU. It occurs in response to a major physiological insult like sepsis, burns or trauma and is initiated by inflammatory mediators. In this condition, the pulmonary microcirculation becomes over-permeable and the lungs become oedematous and rigid requiring high inflation pressures to maintain adequate ventilation. This results in hypoxia, increased shunting and patchy atelectasis. Specific pulmonary support consists of mechanical ventilation with positive end expiratory pressure (PEEP). This prevents atelectasis and improves oxygenation by limiting the areas of ventilation/perfusion mismatch. When hypoxia has continued, in spite of PEEP, other methods of ventilation have been helpful, such as continuous positive airways pressure ventilation (CPAP), high-frequency jet ventilation and reversing the inspiratory-to-expiratory ratio, although these have not been shown to be superior to conventional techniques. Extracorporeal membrane oxygenation (ECMO) is a new technique which may improve survival in patients with ARDS. PGE_1 is a potent vasodilator of the pulmonary microcirculation. It has been given experimentally and clinically to improve pulmonary function by increasing arterial oxygenation. Fibreoptic bronchoscopy with lavage is effective at removing obstructing plugs of mucus.

Necrotizing fasciitis

Severe subcutaneous infections may lead to thrombosis of the vessels leading to the overlying skin, and cutaneous gangrene supervenes. This is necrotizing fasciitis, and tends to complicate cellulitis caused by group A streptococci or a mixed group of anaerobic and aerobic organisms, in which case it is called Meleney's synergistic gangrene. If this occurs in the perineum, it is termed Fournier's gangrene. The presence of devitalized tissue promotes infection by anaerobic organisms. Multiple organ failure occurs rapidly in these severe initially localized infections, particularly renal failure, and the infection rapidly becomes systemic. The treatment is wide surgical debridement of infected and devitalized tissues, and intensive care for organ support, monitoring and antibiotics.

Organ support and monitoring

Cardiovascular

In the hypermetabolic state requirement for IC, tissue oxygen demand is greater than normal. Areas of tissue underperfusion occur with consequent patchy necrosis and eventual organ failure. Oxygen delivery can be maintained by maximizing cardiac output and oxygen saturation, and maintaining haemoglobin at 10–11 g/100 ml. Cardiac output can be increased by ensuring enough fluids are given to maintain the preload, with inotropic agents to maintain blood pressure and systemic vascular resistance. Oxygen saturation should be maintained over 90% with a PaO_2 greater than 60 mmHg. Optimal values in a high-risk patient are a cardiac index of 4.5 l/min/m², oxygen delivery of 600 ml/min/m² and oxygen consumption of 170 ml/min/m². Oxygen demand is reduced by assisting ventilation, preventing excessive feeding and treating elevations in temperature with rectal paracetamol and tepid sponging.

The ECG and CVP are continually monitored. The CVP directly reflects the cardiac preload. Left ventricular function is reflected by systemic arterial pressure, pulmonary artery wedge and occlusion pressures, and cardiac output. Left atrial filling pressure is a better indicator of cardiac function than right heart filling pressure, but this cannot be measured directly. Swann–Ganz catheters measure the pulmonary artery wedge and occlusion pressures (left atrial pressure), and an assessment of left ventricular preload can be made. Cardiac output may be measured using intracardiac temperature-sensitive catheters.

Renal

Urine output via urinary catheter is measured continually and expressed in millilitres output per hour. Normal hourly urine output ranges widely, but levels lower than 30 ml/hour are suggestive of renal underperfusion. If this is allowed to continue, acute tubular necrosis and renal failure may ensue. This is characterized by a period of anuria, which may last up to 24 hours, followed by oliguria as the kidneys regain their function. This is common in the surgical patient with haemorrhagic or septic shock. If urine output drops, prerenal failure is best prevented by first ensuring adequate volume replacement (maintaining the right-sided cardiac pressures) and, if necessary, selectively vasodilating the renal vessels, thus maintaining renal perfusion with low-dose intravenous dopamine at 2–5 µg/kg/min. Nephrotoxic agents are stopped.

Established renal failure is treated with conventional haemodialysis or, more recently, extracorporeal continuous arteriovenous haemofiltration (CAVHF) or continuous arteriovenous haemodialysis (CAVHD). These are not associated with the same cardiovascular instability as traditional dialysis. Renal support is continued until the patient's renal function is seen to improve.

Respiratory

Surgical patients from theatre may be electively ventilated to avoid respiratory depression and pulmonary atelectasis from heavy analgesia, and to ensure optimal tissue oxygenation. Elective postoperative ventilation requires infused sedatives and full ventilatory support through an endotracheal tube. Those requiring prolonged ventilation have a tracheostomy to prevent prolonged endotracheal trauma, and aid suction of the tracheobronchial tree. Patients being weaned off the ventilator may need selective intermittent mandatory ventilation (SIMV), which demands respirations from the patient at intervals. Patients with pulmonary atelectasis or infection, both common in the surgical setting, may need extra ventilatory pressure to ventilate collapsed alveoli and this is achieved in the non-sedated patient using continuous positive pressure ventilation through a face mask, or intermittent positive pressure ventilation (IPPV), if the patient is intubated.

All patients with respiratory difficulties need regular arterial blood gas analysis. An arterial line facilitates collection of arterial blood. The many parameters measured indicate pulmonary and metabolic function. Poor PaO_2 despite a high percentage FiO_2 is indicative of parenchymal pulmonary disease, commonly ARDS, gross pulmonary collapse or consolidation. A base excess reducing progressively from −2.0 indicates a metabolic acidosis.

Cerebrovascular

Head-injured patients may have traumatic cerebral oedema or diffuse brain injury, and no evidence of a surgically correctable abnormality. These need the ICU for ventilation to avoid hypercapnia and reduce cerebral vasospasm, and maintain cerebral perfusion to counter increased intracranial pressure (ICP). Increasing the ICP reduces the cerebral perfusion pressure (CPP), and this is best monitored by the insertion of an extradural pressure bolt through which the ICP may be transduced. Continuous electroencephalography may be used to monitor cerebral activity.

Hepatoenteric

The gut-mucosal barrier is appreciated by many as being contributory to the MOF syndrome by allowing the release of bacteria and endotoxin into the portal circulation. Once these have passed the hepatic reticuloendothelial system, generalized release into the systemic circulation occurs. Inflammatory mediators circulate and act on the gut to produce an ileus and leaking capillaries, which further encourage endotoxin and bacterial translocation, and so on. This cycle of events can be prevented by maintaining enterocyte mass, reducing the upper gastrointestinal microflora and maintaining the normal commensal lower intestinal microflora. Early enteral feeding with the addition of glutamine, the major respiratory fuel of intestinal enterocytes, provides intraluminal bulk and maintains enterocyte mass. The addition of specific nutrients and growth factors to encourage enterocyte proliferation further is still at an experimental stage. Gastrointestinal ileus is not a contraindication to enteral feeding since the stomach can be aspirated hourly before each feeding session. Coagulation factor deficiencies are corrected with vitamin K and FFP. Plasma oncotic pressure may be maintained with 20% albumen or hydroxyethylstarch (HESPAN) infusions.

Peptic ulcer prophylaxis

H_2 receptor antagonists and antacids, frequently used in the ICU, are administered to prevent stress-induced ulceration and bleeding. They also neutralize gastric pH, encourage upper gastrointestinal colonization and increase the incidence of nosocomial pneumonias in ventilated patients. Recent evidence suggests that stress ulcer prophylaxis is best achieved with sucralfate, which coats the gastric mucosa but does not affect its pH. In the same way, early enteral feeding may abolish the need for stress ulcer prophylaxis. Hypopharangeally delivered non-absorbable antibiotics are an alternative way to reduce the incidence of nosocomial pneumonias.

Cutaneous support

Maintenance of skin care is of prime importance if the patient is immobile and ventilated. Prolonged sacral pressure, malnutrition and urinary soiling will inevitably lead to an infected necrotic pressure sore which places a considerable physiological stress on a sick patient. Regular turning, catheterization, adequate protein nutrition and nursing vigilance are minimum requirements in prevention.

Further reading

McCrirrick AB, Nevin M. Intensive care monitoring of the surgical patient. *Current Practice in Surgery*, 1994; **6:** 202–206.

McCrory DC, Rowlands BJ. Septic shock syndrome and multiple system organ failure. *Current Practice in Surgery*, 1993; **5:** 211–215.

Molloy RG, Mannick JA, Rodrick ML. Cytokines, sepsis and immunomodulation. *British Journal of Surgery*, 1993; **80:** 289–297.

Singer M (Ed). ABC of intensive care. *British Medical Journal.*

Stott S. Recent advances in intensive care. *British Medical Journal*, 2000; **320:** 38–361.

Related topics of interest

Assessment of the acute abdomen (p. 41); Burns (p. 62); Head injury (p. 158); Multiple organ failure (p. 227); Nutrition in the surgical patient (p. 233); Trauma management (p. 328).

INTERMITTENT CLAUDICATION

Nick Wilson

This term is derived from the Latin *claudicatio* ('I limp') and refers to pain arising due to inadequate arterial blood flow in exercising muscle which is relieved by rest. Intermittent claudication occurs most commonly in the legs, but can also occur in the arms.

Pathology

Atherosclerosis is the cause in the great majority of patients and the common sites affected include the origin of the common iliac arteries, the superficial femoral arteries, particularly at the adductor hiatus, and the popliteal artery. The principal risk factors are cigarette smoking, hypertension, diabetes, hypercholesterolaemia, and family history. Other causes (trauma, popliteal entrapment syndrome, compartment syndrome) should be considered particularly in younger patients.

Pathophysiology

Patients with intermittent claudication have near normal limb blood flow at rest, but cannot increase blood flow adequately during exercise. According to Poiseuille's Law, flow is proportional to the fourth power of the radius of the tube and thus, increasing degrees of stenosis lead to an exponential decline in flow. Multiple stenoses are effectively resistances in series and have an additive effect.

Natural history

Claudication affects 1.5% of patients under the age of 60 years, 3.7% of patients 60–70 years and 52% of those over 70 years. Claudication remains static in many patients, approximately 20% deteriorating over a 5-year period. Arterial reconstruction for critical ischaemia is required in 5–10% over a similar period and a similar proportion will progress to amputation (this rises to 30% in patients over 75 years). The overall mortality of these patients is higher than that of an age-matched normal population, 5 and 10 year survival being 75% and 40% respectively[c]. The excess mortality is mainly attributable to myocardial infarction and stroke.

Clinical features

1. Symptoms. Patients complain of pain in single or multiple muscle groups which occurs on walking and resolves at rest. Pain occurs at a predictable walking distance which decreases on an incline or in cold weather. Pain usually begins in the calf if there is superficial femoral/popliteal artery involvement, but extends to the thighs and buttocks if there is iliac artery involvement.

2. Signs. Examination may reveal absent or weak pulses and possibly a bruit over the stenotic segment. There may be accompanying manifestations of hypertension, diabetes, hyperlipidaemia, cardiac and neurovascular disease. The differential diagnosis includes venous claudication, degenerative hip disease, lumbosacral disc protrusion and lumbar spinal stenosis.

Investigation

1. *Hand-held continuous wave Doppler.* Ankle:brachial Doppler index is the simplest non-invasive measurement and ratios of 0.4–0.8 are typical in claudicants. The measurement of Doppler indices before and after exercising on a treadmill together with symptomatic correlation is also helpful and will reveal more subtle changes than resting examination alone.

2. *Duplex ultrasound.* This is the standard investigation for defining the anatomy of arterial disease and for selecting patients who may be suitable for angioplasty. Some surgeons will undertake bypass surgery guided only by ultrasound findings. Ideally, duplex ultrasound should be available in the vascular clinic so that patients can be seen and imaged in a 'one stop' setting.

3. *Arteriography.* Arteriography is used mainly to guide the placement of angioplasty catheters/balloons. Diagnostic arteriography has largely been replaced by ultrasound, but where detailed anatomical information is required arteriography is still necessary. Conventional and digital subtraction angiography are used by most radiologists.

4. *Risk factor management.* Assessment of coexisting cardiac and coronary disease is necessary in some patients and polycythaemia, thrombocythaemia, diabetes, hypertension, hyperlipidaemia and bronchial carcinoma should be sought.

Treatment

Many patients whose mild claudication remains stable require only an explanation of the problem and reassurance. All patients should be strongly advised to stop smoking and coexisting conditions (diabetes, hypertension, etc.) should be treated. Obese patients should be advised to lose weight. Beta-blockers should be avoided where possible, particularly in conjunction with calcium antagonists. Oxypentiphylline is reputed to enhance red cell deformability and reduce platelet aggregation, but trials have failed to demonstrate more than mild subjective improvement in some patients.

1. *Exercise programme.* Supervised exercise programmes have been demonstrated to improve walking distance in stable claudicants and are the first line of treatment in the great majority of patients. The results are equal to those of angioplasty in the long term, but the exercise programme must be maintained[c]. The benefits seem greatest for patients with superficial femoral artery disease, predominantly.

2. *Angioplasty.* This has most to offer patients whose symptoms are caused by iliac artery occlusion or stenosis. The role of stent placement is not yet fully defined but most interventionalists reserve this for patients undergoing angioplasty for restenosis. In the superficial femoral artery angioplasty achieves relief of symptoms in only 50% of patients at 1 year[c]. Transluminal and subintimal techniques are used, the latter being more suitable for long occlusions. Laser assisted angioplasty and atherectomy have proved disappointing and cannot be recommended for routine use.

3. *Bypass surgery.* Most surgeons are reluctant to offer bypass surgery to claudicants in view of the relatively benign natural history of claudication and the effectiveness of less invasive treatments. In low-risk patients with iliac or isolated superficial femoral artery disease and good run off whose claudication is disabling, bypass surgery may be appropriate.

Aortofemoral grafting can be performed with 2–3% mortality, low morbidity and 5-year patency rates greater than 90%. Femoropoliteal bypass carries a low mortality (1%) and 5-year patency rates of 75% where vein is used for the conduit or 55% where polytetraflouroethylene (ePTFE) is used. Several series report similar patency rates for vein and ePTFE in the above knee position. Femorotibial bypass is rarely indicated for claudication alone. Extranatomic grafting (femoro-femoral, axillo-femoral, axillobifemoral) may occasionaly be used where there is a good donor vessel and contraindications to anatomic bypass.

Lumbar sympathectomy does not improve muscle blood flow and is of no benefit in most patients with intermittent claudication.

Further reading

Golledge J, Ferguson K, Ellis M, Sabharwal T *et al.* Outcome of femoropopliteal angioplasty. *Annals of Surgery*, 1999; **229:** 146–153.
Walker RD, Nawaz S, Wilkinson CH, Saxton JM, Pockley AG, Wood RI. Influence of upper- and lower-limb training on cardiovascular function and walking distances in patients with intermittent claudication. *Journal of Vascular Surgery*, 2000; **31:** 662–669.

Related topics of interest

Amputations (p. 21); Aneurysms (p. 24); Cerebrovascular disease (p. 76); Critical leg ischaemia (p. 100); Renovascular surgery (p. 284); Vascular imaging and intervention (p. 350); Vascular trauma (p. 357); Vasomotor and vasculitic conditions (p. 360).

INTESTINAL OBSTRUCTION

Deya Marzouk, Christopher Lattimer

Intestinal obstruction accounts for approximately 5% of all acute surgical admissions. Small bowel obstruction accounts for about 85% of these, with large bowel obstruction accounting for the rest.

Pathophysiology

The intestine gradually distends and fails to reabsorb the normal gastrointestinal secretions (7–8 litres per day) and swallowed air. This causes a net fluid deficit of several litres and leads to dehydration, shock and anuria. Enteric bacteria proliferate in the presence of stagnant fluid, with increasing translocation of bacteria and toxins through the bowel wall. Strangulated loops of bowel become progressively distended with fluid, which along with venous obstruction result in oedema of the bowel wall and bleeding. The swelling eventually stops arterial circulation and results in bowel infarction.

Aetiology

1. Luminal. Meconium, gallstones, foreign bodies, Ascaris worms, faecal impaction and bezoars.

2. Mural. Congenital intestinal atresia, imperforate anus, Meckel's diverticulum, tumours, intussusception, inflammatory bowel disease, ischaemic and radiation strictures, intramural haematomas in patients on anticoagulants.

3. Extrinsic. Congenital bands, acquired adhesions and bands, external and internal hernias, volvulus, inflammatory mass, extrinsic tumours, annular pancreas.

Classification

- Acute or chronic.
- Small intestinal, or colonic or gastric outlet.
- Mechanical, adynamic ileus or colonic pseudo-obstruction.
- Partial or complete.
- Closed loop (intestine is obstructed at two points e.g. distal colonic obstruction with competent ileocaecal valve, volvulus and incarcerated hernias) or open loop.
- Simple (occlusion of intestinal lumen without compromise of blood supply) or strangulated (with compromise of blood supply, e.g. in incarcerated hernias, intussusception, volvulus etc.).

The type of obstruction dictates the choice and urgency of initial treatment (surgical versus conservative). An attempt should be made to diagnose the cause of obstruction preoperatively since the cause (when obvious) can also suggest the type of obstruction, e.g. in cases of volvulus.

Clinical picture

The four cardinal features (colicky abdominal pain, vomiting, absolute constipation and abdominal distension) vary according to the level of obstruction.

1.   In high small bowel obstruction   central colicky abdominal pain is followed by frequent vomiting of copious amounts of bile-stained small bowel contents and rapid dehydration. Distension is minimal or absent (frequent vomiting effectively decompresses bowel).

2.   In low small bowel obstruction   central colicky abdominal pain is followed by vomiting after an interval which varies with the level of obstruction. Vomiting is less frequent and less copious than in high small bowel obstruction and usually becomes faeculent. Abdominal distension is a prominent feature.

3.   In large bowel obstruction   marked abdominal distension is seen. Vomiting occurs late and is faeculent. There may be a history of recent change in bowel habits. Colonic obstruction usually presents more gradually than small bowel obstruction except in volvulus and in closed loop obstruction secondary to competent ileocaecal valve, when the caecum is at risk of rupture.

Patients may not exhibit this classic picture. The patient may evacuate the rectum distal to an obstruction, may pass flatus in partial obstruction or may even have diarrhoea. Colicky abdominal pain followed by bouts of explosive diarrhoea also may be a symptom of partial obstruction. Pain, which becomes diffuse, poorly localized or constant and severe, usually indicates the presence of strangulation.

Physical examination early may reveal little. All hernial orifices should be examined carefully for any evidence of incarcerated hernias especially in elderly patients (where occasionally one would find an incarcerated, hardly tender femoral hernia). Auscultation during colic may reveal loud high pitched or metallic intestinal sounds. A succussion splash may be heard in gastric outlet obstruction and occasionally with dilated bowel loops. Visible peristalsis may be seen in thin patients. In the presence of strangulation, intestinal sounds may become quiet, frequently with evidence of localized tenderness or generalized peritonitis. In late cases fever, tachycardia and distension and decreased urine output. Neglected patients may go into renal failure.

Laboratory investigations

In early stages of bowel obstruction, blood tests may be normal, later haemoconcentration, leucocytosis and electrolyte abnormalities occur. Raised white cell count above 20 000 suggests bowel ischaemia. Biochemistry may suggest dehydration or established renal failure in neglected patients. It is prudent to measure arterial blood gases in ill patients. These may show evidence of metabolic acidosis in patients with bowel ischaemia and sepsis.

Radiological diagnosis

Plain abdominal X-rays are very useful in diagnosing the presence of acute intestinal obstruction (dilated gas filled loops of bowel, air–fluid levels) as well as the level of obstruction (pattern and distribution of gaseous distension in bowel). The small bowel is recognized by its valvulae conniventes, while the colon is recognized by its haustral folds. Plain abdominal X-rays may also provide clues to the possible aetiology (e.g. volvulus), complications (e.g. gas under the diaphragm) or potential for complications (dangerously distended caecum more than 10 cm indicating imminent rupture of the caecum). Serial abdominal films are important in conservatively managed patients to assess progress.

Erect chest X-rays may detect free gas under the diaphragm indicating intestinal perforation, show pre-existing chest condition and any possible aspiration (from vomiting).

Emergency (instant) limited barium enema on an unprepared colon distinguishes organic obstruction from pseudo-obstruction. This may be performed using dilute barium or water-soluble contrast (e.g. gastrograffin), the latter is mandatory if there is any suspicion of perforation (possible perforated/perforating cancer or diverticulitis) or gangrenous bowel (possible sigmoid volvulus with abdominal tenderness), as barium will cause severe (usually fatal) peritonitis.

Initial treatment

Patients with intestinal obstruction may look deceptively well early in their obstruction, but many are extremely ill and require prompt resuscitation, frequent or continuous monitoring of their vital as well as abdominal signs. Frequent clinical examination is essential. Initial treatment consists of:

1. Fluid and electrolyte resuscitation, which should take into account the large volume deficit and third space losses and is guided by clinical signs of dehydration, tachycardia and urine output. All anticipated losses should be replaced with normal saline or similar isotonic solutions. Normal daily fluid requirement is given on top of the expected deficit. Patients need a urinary catheter and may need a central venous line to monitor fluid balance.
2. Nasogastric tubes should be aspirated regularly and allowed to drain freely.
3. Broad-spectrum antibiotic prophylaxis (against both aerobic and anaerobic bacteria).
4. Transfer to HDU or ICU may be needed in high-risk patients for optimization before surgery.

Conservative management is usually indicated in pseudo-obstruction, recurrent adhesive obstruction and obstruction secondary to radiation enteritis. Other patients usually need surgery.

Presence of localized tenderness, tachycardia, fever and metabolic acidosis favours (but by no means confirms) strangulation. If there is any doubt about the possibility of strangulating/closed loop obstruction, it is better to operate as soon as the patient is adequately resuscitated. Emergency surgery is necessary in suspected strangulation, closed loop obstruction and volvulus.

Principles of surgical treatment

At surgery if the caecum is distended then the obstruction lies in the colon. If the caecum looks like it is about to perforate, then it must be decompressed first using needle (attached to suction tubing) to decompress the air inside. The rectum is then palpated and traced proximally to the site of the obstruction in the colon. If the caecum is not distended then the obstruction lies in small bowel. The dilated small bowel is followed proximally to the point of obstruction.

The operation may involve division of adhesions, reduction of incarcerated hernia, resection or bypass of diseased bowel, enterotomy and removal of intraluminal obstruction, e.g. gallstone ileus or formation of a proximal stoma.

Intestinal decompression may be done, either by milking the intestinal contents back to the stomach and asking the anaesthetist to suck out stomach contents (the preferred method when the intestinal lumen has not been entered) or with a savage decompressor (if intestinal lumen is entered). The site of savage decompression is best included in the resected intestine when intestinal resection is done otherwise it is closed in one or two layers.

Small bowel obstruction

Adhesive obstruction

This is the commonest cause of small bowel obstruction. Most are secondary to previous abdominal surgery, especially colonic (including appendicectomy) and gynaecological operations. It may also follow previous abdominal inflammatory processes. It may occur weeks or many years following the initial operation. Repeated episodes occur in 10–30% of patients[c].

The mere presence of an abdoimnal scar does not exclude other causes of obstruction and more importantly does not guarantee that the obstruction is a simple one, since strangulation may occur if bands cause closed loop obstruction, an internal herniation or a volvulus.

Treatment is either surgical (division of adhesions or adhesiolysis) or conservative (nasogastric suction and i.v. fluids). Surgery is preferred except in patients with recurrent typical previous similar episodes, who underwent laparotomy for adhesions before and those patients with partial obstruction who settle quickly on conservative management.

Laparotomy for adhesions can be difficult and needs patience. The old scar is opened (unless it was a transverse incision) and the peritoneum is entered with care. Adhesions should be divided sharply and all small bowel is freed from D–J flexure to ileocaecal valve, as one is not always sure which adhesion is really the cause (or the only cause) of obstruction. Division of all adhesions may be less desirable if it appears that obstruction is caused by another mechanism (e.g. a tumour or an internal herniation) since they have a tendency to reform again. Following adhesiolysis and checking abdominal viscera for other pathology, the small bowel is replaced in anatomical position without twists. Recurrent adhesive obstruction may be treated by adhesiolysis and intraluminal stenting with a Baker tube left in situ for 3 weeks.

Obstruction secondary to incarcerated hernia

Incarcerated femoral, inguinal, paraumbilical, Spigelian or incisional hernias may be missed, unless all hernial orifices are examined carefully. Occasionally obstruction can be colonic in case of incarcerated sliding hernias. Very rarely obturator and gluteal hernias may present with obstruction and are only diagnosed intraoperatively.

Treatment is surgical by reduction (with resection anastomosis for non-viable intestine) and appropriate repair of the hernial defect. In cases of incarcerated incisional hernia, it is advisable to open the peritoneum and check for intraperitoneal adhesions and bands as the real cause of symptoms, as occasionally the patient is symptomatic from intraabdominal adhesions or bands rather than the hernia.

Obstruction secondary to internal herniation

They are rare and may occur near the D–J flexure (superior and inferior duodenal fossae, right and left duodenojejunal fossae), ileocaecal junction (superior and inferior ileocaecal fossae, retrocaecal fossa), foramen of Winslow, holes in the mesentry or omentum (congenital or from previous surgery) or lateral to stomas or through defects in pelvic floor following abdominoperineal resection of the rectum.

The diagnosis is usually made intraoperatively. Diagnosis may be suggested preoperatively by presence of a ball-shaped mass of small bowel loops on plain abdominal films (this may correspond to a localized spherical tender abdominal mass).

Treatment is by an operation. The first step is to identify the anatomical relations at the neck of the sac, which may contain vital structures, which should not be divided. In most cases the hernia can be reduced by gentle traction. Division of the neck of the sac must not be done in cases of hernias to the foramen of Winslow (portal triad) and in right duodenojejunal fossa hernias (superior mesenteric artery).

Early postoperative obstruction (within 1 month)

In most cases this is secondary to fibrinous adhesions[b] and resolves on conservative management. Prolonged adynamic ileus is another important cause and again responds to conservative treatment and correction of any underlying cause (e.g. electrolyte disturbance or sepsis). Should conservative management fail to lead to resolution after several days, then serious consideration must be given to re-exploration. It is important not to miss leakage or postoperative infected collections (interloop, pelvic or subphrenic abscess) as the real cause in these situations. The third possibility is mechanical bowel obstruction. This should be suspected in the presence of high-pitched bowel sounds and plain X-ray evidence of proximal dilatation of small bowel (occasionally seen in CT scans ordered to exclude postoperative collections which may show dilated as well as collapsed loops of bowel). The last possibility is especially suspected when the nature of the previous operation suggests the possibility of internal herniation, e.g. hernia in the space lateral to an abdominal stoma, prolapse of small bowel through pelvic floor after abdominoperineal resection of the rectum.

Gallstone ileus

This usually occur in elderly ladies. Intermittent episodes of colicky abdominal pain eventually culminate in acute intestinal obstruction.

Characteristically there is air delineating the biliary tree. The stone obstructing the ileum may or may not be seen in the right iliac fossa.

Treatment is by an enterotomy, proximal to the site of obstruction. It is imperative to examine the whole of the duodenum and small bowel (there may be more than one stone in the intestine). Recurrent gallstone ileus occurs in 5–10% of patients, half within a month (stones missed in the first operation).

Rarely pressure necrosis in the obstructed part of intestine may need resection anastomosis. The choledochoduodenal fistula is best undisturbed.

Radiation enteritis

Radiation damage to the small bowel may present months or more commonly years after pelvic radiotherapy. This results in progressive fibrosis of intestinal wall with narrowing, strictures, dense adhesions and impaired intestinal motility. Irradiated bowel is usually thick, fibrotic, friable and bound by thick adhesions. The serosa is usually greyish white, lustreless and avascular. Scattered telangiectatic serosal lesions are characteristic. The mesentery is often thickened and contracted.

Patients usually present with partial small bowel obstruction. Initial treatment is conservative. If obstruction does not settle then surgery is indicated. Surgery is hazardous with a higher risk of postoperative leakage. Resection if feasible should be wide as radiation changes are always more extensive than macroscopic appearance, with intestine brought from outside the field of irradiation for at least one end of the anastomosis. Bypass is the only option if resection would result in loss of most of the distal small bowel or if intestines are densely adherent to vital structures.

Small bowel obstruction secondary to Crohn's disease

These patients may present with a long history of intestinal colics, vomiting and weight loss. Initial treatment is conservative. Steroids may help by controlling the inflammation, reducing the oedema and re-establishing a working lumen. Surgery is needed if conservative treatment and steroids fail or in the presence of septic complications such as an interloop abscess. It is important not to continue with unsuccessful conservative management over long periods while the patient loses weight and become nutritionally worse.

A combination of limited intestinal resection and stricureplasty is usually required. Stricureplasties should be limited to areas of short fibrotic strictures (use in areas with apparent active disease can be complicated by postoperative leakage).

Anticoagulant-induced intestinal obstruction

Spontaneous small intestinal intramural haematoma may occur in patients on warfarin therapy. It frequently affects the proximal jejunum and most resolve spontaneously within 2–3 days. The diagnosis is suggested by INR value beyond the therapeutic range and the presence of bleeding elsewhere such as ecchymoses and haematuria. A small bowel enema shows a narrowed segment with a characteristic picket fence appearance. Treatment is conservative, stopping warfarin and occasionally vitamin K. If patient is explored because the diagnosis was not considered preoperatively or because of concern about the cause of the obstruction, the haematoma is best left alone as it usually resolves spontaneously.

Intussusception

These patients present with intermittent symptoms before an acute obstruction. They may have a mobile abdominal mass which may appear and disappear from time to time and may have the characteristic mucocutaneous pigmentations of Peutz-Jeghers syndrome. Five per cent of intussusception occurs in adults. This affects both small and large bowel with equal frequency and in 90% they are secondary to malignant or benign lesions. Malignancy is commoner in colonic intussusceptions in adults and thus the treatment of choice is by resection, not reduction. Partial reduction may need to be done if the intussusception involves a large part of the distal small bowel. Peutz-Jeghers syndrome causes many of the intussusceptions seen in the small bowel and these can be treated by reduction, with open polypectomy of the larger polyps.

Large bowel obstruction

Large bowel cancer accounts for up to 80–90% of cases of large bowel obstruction; most occur at or distal to the splenic flexure. Other causes include diverticular stricture, diverticulitis involving small bowel, volvulus and other rare causes (incarcerated sliding hernia, radiation or ischaemic strictures).

Colonic and rectal malignancies

Treatment depends on the condition of the patient, condition of the bowel to be used in anastomosis and the skill of the surgeon. Shock, circulatory instability of the patient and peritonitis may dictate a staged procedure, e.g. Hartmann's procedure. Likewise a staged procedure may be indicated if there is potential tension of the anastomosis or surgeon's inexperience.

Obstructing right-sided lesions (proximal to the splenic flexure) are treated by resection with primary anastomosis. Unresectable tumours should be treated by internal bypass or a proximal stoma.

Obstructing left-sided lesions, including high rectal cancers, are treated by resection with primary anastomosis, with or without on-table antegrade colonic lavage, with or without a covering stoma. Alternatively a Hartmann's procedure or a subtotal colectomy with ileorectal anastomosis may be performed. If left-sided obstructing lesions present with caecal perforation this usually mandates a subtotal colectomy, unless it is not deemed safe for primary anastomosis, in which case resection is carried out with the formation of a terminal ileostomy and a mucous fistula.

Obstructing low rectal cancers may be treated most appropriately by diverting colostomy. This allows time for preoperative radiotherapy as these lesions are usually locally advanced and also allows for a primary resection and anastomosis. Alternatively it may be possible to re-establish a lumen by means of laser to allow time before elective definitive treatment.

Sigmoid volvulus

Sigmoid volvulus is predisposed to by the presence of a long, narrow mesocolon and chronic constipation. Radiological appearance is characteristic. Plain abdominal X-ray is diagnostic in 70–80% of patients, showing a massively dilated kidney-shaped single loop of bowel arising from the pelvis with its concavity towards the left iliac fossa. Instant barium enema may show a characteristic tapered spiral twist (bird's beak) in cases when plain radiography is inconclusive. It may also reduce the volvulus.

Treatment initially should involve deflation using a rigid sigmoidoscope and the passage of a flatus tube. This succeeds in up to 90% of the patients. The flatus tube should be left in situ for at least 48 hours, otherwise early recurrence is common. An elective sigmoid colectomy is advisable before the patient is discharged home.

If sigmoidoscopic deflation fails or if there are signs of bowel infarction, perforation or peritonitis, then emergency sigmoid colectomy with or without anastomosis (double-barrel colostomy) is the only option.

Endoscopic sigmoidoplexy using a combined colonoscopy and percutaneous insertion of 'colostomy' tubes to fix the sigmoid to the lateral abdominal wall has been successful in unfit patients. These may be changed to flatus tubes, which are left in situ indefinitely to prevent recurrence.

Caecal volvulus

Plain abdominal X-ray may show a large kidney- or comma-shaped gas-filled loop of bowel with its concavity towards the left hypochondrium. The right iliac fossa is seen to be free of gas. Later on the small bowel becomes dilated with fluid filled loops seen.

Colonoscopic decompression and detorsion has been tried, but is rarely successful.

Right hemicolectomy is the preferred treatment in many patients (essential if the caecum is not viable). Alternatively detorsion followed by caecopexy, using nonabsorbable sutures to lateral peritoneum with tube caecostomy. The tube is normally removed after 10 days and most close spontaneously afterwards.

Further reading

Baker S. Plain film radiography of the intestines and appendix. In Baker S, ed. *The Abdominal Plain Film*. East Norwalk. Appleton and Lange, 1990; 155–242.

Daniels IR, Lamparelli MJ, Chave H, Simson JNL. Recurrent sigmoid volvulus treated by percutaneous endoscopic colostomy. *British Journal of Surgery*, 2000; **87:** 1419.

Sinanan M, Pellegrini. Large bowel obstruction: Operative procedures. In Zinner M, Schwartz S, Ellis H, eds. *Maingot's Abdominal Operations,* 10th edition. London: Prentice Hall International (UK) Limited 1997; 1391–1413.

INTESTINAL PSEUDO-OBSTRUCTION AND ILEUS

Nick Lagattolla

The musculature within the gastrointestinal system may develop temporary focal paralysis, resulting in a functional obstruction. This can follow major abdominal surgery or any intraperitoneal infection or event. Any segment of the gastrointestinal system may become paralysed, though some segments are prone.

Acute colonic pseudo-obstruction

Acute colonic pseudo-obstruction (ACPO) is a condition that closely mimics acute large bowel obstruction, both clinically and radiologically, but for which there is no apparent mechanical cause. Despite the accurate description of this syndrome, diagnosis is often delayed and patients are often managed inappropriately. This leads to increased morbidity and mortality, as early diagnosis and correct management of these patients is essential in reducing complications. It is also known as Ogilvie's syndrome. Chronic colonic pseudo-obstruction also occurs.

Pathogenesis

The pathogenesis of this condition remains unclear but ACPO occurs in two broad groups of patients. In 80% of cases it appears to be a complication of other clinical conditions and these can be local or systemic. Common local factors include postpartum, Caesarean section, pelvic surgery or trauma but ACPO has been documented after a very wide range of abdominal or remote surgery, intra-abdominal sepsis/inflammation and retroperitoneal malignancy. Many systemic conditions (metabolic, sepsis, drugs) are also associated with ACPO. In 20% of patients no underlying disorder can be found. Colonic dysmotility is probably the final common pathway in all cases, although it may be produced by a variety of biochemical and physiological disturbances.

Clinical features

Many of these patients are already in hospital and have a concomitant systemic illness or are recovering from surgery or skeletal injury. Colicky abdominal pain may be absent. Enormous abdominal distension is the most dramatic physical finding. Abdominal tenderness is less than expected but its presence, particularly in the right iliac fossa, can indicate incipient caecal perforation. Bowel sounds are rarely absent and digital examination may reveal an empty ballooned rectum.

Investigations

There are no diagnostic laboratory investigations but electrolyte abnormalities or uraemia may indicate a cause for the pseudo-obstruction. Plain abdominal radiography is the single most useful investigation, revealing dilatation of the entire colon, but not the small bowel. The colonic gas pattern may have a cut-off point, mimicking the appearance of a mechanical obstruction.

Complications

Colonic perforation may supervene, and this usually occurs in the caecum. It is unlikely with caecal diameters of less than 12 cm but the risk increases significantly with measurements of 14 cm or greater. Plain radiographs will detect a pneumoperitoneum if perforation has occurred. An already perforated caecum may of course appear collapsed on plain X-rays.

Management

1. **Diagnosis.** Prompt diagnosis of this condition is essential before any inappropriate measures are undertaken. The clinical picture can be difficult to differentiate from malignant large colonic obstruction, particularly with idiopathic ACPO. An accurate diagnosis can usually be made by an instant unprepared contrast enema or if this is equivocal, by emergency colonoscopy, which can also be used to achieve colonic decompression. An urgent limited contrast enema has a well established place in the management of patients with acute large bowel obstruction, as the differentiation of ACPO from acute colonic mechanical obstruction carries important therapeutic considerations.

2. **Conservative treatment.** The initial management is conservative with nasogastric decompression, minimal oral intake, correction of fluid and electrolyte abnormalities and treatment of any associated conditions or infections. Opiates and anticholinergic drugs should be stopped. If there is distal colonic distension, then passage of a flatus tube via a sigmoidoscope under direct vision will temporarily achieve decompression. Pharmacological treatment with anticholinesterases such as neostigmine and gastrointestinal pro-motility agents have been used with some success. Motility stimulation is contraindicated if there is gross caecal distension. Repeated clinical assessment is essential. Repeated plain X-rays may be used to monitor the caecal diameter. This conservative regimen can be continued for 48–72 hours as long as the patient does not develop right iliac fossa signs or progressive caecal distension. Absence of resolution, progressive caecal dilatation or signs of peritonism are indications for prompt colonic decompression to avoid the risk of caecal ischaemia and perforation.

3. **Colonoscopy.** Successful decompression is achieved in approximately 80% of patients. Recurrence can occur in up to 15% of cases but the procedure can be repeated in such cases. Colonoscopy has also been used to aid placement of vented transanal tubes in the caecum, which can be left to prevent or treat recurrent distension. If the distension remains, a decompressive caecostomy should be considered.

4. **Surgery.** In the absence of ischaemic or perforated bowel, caecostomy is the decompressive procedure of choice. This can be performed either as a tube or a formal caecostomy. Caecostomy is a better option than colostomy as the latter may result in relatively poor decompression of the caecum. A localized area of caecal ischaemia or a small caecal perforation can be treated by excision and exteriorization or intubation as a caecostomy. Extensive caecal necrosis will necessitate formal resection. An anastomosis may not be appropriate, and the two ends are best brought out as a double-barrelled stoma with a spouted ileal end.

Outcome

ACPO carries a significant mortality rate even when adequate colonic decompression is achieved as patients are often already sick from an underlying illness. The overall mortality rate in patients undergoing surgery is 30% compared to 14% for conservative treatment. In the presence of a faecal peritonitis from caecal perforation the mortality rate rises to over 90%. Early diagnosis of ACPO is one of the most important aspects of the management of this condition, before inappropriate action is taken.

Paralytic ileus

This relates to the muscular atony that can paralyse the small bowel following any type of intraperitoneal event. Ileus may be generalized or localized. Local loops of paralysed small bowel are commonly found adjacent to septic foci such as a suppurating appendix or sites of inflammation. A generalized ileus may complicate generalized peritonitis, or follow from a laparotomy. Ileus commonly complicates surgery to the retroperitoneum, for example aortic aneurysm repair.

The duration is variable, but typically a generalized ileus lasts for up to three days, unless there is continued sepsis or electrolyte imbalance which would inhibit normal gastrointestinal motility. The treatment is continued nasogastric suction and fluid restriction until normal bowel motility is appreciated by means of ascultation or the passage of flatus and motion.

Gastric atony may follow upper gastrointestinal surgery, or pancreatitis. It is managed similarly to generalized ileus. Of note is that restoration of normal gastric motility in some patients can be particularly delayed, though often there is no dysfunction at all.

Further reading

Dorudi S, Berry AR, Kettlewell MGW. Acute colonic pseudo-obstruction. *British Journal of Surgery*, 1992; **79**: 99–103.

Related topics of interest

Anorectal investigation (p. 28); Colorectal carcinoma (p. 91); Intestinal obstruction (p. 190).

IRRITABLE BOWEL SYNDROME

Nick Lagattolla

IBS is a commonly diagnosed condition. Generally, this is a diagnosis of exclusion, once organic pathology has been positively ruled out; however, the diagnosis may be reached with greater confidence much sooner when all the clinical features are considered.

Clinical features

IBS constitutes a mixed collection of symptoms including abdominal pain, abdominal distension, alteration in bowel habit, sensation of incomplete evacuation, relief of abdominal pain on opening bowels, and dyspeptic symptoms, the motions often alternating between periods of constipation and looseness. Symptoms may be exacerbated by stressful events, and are recurrent, but there are no worrying features such as loss of weight or appetite, or bleeding per rectum. Associated symptoms may include chronic lower back pain, fatigue, lethargy, urinary problems or depression.

Individually, the abdominal symptoms may suggest underlying pathology. However, patients with irritable bowel syndrome will have many of these symptoms together, and the diagnosis can usually be established following a normal full clinical examination including a sigmoidoscopy. It may be wise to arrange either a barium enema or a colonoscopy in older patients to exclude colonic pathology.

Any age group may be affected, although it is most commonly diagnosed in the third and fourth decades. The aetiology is unknown, but it is probable that there is an element of overactivity of colonic musculature. This is based on the nature of the pain, which is usually lower abdominal and cramping, and the fact that antispasmodic medication often relieves it.

Management

The patient should be told they have irritable bowel syndrome and that this is caused by an overactive colon. The association between the symptoms and stress should be reinforced, as stress-avoidance may lead to an improvement.

Frequently, patients already suspect the diagnosis, and reassurance that there is no serious pathology and a positive diagnosis of irritable bowel syndrome is all that is required. However, a trial of an antispasmodic drug or stool-modifying agent is usually necessary.

Referral to a dietitian can be of great help. This may help in two ways. Firstly, a high fibre diet, which is the most frequent requirement in IBS, can be positively reinforced. Secondly, there is some evidence that exclusion diets can help. Whilst difficult to maintain as many food types are excluded, a tyramine-free diet has been found useful.

Pharmacotherapy

1. Stool-modifying preparations. The effect of either stool bulking and softening can be highly successful in those with a tendency to constipation as part of the symptomatology. Dietary modifications will also be required to ensure a high-fibre diet. Conversely, in those with a tendency to loose and frequent motions, these should be avoided, and the pharmaceuticals outlined below may be of greater benefit. Foods aggravating diarrhoea may be identifiable and should be avoided.

2. Antispasmodic drugs. The predominant symptom is usually abdominal pain and a variety of antispasmodic agents are available that may have an effect. The simplest is peppermint oil, which is available in capsules. This has a direct action on intestinal smooth muscle, and one or two capsules are taken three times a day. Other agents acting directly to inhibit smooth muscle are mebeverine hydrochloride (135 mg tds) and alverine citrate (60–120 mg tds).

3. Anticholinergic drugs. These will reduce motility, with a dry mouth and difficulty with near vision as unwanted effects. Anticholinergic drugs that may be of use include hyoscine butylbromide (20 mg qds) and dicyclomine hydrochloride (10–20 mg tds).

Resistant cases

Psychotherapy and hypnotherapy may be of help. Referral to a psychiatrist is unhelpful in the absence of a psychiatric disorder such as depression. Should symptoms persist despite reassurance and courses of antispasmodic agents, then the possibility of a diagnostic error should be considered. Rare causes of abdominal pain may need to be excluded, particularly if symptoms worsen.

Related topics of interest

Anorectal investigation (p. 28); Colorectal carcinoma (p. 91); Diverticular disease (p. 116).

JAUNDICE – INVESTIGATION

Nick Lagattolla

The jaundiced patient must be investigated urgently. A complete history and examination are mandatory and may distinguish obstructive (or cholestatic) jaundice from haemolytic (pre-hepatic) or hepatic causes. Biliary obstruction, as opposed to the other types of jaundice, is the province of the surgeon. Some hepatic disorders may cause intrahepatic cholestasis, which can produce an obstructive picture; however, most cases of obstructive jaundice result from obstruction of the extrahepatic biliary tree, most commonly by gallstones or malignancy.

Principles

Three stages are mandatory in the investigation of jaundice: a full history including travel abroad, a meticulous examination, which may be particularly revealing, and special investigations, of which there are numerous.

History

The passage of dark urine and pale stools is indicative of obstructive jaundice. Inter-mittent jaundice suggests common bile duct calculi, whilst progressive jaundice points to an underlying malignancy causing biliary obstruction. Jaundice associated with pain suggests calculous disease, and painless jaundice suggests malignancy. There are exceptions: carcinoma of the pancreas causes back pain if posteriorly related structures are invaded, and some tumours obstructing the common bile duct can necrose and diminish in size, temporarily relieving obstruction and jaundice. Weight loss and loss of appetite suggest malignancy.

Examination

General examination may show stigmata of chronic liver disease, pointing to a hepatic rather than obstructive jaundice. Charcot's triad suggests cholangitis (pyrexia and rigors, jaundice and an enlarged, tender liver), which is rare in malig-nant but common in calculous biliary obstruction. Cachexia suggests a malignant cause. Spontaneous migrating superficial thrombophlebitis (thrombophlebitis migrans or Trousseau's sign) may indicate an underlying pancreatic carcinoma. Rectal examination may reveal malignant infiltration of the pelvic peritoneum, pal-pable as a mass jutting backward above the prostate (rectal shelf of Blummer), from transcoelemic spread of pancreatic carcinoma. Stools are typically putty coloured in obstructive jaundice. The superimposition of melaena produces a silvery 'gun-metal' stool, which is rare but suggestive of ampullary carcinoma causing both blood loss and obstructive jaundice. The abdominal examination may reveal ascites, hepatomegaly from metastases, a pancreatic mass, or a palpable gallbladder caused by biliary dilatation.

Courvoisier's Law

This states that in the presence of jaundice, if the gallbladder is palpable, then the jaundice is unlikely to be due to gallstones. This is because calculous gallbladders are usually small and fibrotic and impalpable. However, the gallbladder may be palpable if a mucocele arises following impaction of a stone in the neck of the gallbladder.

Blood and urine tests

FBC, U&E, liver function test and a clotting screen are mandatory. In the presence of hepatic disease or obstructive jaundice, urinalysis will detect conjugated bilirubin in the urine. If urobilinogen is detected in the urine, then the jaundice cannot be obstructive, because conjugated bile cannot enter the intestine through an obstructed biliary system, and thus there is no conversion to urobilinogen for reabsorption and urinary excretion.

Liver function tests

These provide a useful picture of the underlying hepatobiliary disorder. Jaundice can become clinically evident if serum bilirubin exceeds approximately 60 mg/dl. The association of a raised alkaline phosphatase and a raised gamma glutamyl transferase points to the hepatic alkaline phosphatase isoenzyme (as opposed to the bone or gastrointestinal isoenzymes), and this is the usual pattern in both hepatic and obstructive jaundice. Obstructive jaundice is often associated with a greatly raised alkaline phosphatase and high levels of bilirubin. In hepatocellular disorders, the transamin-ases are usually grossly elevated, but the bilirubin may only be mildly raised.

Ultrasound

This should be the first investigation requested. The intrahepatic bile ducts become distended before the extrahepatic biliary tree if there is a distal biliary obstruction. The maximum diameter of a normal common bile duct is 8 mm but distension rapidly occurs if there is distal obstruction. Following a cholecystectomy the common bile duct frequently dilates, and this can cause confusion if a complete medical history is not obtained. Gallbladder calculi are easily seen on ultrasound, but calculi are rarely seen in the common bile duct due to overlying gas in the duodenum. However, common bile duct calculi usually result in biliary dilatation on ultrasound. The liver is scrutinized for metastases, and the pancreas is examined for the presence of tumour.

Endoscopic retrograde cholangiopancreatography (ERCP)

A side-viewing gastroscope is used to identify and cannulate the ampulla of Vater. Contrast is injected and radiographs outlining the biliary tree are obtained. The pancreatic duct is usually also outlined. A sphincterotomy can be performed, through which bile duct calculi may be extracted. Pancreatic or distal bile duct malignancies may be biopsied. Stents may also be placed to relieve obstructing lesions. If available, ERCP is the investigation of choice following ultrasound in jaundiced patients.

CT cholangiography

This is a sensitive investigation of the biliary tree. The outcome is a combination of CT, which will detect hepatic lesions and tumours obstructing the extrahepatic biliary tree, with a detailed contrast study of the bile ducts. Being essentially a series of X-rays, CT cannot detect gallstones unless they are calcified, though the detail afforded by intrabiliary contrast will detect filling defects.

Magnetic resonance cholangiopancreatography (MRCP)

This investigation is effectively similar to the above, using MR rather than CT. Meticulously detailed reconstructions of the extrahepatic biliary tree may be obtained. With increasing availability of MR, this is becoming the non-invasive extra-hepatic biliary investigation of choice, though CT cholangiography may be equally sensitive.

Percutaneous transhepatic cholangiography (PTC)

A needle is inserted into the hepatic parenchyma. A dilated intra-hepatic biliary radicle is entered, and contrast is injected. The views obtained of the biliary tract are as good as with ERCP, although the pancreatic duct is not seen, and biopsies cannot easily be taken. PTC is the preliminary step during the insertion of percutaneous transhepatic temporary and permanent biliary stents and drains. A guidewire can be inserted into the dilated duct system, and an external biliary drain is passed over it. Obstructed bile may be drained internally by placing a stent over the guidewire and across the obstruction.

Intravenous cholangiography

This concentrates contrast in the extrahepatic biliary tree, and may be used to assess biliary obstruction. It is a rather dangerous procedure with a recognized incidence of fatal hypersensitivity reactions. For this reason, a test dose is always given. It will not succeed in the presence of jaundice, as the hepatocytes will fail to excrete the contrast. It has largely been superseded by CT and MR cholangiography, and by ERCP.

Radionucleotide scans

Cholecystoscintigraphy (HIDA) and technetium scans may be used to assess both the hepatic parenchyma and bile ducts. The radiolabelled molecules are excreted by the liver into the bile even in the presence of mild jaundice.

Liver biopsy

Primary hepatic disease, or secondary malignant infiltration may require biopsy for confirmation of the diagnosis. This may be performed under ultrasound or CT control, or as a 'blind' procedure, or under general anaesthetic using a laparoscope. The latter allows a particular hepatic lesion to be targeted, and may be the procedure of choice if the liver is not diffusely infiltrated. The liver may also be biopsied via the transjugular route. A fine biopsy wire is passed through a cannula in the right internal jugular vein and the right heart is traversed to enter the hepatic veins under image intensifier control. The hepatic vein wall is breached, and the liver parenchyma can be biopsied.

Further reading

Beckingham IJ, Ryder SD. Investigation of liver and biliary disease. *British Medical Journal*, 2001; **322**: 33–36.

Howard ER, Peel ALG. Surgical studies. In: Burnand KG, Young AE (eds) *The New Aird's Companion in Surgical Studies*. Edinburgh: Churchill Livingstone, 1992; 1129.

Related topics of interest

Gallstones and their complications (p. 130); Pancreatic cancer (p. 248); Portal hypertension (p. 262).

LOWER GASTROINTESTINAL HAEMORRHAGE

Nick Lagattolla

Bleeding may occur from any part of the gut. Blood loss may be chronic and occult resulting in anaemia. Overt blood loss varies widely in presentation. Excluding haemorrhoidal bleeding, the lower gastrointestinal tract is less commonly a source of overt major haemorrhage than the stomach or duodenum.

Clinical examination

Blood originating from the sigmoid colon or distally may be dark or usually bright red and copious; that from more proximal sites in the colon or in the distal small intestine is usually dark red or black, although it does not have the sticky consistency or typical offensive smell of partially digested blood that characterizes the melaena of upper gastrointestinal bleeding. Occasionally, upper gastrointestinal haemorrhage may be brisk enough to cause the passage of unaltered blood per rectum, thus mimicking a colonic bleed.

There may be a history of previous episodes, or patients may be known to suffer from haemorrhoids or ulcerative colitis. Clinical examination is usually unremarkable in terms of localizing the source of the bleed. A digital rectal examination is essential, as this provides the best clue to the origin of the bleed. Tachycardia may be the only sign, though haemorrhagic shock may be present in extreme cases.

Causes

1. Haemorrhoids. These may bleed profusely. The blood is bright red and there is usually a history of blood passed per rectum after passing a motion. First-degree (non-prolapsing) haemorrhoids are impalpable and present with bleeding only, and thus a rectal examination may be entirely normal apart from blood staining of the glove. The bleeding will usually cease, and the diagnosis can be established by proctoscopy, at which time the haemorrhoids can be injected with 3% phenol.

2. Colitis. This is an important cause of bleeding per rectum. Any cause of colitis may result in blood loss, including ulcerative, infective or ischaemic colitis. Infective colitis with *Campylobacter* species often presents with lower abdominal pain and the passage of frank blood per rectum. Ulcerative or Crohn's proctitis or colitis will result in diarrhoea, which may be blood stained. Ischaemic colitis, which usually affects the splenic flexure, may present with blood passed per rectum. The blood tends to be dark, and represents the sloughing of the mucosa resulting from the ischaemia. Rarely, radiation enteritis may cause bleeding. If this is so, then there will be a clear history of radiotherapy, usually for a pelvic malignancy like cervical or prostatic carcinoma. Innocent bowel may be inadvertently irradiated, and this results in increased vascularity.

3. Diverticular disease. A diverticulum can bleed when it is not inflamed. The perforating blood vessels penetrate adjacent to the neck of the diverticulum, where they can easily be eroded by impacted faecoliths. If there is inflammation, bleeding does not result, as mural oedema distances the vessels from the impacted faecoliths. The bleeding may be brisk and bright red, and there are usually no symptoms or signs in the abdomen. Diverticula at any site of the colon may bleed.

4. Angiodysplasia.   The colonic mucosa may have small flat patches of telangiectatic vasculature, rarely greater than one centimetre in diameter. These are termed angiodysplasia, and they probably account for the majority of cases of acute and chronic colonic bleeds. They are often multiple and are most commonly found in the right colon, but may occur at other sites in the gastrointestinal tract.

5. Meckel's diverticulum.   A Meckel's diverticulum may be the site of ectopic gastric mucosa. This will produce gastric acid, and whilst the acid-tolerating mucosa within the diverticulum will be relatively protected, the adjacent ileal mucosa will be intolerant, and a peptic ulcer may develop next to the neck of the diverticulum. This ulcer may bleed, like its counterparts in the duodenum, and will present with the passage of (often copious) dark blood per rectum.

6. Tumours.   Carcinoma of the colon very rarely presents as massive haemorrhage, but frequently causes anaemia from chronic occult blood loss. However, the passage of dark blood per rectum may indicate a carcinoma. Colonic polyps lymphomas, leiomyomas and haemangiomas of the small bowel or colon may bleed.

7. Bowel ischaemia.   Intestinal ischaemia, including ischaemic colitis, results in intraluminal blood, and may present with dark blood passed per rectum. Causes include mesenteric arterial or venous infarction or mesenteric embolism. Ischaemia as a result of bowel strangulation or obstruction may result in blood loss, as seen with intussusception. Acute hypovolaemic shock may cause sloughing of the intestinal (usually colonic) mucosa, resulting in blood passed per rectum.

Investigations

The pulse rate and blood pressure are measured hourly, and if possible, the central venous pressure is measured. Blood is sent for haemoglobin estimation and cross matching.

1. Endoscopy.   Patients suspected of having a lower gastrointestinal tract bleed must undergo proctoscopy and sigmoidoscopy. These may be difficult to perform during the bleeding, as the blood will tend to obscure the field of view. Occasionally, one can 'get above' the bleeding point, and blood no longer obscures the view, suggesting that the origin of the bleed is distal to that site. Proctocolitis may be evident and biopsies confirm the diagnosis. It is rare for colonic carcinoma to result in frank haemorrhage, though polyps are more likely to do so, and if these are present in the rectum, sigmoidoscopy will provide an occasion to biopsy these and to establish a diagnosis. Angiodysplasia may be seen on colonoscopy as bright red patches of dilated vessels in the colonic mucosa, and they may be treated by colonoscopic laser or diathermy.

2. Radiolabelled red cell scanning.   Patients actively bleeding may be investigated using a radiolabelled red blood cell scan. An aliquot of the patient's own blood is returned after labelling of the red blood cells with technetium-99. The patient is scanned by gamma camera and the site of any pooling of the isotope is seen as a 'hot spot' on the scan. Sites of blood loss as low as 0.1 ml/min may be identified.

3. *Selective mesenteric angiography.* Continued dramatic bleeding in the absence of a known cause warrants mesenteric angiography. The femoral artery is cannulated, and, in sequence, the coeliac axis, superior and then inferior mesenteric arteries are selectively cannulated and injected with contrast. The site of bleeding can be accurately located if blood loss is at least 1 ml/min, and surgery may be confidently undertaken. Selective mesenteric arteriography will also detect angiodysplasia.

Management

Generally, bleeding from the lower gastrointestinal tract ceases spontaneously, and thus most cases can be managed conservatively by blood transfusion and close observation of vital signs. Proctosigmoidoscopy should be performed, and unless an obvious lesion to account for the blood loss is seen, colonoscopy should be requested the following day. If bleeding continues, a radiolabelled red cell scan should be undertaken, though this is not available out of normal hospital hours. If this test fails to demonstrate the source, or frank bleeding continues, mesenteric angiography should be performed.

Should bleeding be copious and with no available diagnosis, 'blind' emergency surgery may be necessary. This is a most unfortunate scenario, as the bleeding source is not necessarily evident at laparotomy. The patient will almost certainly end up having had either a right hemicolectomy on the suspicion of caecal angiodysplasia, or a sigmoid colectomy on the suspicion of diverticular bleeding, or possibly a subtotal colectomy if no clues at all are encountered intraoperatively. Furthermore, a proportion of those who end up with a 'blind' bowel resection continue to bleed.

Further reading

Ambrose NS, Wedgewood KR. Bleeding from the lower gastrointestinal tract. *Surgery*, 1990; **85:** 2027–2033.

Related topics of interest

Blood transfusion (p. 53); Colorectal carcinoma (p. 91); Gastrointestinal polyps (p. 142); Haemorrhoids (p. 153); Ulcerative colitis (p. 331); Upper gastrointestinal haemorrhage (p. 338).

LYMPHOEDEMA AND THE MANAGEMENT OF THE SWOLLEN LIMB

Nick Wilson

Lymphoedema is swelling of the tissues as a result of tissue fluid accumulation caused by abnormalities of the lymphatic system. The legs are affected principally (80%) but the arms, genitalia and face can be affected.

Differential diagnosis of the swollen leg

Causes of leg swelling other than lymphoedema are common and should be excluded before lymphoedema is diagnosed. Heart failure, renal failure and liver failure all cause leg oedema which is usually bilateral. Allergic conditions, angiooedema, venous obstruction, lipodystrophy and factitious oedema and gigantism should be considered.

Primary lymphoedema

Impaired lymphatic drainage caused by an abnormality of lymphatic drainage channels is the mechanism, but the underlying cause remains obscure. Having excluded other causes of leg swelling and lymphoedema, a clinical diagnosis of primary lymphoedema may be made. Primary lymphoedema may be classified according to its time of onset (congenital, praecox, tarda), or its lymphographic appearance (aplastic, hyperplastic, megalymphatics). Patients with distal swelling of the foot, ankle and lower leg tend to have distal, obliterative, aplastic lymphatics, whereas those with lymphatic vesicles and associated chylous ascites or chylothorax tend to have megalymphatics.

Secondary lymphoedema

Secondary lymphoedema is much commoner and usually the result of either malignant infiltration of regional lymph nodes or damage to lymph nodes as a result of surgery or radiotherapy or both. Arm involvement is much commoner than in primary lymphoedema. World-wide, infection with the *Wunchereria bancrofti* worm and silica infiltration of the lymphatics, both causing chronic inflammatory changes in the lymphatics, are of far greater significance.

Clinical features

Swelling of one lower leg is the commonest presentation and in the early stages this usually pits. Fibrosis occurs with chronicity and the swelling may no longer pit. The ankle contour is lost at an early stage and if the toes are involved, they adopt a square profile and develop lichenified filiform fronds, particularly on the dorsal surface. The increased fluid and protein content of the skin and subcutaneous tissues renders affected limbs more prone to cellulitis, which may be severe. Such episodes destroy residual lymphatics and may exacerbate swelling. In gross lymphoedema, the swelling may affect the thigh such that walking may become difficult.

Investigation

In many cases the diagnosis of lymphoedema can be made clinically. Where doubt exists, investigations to exclude other causes of oedema (renal function, liver function, cardiac function tests) should be performed.

1. Isotope lymphogram. This should be performed where the nature of the oedema remains unclear. The rate of isotope uptake by the groin lymph nodes is measured by gamma emission. Levels diagnostic of venous oedema and lymphoedema are established by individual laboratories.

2. Contrast lymphangiogram. Lymphatic vessels are first identified by injection into the foot web spaces of a vital dye such as patent blue and then cannulated so that Lipiodol can be infused slowly. Radiographs are then taken to reveal the lymphatic morphology. This investigation is now used only if isotope lymphography indicates an isolated lymphatic block at the groin or pelvic nodes and will indicate whether mesoenteric lymphatic bypass is possible.

3. CT and MRI. These techniques demonstrate abnormalities of skin (thickening) and subcutaneous tissues ('honeycombing'), which occur in lymphoedema.

Treatment

1. Elevation, massage and compression stockings. The great majority of patients are best treated with mechanical means to reduce the oedema. Massage milks the oedema proximally and can be performed by pneumatic compression devices having chambers which inflate from distal to proximal. Elevation reduces the intravascular and lymphatic hydrostatic pressure, whilst grade III graduated compression stockings increase the extravascular hydrostatic pressure, reducing the pressure gradient across the microcirculation. Multilayer bandaging using low-stretch bandages prior to compression hosiery further enhances the reduction in limb volume. Massage with aqueous cream or light vegetable oils helps to keep the skin in good condition. Skin care to avoid the ingress of bacteria resulting in cellulitis is important and early treatment of cellulitis with elevation, hydration and antibiotics is vital. Diuretics are generally unhelpful.

2. Reduction operations. Most patients with lymphoedema do not require surgery. Where the leg becomes unmanageable by conservative means, a debulking procedure may be considered. If the skin is in good condition, Homan's operation may be performed. Flaps are raised and a central strip of skin and subcutaneous tissue is excised. The flaps are then sutured back together. This is usually performed on the medial side of the leg first, but may be repeated on the lateral side if further debulking is required. Above and below knee procedures may be performed.

Where the skin is in poor condition, Charles' operation is more suitable. All of the skin and subcutaneous tissue is excised. Split skin grafts are applied to the deep fascia.

3. Ileal mesoenteric bridge operation. This is the only successful lymphatic bypass operation, but it is suitable only for a small number of patients who have an isolated lymphatic block in the groin or pelvic nodes. Only 50% of these patients have a good result. A segment of ileum is taken out of circuit on its mesentery and the proximal and distal free ends anastomosed to restore bowel continuity. The isolated segment is opened along its long axis and stripped of its lymphatics to expose the rich network of submucosal lymphatics. This segment is then tunnelled into the pelvis or groin where the lymph nodes just distal to the obstruction are bivalved. The segment of bowel is sewn onto the lymph nodes and lymphatic connections between the two surfaces form.

Lympho-lymphatic and lymphovenous anastomoses have been attempted but results are disappointing.

Further reading

Badger CM, Peacock JL, Mortimer PS. A randomised, controlled, parallel-group clinical trial comparing multilayer bandaging followed by hosiery versus hosiery alone in the treatment of patients with lymph-oedema of the limb. *Cancer*, 2000; **88:** 2832–2827.

Kinmonth JB. *Lymphatics, Surgery, Lymphangiography and Diseases of the Chyle and Lymph Systems*, 2nd edn. London: Edward Arnold, 1982.

Mortimer PS. Swollen lower limb – 2: lymphoedema. *British Medical Journal*, 2000; **320:** 1527–1529.

Related topics of interest

Calf pump failure and venous ulceration (p. 66); Deep vein thrombosis (p. 113); Vascular malformations and tumours (p. 353).

MALIGNANT MELANOMA

Prakash Sinha, Christopher Lattimer

Malignant melanoma is a neoplasm arising from epidermal melanocytes. It is a neoplasm with unpredictable behaviour – ranging from spontaneous regression to rapid progression and death. The incidence of melanoma is increasing at an alarming rate of 2–5% annually and doubling every decade. Queensland, Australia harbours the highest incidence. The increase in incidence could be related to the decreasing ozone layer (1% per year).

Risk factors

Increase in sun exposure, fair skin, blue eyes, red or blond hair all predispose to increase in risk. The pattern of exposure is important and intermittent exposure such as on holidays, weekends, and during sports is more closely associated with melanoma than continuous and regular exposure in outdoor workers. Use of sunbeds is also harmful. Sun exposure is supposed to decrease the number of T lymphocytes in the skin. Other risk factors include the dysplastic naevus syndrome, albinism, Xeroderma pigmentosum, prior history of melanoma, congenital giant hairy naevus and Hutchison's freckle.

Prevention

1. Avoidance of direct sunlight exposure.
2. Use of sun shades where possible.
3. Wearing sun-protective clothes (long sleeve) – SLIP.
4. Wearing of hats – SLAP.
5. Application of sun protection factors (with high UVA protection) – SLOP. Reapplication is necessary as they get rubbed off or sweated off.
6. Avoid sunbeds, tanning booths and lamps.
7. Avoid sun exposure from childhood and teenage years.
8. In Australia there is compulsory head protection in school.

Screening

Screening clinics with surface microscopy of suspicious moles is run in Australia. Patients with high risk such as previous history of melanoma, large number of naevi, and multiple dysplastic/atypical naevi need surveillance. Familial melanoma is rare and family members are not at high risk unless they have multiple atypical or dysplastic naevi.

Detection

Detection of early disease is of paramount importance because early lesions are curative and advanced lesions have an appalling prognosis. Most melanomas develop in a pre-existing mole. Changes to recognize in a suspicious mole are: increase in growth, change in colour, bleeding, ulceration, itching, crusting and inflammation (**A**symmetry, **B**order, **C**olour, **D**iameter, **E**nlarging). Removal should be considered for all moles larger than the back end of a pencil. Melanoma may arise in previously clear skin and present as a recent development of a pigmented lesion that looks different.

Classification

Five types of malignant melanoma are recognized.

Type	Characteristics	Incidence	Prognosis
Superficial spreading	Horizontal growth	64%	–
Nodular	Vertical growth	12–25%	Poor
Lentigo maligna	Flat, slow growing	7–15%	Good
Acral lentigenous	Palms, soles, sublingual, retina, genital	10–13%	Poor
Amelanotic	Pink with little pigment		Poor

Truncal melanoma (commoner in men), melanomas occurring in the BANS region (*B*ack, back of *A*rms, *N*eck, *S*calp) and ulcerated melanomas have a poorer prognosis, stage for stage. The incidence of acral lentigenous melanoma is increased in Asian and black populations. Production of MSF (Melanocytes Stimulating Factors) may explain the appearance of malignant melanoma in remote sites[c].

Microstaging

Tumour thickness (Breslow microstaging) is the single most important prognostic factor[b]. It is measured histologically with an optical micrometer from the granular surface to the deepest penetration.

Breslow thickness and relative 5-year risks

Tumour thickness (mm)	Risk of local recurrence (%)	Risk of node metastasis (%)	Risk of distant metastasis (%)
<0.76	0.2	2	2
0.76–1.5	2	25	8
1.5–4	6	57	15
>4	13	62	72

The level of tumour invasion into the various subdivisions of the dermis forms the basis of the Clark microstaging.

Clark microstaging

Level	Description
I	Intraepithelial
II	Into papillary dermis
III	Papillary/reticular junction
IV	Into reticular dermis
V	Penetration into subcutaneous fat

Both methods are complimentary but have their drawbacks. Ulcerative lesions and regressed lesions may be relatively thin yet have a poor prognosis. Similarly, a thick lesion on the sole or back may only reach Clark level I. A high mitotic rate carries a poor prognosis.

Spread

Malignant melanoma spreads by local extension, by lymphatics or by the blood stream. The disease remains confined to the epidermis for a period of time and grows radially (radial growth phase) before it invades the dermis and enters a vertical growth phase. Lymphatic spread is by embolism to the nodes or by lymphatic permeation producing in-transit or local satellite deposits. Blood borne metastasis are seen in the lungs, liver, brain, skin and rarely bones, small intestines, heart and breast.

Biopsy

Diagnosis of a suspicious lesion is confirmed on an incisional or excisional biopsy. Excision biopsy is preferable but incisional biopsy may be necessary for large lesions.

Excision biopsy should be complete excision of the suspected lesion, including full thickness of skin with a 2 mm lateral margin. There is no place for punch biopsy.

Investigations

A baseline full blood count, liver function test and chest X-ray are undertaken. Ultrasonography is a useful tool to investigate liver metastasis. Staging CT scan of chest, abdomen and pelvis is undertaken routinely before treatment in some centres. A MIBI nuclear medicine scan is occasionally useful in detecting occult metastasis. PET (positron emission tomography) scan and immunoscintigraphy (ISG) using tumour-specific antibodies labelled with a γ-emitting radioisotope (technetium-99m) are highly sensitive as well. These scan the whole body.

Treatment

Treatment is primarily surgical. For adequate surgical excision a good rule of thumb is that impalpable lesions require a 1-cm margin and palpable lesions a 2-cm margin[c]. If indicated subsequent wide re-excision requires removal of all the underlying subcutaneous tissue till the fascia. Orientation of any elliptical incision, required for primary closure, should be along the axis of lymphatic drainage. Subungual melanomas require partial amputation with level of bone section just proximal to the middle phalangeal head.

Treatment of lymph nodes

Clinically palpable nodes should be assessed preferably by fine needle aspiration cytology rather than open biopsy as there is a risk of tumour spillage in the latter. The aspiration of black particles often indicates nodal involvement before a definite cytology report has been prepared[c]. Elective node dissection is not recommended for large majority of the patients due to the morbidity of the procedure (seroma formation, lymphoedema, infection and neuralgia). Clinically involved nodes require radical therapeutic lymph node dissection. Adequate clearance gives a good prognosis with a 10-year survival of 50% when one node is involved[b]. If more nodes are involved regional radiotherapy may be considered.

Sentinel node biopsy is under trial to identify early lymph node metastasis (micrometastasis). This is done by injecting radioactive colloid and/or blue dye around the site of primary lesion and the first echelon lymph node draining this area is identified by lymphatic mapping with lymphoscintigraphy, hand-held gamma probe and the blue colour of the node. This lymph node is removed for biopsy and if found positive lymph node dissection can be recommended.

Isolated limb perfusion

Isolated lymph perfusion with alkylating agents, indicated for local recurrence and 'in-transit' disease, is effective at reducing lesion size and, on occasion, healing them completely[b]. The procedure is usually combined with a modified lymph node dissection. Enthusiasts also use this technique as adjuvant therapy for primary lesions greater than 1.5 mm thick.

Other therapy

Adjuvant therapy are often expensive, toxic and of no benefit. Carbon dioxide laser ablation may be used for multiple small cutaneous lesions. Malignant melanoma is refractory to chemotherapy but radiotherapy plays a major role in treatment of symptomatic brain, bone and spinal metastasis. Single deposits, like peripheral pulmonary deposits or cerebral lesions, are often removed surgically to good effect. Chemo-immunotherapy using antimelanoma monoclonal antibodies conjugated with toxins (ricin), α-interferon and interleukin-2 have been disappointing[b]. Use of leukine (GM-CSF), levamisole and tumour vaccines are at experimental stage with encouraging results in some studies. Unfortunately there is a tendency to positive reporting bias and negative trials are not published.

Prognosis and survival

Prognosis depends largely on two factors: thickness of the lesion (Breslow thickness) and lymph node or distant metastasis at presentation. Site, ulceration and mitotic index may have prognostic significance. The 5-year survival according to the thickness is shown in a table above, whereas the 10-year survival is 40%–50%, 26% and 15% in patients with 1, 2–4 and 5 or more regional lymph nodes involvement, respectively[b]. The importance of early diagnosis and appropriate treatment cannot be re-emphasized. Malignant melanoma still remains an unpredictable disease and spontaneous regression even after liver metastasis can occur. If such a patient received adjuvant therapy it would be considered a success!

Further reading

Breslow A. Thickness, cross-sectional areas and depth of invasion in the prognosis of cutaneous melanoma. *Annals of Surgery*, 1970; **172**: 902–908.

Garbe C, McLeod GR, Buettner PG. Time trends of cutaneous melanoma in Queensland, Australia and Central Europe. *Cancer*, 2000; **89**(6): 1269–1278.

Hughes TM, A'Hern RP, Thomas JM. Prognosis and surgical management of patients with palpable inguinal lymph node metastases from melanoma. *British Journal of Surgery*, 2000; **87**(7): 892–901.

Soutar DS. The surgical management of cutaneous malignant melanoma. In: Johnson CD, Taylor I. *Recent Advances in Surgery – 19*. Churchill Livingstone, Edinburgh; 1996: 215–234.

Related topic of interest

Sentinel node biopsy (p. 296).

MECKEL'S DIVERTICULUM

Deya Marzouk

Introduction

Meckel's diverticulum is the commonest congenital diverticulum of the gastro-intestinal tract, occurring in approximately 2% of the population. It results from incomplete closure of the omphalomesenteric (vitellointestinal) duct. It is located approximately 2 feet proximal to the ileocaecal valve. It is approximately 2 inches long and usually has a wide base arising from the antimesenteric border of the ileum. Variations do occur depending on the degree of atrophy of the remnants of the omphalomesenteric duct and can result in a shorter or longer diverticulum, a narrow base and connection to the umbilicus by a fibrous cord or even a fistulous communication. It may also have a separate vitellointestinal artery running in a small mesenteric fold, the mesodiverticular band. Ectopic gastric, fundic or pancreatic mucosa is commonly found within the diverticulum.

Clinical picture

Meckel's diverticulum is asymptomatic in the vast majority of people. Symptoms occur in approximately 4% of all patients with Meckel's diverticula (2% or less in adults) when complications such as obstruction, inflammation, peptic ulceration with pain, bleeding or perforation develop. The great majority of symptom-atic Meckel's diverticulae occur in children and young adults[b]. Symptoms caused by Meckel's diverticula are mainly due to the presence of bands or ectopic gastric mucosa within the diverticulum (the latter cause hemorrhage and perforation).

Complications

These include intestinal obstruction, lower GI bleeding, acute diverticulitis and development of tumours.

1. **Intestinal obstruction.**   Intestinal obstruction may occur secondary to small bowel volvulus around a band extending from the tip of the diverticulum to the umbilicus, torsion of the diverticulum or secondary to ileoileal or ileoileocolic intussusception. Rarely, this may be secondary to internal herniation behind a mesodiverticular band or obstruction within a hernia (Littre's hernia).

2. **Lower GI bleeding.**   Haemorrhage from Meckel's diverticulum usually results from acid-induced peptic ulceration involving the ileum just distal to the diverticu-lum. Bleeding is usually painless and episodic and occasionally is brisk. The diagnosis may be confirmed by Tc-99m pertechnetate radionucleide scanning.

3. **Meckel's diverticulitis.**   Meckel's diverticulitis is clinically indistinguishable from appendicitis. The correct diagnosis is rarely made preoperatively[b]. Perforation occurs in up to 50% of cases, with resultant peritonitis. Diverticulitis usually occurs in long diverticulae with a narrow base.

4. *Umbilical anomalies.* An umbilical fistula (patent omphalomesenteric duct) may be the presenting feature of some patients.

5. *Tumours.* Rarely various tumours including leiomyomas, leiomyosarcomas, carcinoids and adenocarcinoma develop in Meckel's diverticula.

Diagnosis

A complicated Meckel's diverticulum should be considered in the differential diagnosis of children with lower GI bleeding, patients with signs of peritonitis or mechanical small bowel obstruction. The diagnosis is usually made intraoperatively especially in cases with obstruction or diverticulitis. Occasionally, the diagnosis is suggested by preoperative sonography, CT or small bowel enema.

Diagnosis may be made using Tc-99m pertechnetate radionucleide scanning (to detect heterotopic gastric mucosa within the diverticulum) in patients with lower GI bleeding (usually after negative gastroscopy and colonoscopy). Rarely, preoperative angiography may reveal a persistent vitellointestinal artery or other angiographic abnormalities at the site of the Meckel's diverticulum such as vascular blush, early venous return, and arterial irregularity.

Treatment

Treatment of symptomatic Meckel's diverticulum is by resection, either diverticulectomy only or segmental ileal resection including the diverticulum. The latter is performed for wide-based diverticulae or gangrenous diverticulae[b]. Segmental resection should be performed for bleeding Meckel's diverticula. It is important to remove the ectopic mucosa and site of ulceration to prevent rebleeding episodes (the bleeding site is usually in the ileum distal to the diverticulum).

When a Meckel's diverticulum is encountered at operation, division of its mesentery, the mesodiverticular band, rather than diverticulectomy, to relieve the volvulus might devitalize the Meckel's diverticulum and should be avoided.

Recently, laparoscopic removal has been reported. This involves either diverticulectomy by means of ligation with an 'endoloop' in a similar manner to laparoscopic appendicectomy or laparoscopic resection using 'endo-staplers' with extracorporeal or intracorporeal anastomosis.

Meckel's diverticulum encountered incidentally during laparotomy

The current opinion favours leaving wide-mouthed thin-walled unattached diverticulae well alone[b]. The likelihood of Meckel's diverticulum becoming symptomatic in an adult is 2% or less, which does not justify the possible complication rate associated with its resection. On the other hand if there is a fibrous band or a patent fistula to the umbilicus these should be divided. The presence of mesodiverticular band calls for some judgement. If the band is fibrous it may be divided, but if it contains blood vessels, it is best to leave it, as its division may devitalize the Meckel's diverticulum postoperatively. Alternatively, diverticulectomy may be performed if it is judged that the vascular mesodiverticular band poses risk of future internal herniation. Thickening on palpation suggests ectopic tissues or tumours and also favours resection.

Further reading

Peoples JB, Lichtenberger EJ, Dunn MM. Incidental Meckel's diverticulectomy in adults. *Surgery*, 1995; **118:** 649–652.

Schmid SW, Schafer M, Krahenbuhl L, Buchler MW. The role of laparoscopy in symptomatic Meckel's diverticulum. *Surgical Endoscopy*, 1999; **13:** 1047–1049.

Soltero MJ, Bill AH. The natural history of Meckel's diverticulum and its relation to incidental removal. A study of 202 cases of diseased Meckel's diverticulum found in King County, Washington, over a fifteen year period. *American Journal of Surgery*, 1976; **132:** 168–173.

St-Vil D, Brandt ML, Panic S, Bensoussan AL, Blanchard H. Meckel's diverticulum in children: a 20-year review. *Journal of Pediatric Surgery*, 1991; **26:** 1289–1292.

MESENTERIC ISCHAEMIA

Nick Lagattolla

Mesenteric ischaemia is a condition where segments of the intestine become ischaemic secondary to vascular insufficiency. The ischaemia may be acute or chronic. Acute ischaemia is either focal or diffuse.

Acute focal ischaemia

Focal ischaemia most frequently results from mechanical intestinal obstruction, for example bowel strangulation caused by hernia, adhesive bands or volvulus. The wall of obstructed bowel is relatively ischaemic compared to normal bowel, and thus perforation may supervene. Perforation follows the development of necrosis as a result of the ischaemia, and this will occur at the site of any obstruction, due to a pressure necrosis, or at the site of the bowel most distal from the point at which the arterial supply is obstructed; for example, in a strangulated femoral hernia, the bowel may necrose and perforate at the neck of the hernia, or at the apex of the herniated bowel loop. Rarely, focal ischaemia may result from an embolus lodging and blocking a mesenteric arterial arcade, or focal vasculitides like rheumatoid disease and polyarteritis nodosa.

Clinical signs suggesting there are ischaemic changes in bowel are a change in the nature of the pain from colicky to constant, and the presence of signs of peritonism, if not frank peritonitis. These signs warrant surgery, and if any ischaemic bowel is encountered that fails to recover after envelopment in warm packs, then it should be excised. Telltale signs that bowel is no longer viable include the loss of the usual serosal lustre, lack of peristalsis, and absence of mesenteric arterial pulsation. Unless the bowel is frankly black, the colour is not a particularly good indicator. Doubtful viability bowel should be considered viable, and returned to the peritoneum to be explored the next day at a planned second-look laparotomy.

Acute diffuse ischaemia

Aetiology

Acute diffuse ischaemia usually results from thrombosis or embolism in a major mesenteric artery, usually the superior mesenteric. Thrombosis is more common than embolism. Embolism is usually cardiogenic, arising from either post-myocardial infarction mural thrombus or atrial fibrillation. Thrombosis of a main mesenteric vein may also result in diffuse ischaemia. More rarely acute diffuse ischaemia occurs as a result of severe systemic hypotension with compensatory reduced splanchnic blood flow. This is non-mesenteric ischaemia that is caused by a critical reduction of intestinal perfusion due to extramesenteric factors, including cardiac failure and septic or hypovolaemic shock. Splanchnic vasoconstriction is a predictable secondary response in this setting. Many of these patients are either digitalized for cardiac failure or receiving vasopressor therapy. Acute diffuse ischaemia can lead to frank multifocal or generalized bowel infarction and gangrene.

As an indication for urgent laparotomy, diffuse ischaemia will account for less than 5% of operations but it continues to carry a very high mortality – between 80 and 90% depending on the underlying cause. Non-occlusive infarction accounts for approximately one third of all cases.

Clinical course

The clinical picture will depend on the extent and severity of the initial problem. Pain is almost always present and is the earliest symptom. The pain is typically very severe. Vomiting, diarrhoea and rectal urgency may occur, reflecting the disturbance in intestinal function. Blood may be lost into the lumen as the infarction progresses resulting in occult or frank blood in the faeces. Extensive infarction eventually produces systemic effects including hypovolaemia, metabolic acidosis and endotoxic shock. Perforation and ensuing peritonism ensue as the final stages of the condition.

Diagnosis and treatment

1. At presentation. The early diagnosis of acute mesenteric ischaemia remains elusive. The only consistent symptom is severe generalized abdominal pain. Additional clinical information that should raise the index of suspicion includes the presence of peripheral vascular disease, recent myocardial infarction or a recent intra-aortic procedure, such as cardiac catheterization. There is a paucity of physical findings before the onset of perforation. Laboratory investigations are not diagnostic but may be useful in excluding other diagnoses such as acute pancreatitis. However, acute mesenteric ischaemia is one of many causes of the acute abdomen that can cause an elevated serum amylase, and there is often a very high leucocytosis. Arterial blood gases will confirm an increasingly severe metabolic acidosis. Plain abdominal radiography may reveal a non-specific ileus. Intramural or intraportal gas occurs only in late stages. Angiography is not of value in acute mesenteric ischaemia.

2. At operation. Adequate resuscitation prior to surgery is essential, as in all acute abdominal cases. The principles are accurate assessment of bowel viability, revascularization if indicated and/or resection. Clinical assessment relies on colour, contractility and bleeding, all of which are highly subjective criteria. The use of a Doppler ultrasound probe and systemic fluoroscein dye perfusion are more objective but are either seldom available or rarely used. Appropriate treatment will be dictated by the cause of the original insult. In occlusive ischaemia embolus or thrombus formation in the superior mesenteric artery should be treated by embolectomy and thromboendarterectomy/bypass grafting respectively. As much as 70% of the small intestine can be resected without long-term nutritional consequences, but a careful record of the length and type of remaining bowel should be made. More small bowel can be resected, but the patient is likely to require permanent parenteral nutrition. If after resection the viability of remaining bowel is in doubt, then anastomosis should be deferred until a second-look laparotomy (24 hours later) when further resections can be performed and/or intestinal continuity restored. In acute colonic ischaemia, the general condition of the patient and local factors such as peritoneal contamination will dictate whether an immediate anastomosis is performed or a stoma is constructed in a staged resection. These patients require careful postoperative monitoring, preferably in a high-dependency unit. Continued fluid depletion and the release of toxic vasoactive mediators into the circulation following resection or successful vascular reconstruction can cause circulatory collapse.

3. Non-operative measures. With non-mesenteric causes of reduced intestinal perfusion, management clearly is directed at correction of the primary problem. Transthoracic/transoesophageal echocardiography may determine the source of emboli requiring long-term anticoagulation. Atrial fibrillation and other cardiac dysrhythmias require treatment, with referral to a cardiologist. The use of vasopressor agents that increase mesenteric vascular resistance should be avoided. However, such measures may indeed supplement surgery, as infarcted bowel will result in systemic sepsis and cardiovascular collapse.

Prognosis

In occlusive cases, thrombosis carries a higher mortality than embolism (50–80%). Non-occlusive ischaemia has a uniformly high mortality rate (80%), reflecting that intestinal ischaemia is often a pre-terminal event in the course of a serious illness.

Chronic mesenteric ischaemia

The predominant symptom arising from chronic mesenteric ischaemia is post-prandial abdominal pain, usually central, which is often referred to as mesenteric claudication. There is also always considerable weight loss. There are no signs. Selective mesenteric intra-arterial digital subtraction arteriography remains the definitive investigation. Angiography can reveal the site of arterial occlusion or stenosis of a major artery and is mandatory in planning revascularization. It is usually considered necessary for two of the three gastrointestinal arteries (coeliac, superior and inferior mesenteric arteries) to be occluded, and the remaining artery to be severely stenotic before symptoms can occur. Therefore no attempt at revascularization should be undertaken unless it is established that all three arteries are compromised. Re-implantation of a proximally occluded artery, or a jump graft to a patent segment comprise the arterial reconstructions possible, usually to the inferior or superior mesenteric. It follows that only one artery need be revascularized. Angioplasty may be possible if there is an accessible stenosis.

Further reading

Croft RJ, Menon GP, Marston A. Does intestinal angina exist? A critical study of obstructed visceral arteries. *British Journal of Surgery*, 1981; **68:** 316–318.

Ottinger LW. The surgical management of acute occlusion of the superior mesenteric artery. *Annals of Surgery*, 1978; **188:** 721–731.

Related topic of interest

Assessment of the acute abdomen (p. 41).

MINIMAL ACCESS SURGERY

Nick Wilson

Diagnostic and therapeutic endoscopy have been commonplace in gynaecological and urological practice for many years, but even diagnostic laparoscopy was not widely practised by general surgeons until the first laparoscopic cholecystectomies were performed in 1988. Since then laparoscopic surgical practice has exploded with surgeons learning and practising the techniques at a hitherto unseen rate. Demand for the new techniques was driven by public demand although this was latterly tempered by several well publicized complications and deaths that emphasized inherent problems with the new two dimensional, tactileless techniques together with deficiencies in training and the regulation of minimal access surgery. There were few large studies initially, but more commonplace procedures have now been assessed in randomized trials. The advent of high-quality video equipment and other instrumentation has led to the development of many endoscopic operations but only a small proportion of these have been adopted in mainstream general surgical practice. Trainees are encouraged to attend basic and advanced training courses nowadays and many hospitals have training rooms with laparoscopic simulators available.

The advantages of minimally invasive surgery are:

- The avoidance of a long incision.
- Reduced post-operative pain.
- Less impairment of respiratory function.
- Reduced metabolic disturbance.
- Reduced hospital stay.
- Quicker return to normal activities and work.

General principles

Intracavitary abdominal procedures require the creation of a pneumoperitoneum by introduction of a cannula under vision through which carbon dioxide is introduced. A 0° or 30° laparoscope is introduced and subsequent trocars must all be introduced under direct vision. Basic instruments include fine-grasping forceps for retracting, suction/irrigation cannulas, curved dissecting forceps and diathermy scissors or hook. Electrocoagulation is generally preferred to laser as the overshoot phenomenon, which can damage distant tissues, is avoided. Various clip devices are used to ligate small vessels and ducts and more sophisticated staple devices are available to close bowel and perform anastomoses. Roeder slip-knots can be used to ligate vessels and ducts. Instrumentation to extend the armamentarium of endoscopic techniques is developing rapidly.

Complications

- Diagnostic laparoscopy: mortality $< 0.03\%$, major complications 0.6%, minor complications 4%.
- Abdominal wall/omental emphysema.
- Circulatory/respiratory collapse from tension pneumoperitoneum.
- Trocar puncture of bowel or bladder.

- Trocar puncture of major vessel (aorta, iliac vessels, cava).
- Carbon dioxide embolus.
- Diathermy, laser, clip injury (e.g. to bile duct).
- Haemorrhage.

Specific general surgical procedures

1. Biliary surgery. Cholecystectomy remains the most widely practised and acknowledged procedure and is clearly superior to the open operation[b]. Management of the common bile duct varies from ignoring the possibility of duct stones to endoscopic retrograde cholangiopancreatography or peroperative cholangiography routinely or selectively. Bile duct stones may be cleared laparoscopically using a fine-bore flexible choledochoscope, baskets and balloon catheters. Bile duct injury is the most significant complication and there is evidence that this occurs more commonly than in the open operation. Conversion to the otherwise rarely performed open procedure is required in 5–10% of cases.

2. Appendicectomy. Laparoscopy can be used to verify the diagnosis, particularly in young women. Where acute appendicitis is confirmed, laparoscopic or laparoscopic-assisted appendicectomy is logical. A good view of the peritoneal cavity is obtained allowing diagnosis of other causes of acute abdominal pain. The operation often takes longer than the conventional procedure and involves three or four trocar sites. Recovery is slightly quicker than for the open procedure and wound infection rates are lower[b]. The necessary equipment and appropriately trained staff must be available for emergency operating. Several large series have reported satisfactory results.

3. Hernia repair. The laparoscopic procedure changes a simple body wall operation that can be performed as a day case under local anaesthetic to an intra-abdominal or properitoneal procedure performed under general anaesthetic. Transabdominal preperitoneal (TAPP) hernia repair is the most widely used technique[b]. Patients recover more quickly than following open repair and recurrence rates are low at around 2%[b] but the technique is more expensive[b]. The National Institute for Clinical Excellence (NICE) has recommended that laparoscopic repair be used only for recurrent and bilateral hernias.

4. Antireflux surgery. The Nissen procedure has been developed for laparoscopy. A loose short wrap of gastric fundus around the gastro-oesophageal junction is performed with a crural repair where appropriate. Early results appear favourable with low morbidity and mortality. The procedure is time consuming and a high degree of operator expertise is required, but it has the ability to resolve symptoms and reflux such that long-term medication can be avoided. Recovery is quicker than following the open procedure[b].

5. Sympathectomy. Thoracoscopic sympathectomy is a welcome alternative to the open operation performed via the difficult anterior supraclavicular route. Palmar hyperhydrosis is the prime indication. Unilateral or bilateral procedures can be performed. The thoracoscope is introduced through the fifth intercostal space in the anterior axillary line. The risk of Horner's syndrome is lower than in the open operation. Compensatory hyperhydrosis of the trunk or thighs occurs to some extent in 50% of patients and is commoner where hands, axillae and feet are affected.

6. *Peptic ulcer surgery.* Posterior truncal vagotomy with anterior seromyotomy is currently the preferred technique for the treatment of patients with refractory duodenal ulcer disease. Patching of perforated duodenal ulcer and gastroenterostomy can also be performed. Relatively few patients now require elective peptic ulcer surgery and few series have been performed.

7. *Colectomy.* Series of resections for benign and malignant disease have been reported. Early results indicated that hospital stay and complications are not significantly reduced by using laparoscopic techniques. The possibility of inadequate clearance of malignant disease and the occurrence of port site metastases have tempered enthusiasm for the use of laparoscopic techniques in the treatment of bowel cancer, but resections for inflammatory bowel disease can be performed effectively.

8. *Splenectomy.* Normal-sized or small spleens can be removed laparoscopically and idiopathic thrombocytopenic purpura is the commonest indication. No randomized trials have been reported.

9. *Adrenalectomy.* This is undertaken for a wide range of abnormalities including Cushings syndrome, adenoma and phaeochromocytoma. The technique is not yet widely available.

Further reading

Pederson AG, Peterson OB, Wara P, Ronning H, Qvist N, Laurberg S. Randomised clinical trial of laparoscopic versus open appendicectomy. *British Journal of Surgery*, 2001; **88**: 200–205.
The MRC Laparoscopic Groin Hernia Trial Group. Laparoscopic versus open repair of groin hernia: a randomised comparison. *Lancet*, 1999; **354**: 185–190.

Related topics of interest

Acute appendicitis (p. 4); Adrenal tumours (p. 13); Endoscopy (p. 119); Gallstones and their complications (p. 130); Gastro-oesophageal reflux (p. 146); Inguinal hernia (p. 179); Peptic ulceration (p. 255).

MULTIPLE ORGAN FAILURE

Chris Perera, Christopher Lattimer

Multiple organ failure (MOF) is the leading cause of death in the surgical ICU. It was first recognized in 1973. It can be defined as the result of a severe physiological insult which leads to the failure of several organs not necessarily involved in the original insult. The realization that the organs involved become hypermetabolic rather than actually failing has led some to change the name to the multiple organ dysfunction syndrome (MODS). Similarly, the host response of disseminated inflammation to the powerful physiological insult has been termed the systemic inflammatory response syndrome (SIRS).

Aetiology

MOF typically occurs after shock, infection, massive tissue injury, and in the presence of large amounts of necrotic tissue. Depending on the physiological reserve of the organs concerned the order of failure commences with pulmonary, followed by hepatic, intestinal and lastly, renal failure. There is a direct relationship between the number of organs failing and the length of time the patient is in organ failure with the mortality of the patient. Unfortunately, there remains a grey area where it is impossible to predict which patients will develop MOF prior to the insult and to predict with accuracy the outcome. This problem of patient assessment is a major factor limiting the value of various therapeutic trials. To date, IL-6 levels appear to be the best single predictor of outcome in the MOF syndrome.

Pathogenesis

The current hypotheses of MOF include a persisting focus of infection, uncontrolled generalized inflammation (SIRS), gut mucosal failure, reticuloendothelial system failure and the production of oxygen free radicals. The contribution of each of these to MOF will be examined.

Sepsis

The observation that the organs which fail are often remote from the disease process led to the suggestion that an endogenous or exogenous circulating factor acts as a mediator. Whilst in the majority of patients infection is the initiating cause, in a third of patients with MOF there has been no evidence of an infective focus. The concept of an empiric laparotomy to identify this infective focus is now outdated as these operations rarely discover occult sepsis that has been missed on less invasive investigations like ultrasound and CT.

Systemic inflammatory response syndrome and sepsis syndrome: relevant definitions

Systemic inflammatory response syndrome (SIRS)

Systemic inflammatory response to a variety of severe clinical insults. The response is manifested by two or more of the following conditions:

- Core temperature, $< 36°C$ or $> 38°C$
- Tachycardia, > 90 beats/min
- Tachypnoea, > 20 breaths/min while breathing spontaneously or $PaCO_2$ < 4.3 kPa
- White blood count, $> 12\,000$ cells/mm^3, < 4000 cells/mm^3 or $> 10\%$ immature forms

And at least one of the following manifestations of inadequate organ function or perfusion:

- Altered mental state
- Hypoxaemia, $PaO_2 < 72$ mmHg breathing ambient air
- Oliguria, urinary output < 30 ml or < 0.5 ml/kg for at least 1 hour

With clinical evidence of infection:

- *Infection*: microbial phenomenon characterized by an inflammatory response to the presence of micro-organisms or the invasion of normally sterile tissue by those organisms
- *Bacteraemia*: the presence of viable bacteria in the blood

Sepsis

The systemic response to infection. This systemic response is manifested by three or more of the conditions described above (SIRS) and presented clinical or micro-biological evidence of infection.

Severe sepsis

Sepsis associated with organ dysfunction, hypoperfusion or hypotension. Hypoperfusion and perfusion abnormalities may include, but are not limited to lactic acidosis, oliguria or an acute alteration in mental status.

Septic shock

Sepsis with hypotension, despite adequate fluid resuscitation, together with the presence of perfusion abnormalities that may include, but are not limited to lactic acidosis, oliguria or an acute alteration in mental status. Patients who are on inotropic or vasopressor agents may not be hypotensive at the time that perfusion abnormalities are measured.

Sepsis-induced hypotension

A systolic blood pressure of < 90 mmHg or a reduction of > 40 mmHg from baseline in the absence of other causes for hypotension.

Multiple organ dysfunction syndrome

Presence of severely altered organ function in an acutely ill patient such that homeo-stasis cannot be maintained without intervention.

Inflammatory mediators

The similarity between systemic infection and a septic state in which no infection has been identified suggests that common mediators are responsible. These have been isolated and include bacterial endotoxin, TNF-α, IL-6, IL-1 and oxygen free radicals. The injection of TNF-α or endotoxin into healthy human volunteers can accurately reproduce the septic response. TNF-α specifically is believed to participate in the muscle proteolysis that accompanies sepsis and it is enhanced by glucocorticoids.

Gut mucosal barrier

Recent interest has implicated the gut, with its reservoir of bacteria, as the driving force behind MOF. Loss of the gut mucosal barrier leads to the translocation of Gram-negative bacteria and endotoxin into the portal circulation, which is believed to initiate MOF. This situation is potentiated if the natural defences of the gut (the intestinal microflora, a host immune response and adequate functional enterocyte mass) are compromised, which is a common feature of a septic patient. Sepsis encourages immunosuppression and antibiotic regimes displace the normal intes-tinal flora with an overgrowth of potentially pathogenic flora. The upper intestinal tract becomes colonized if medication is given to reduce gastric acidity. Parenteral or hyperosmolar enteral feeds lead to disuse atrophy of the mucosa, further decreasing the gut's defence against invasion. If healthy human volunteers receive a single dose of enterotoxin, they develop a hypoalbuminaemic and capillary leak syndrome. The intestines become oedematous, form an ileus and exhibit increased permeability to bacteria.

Intestinal ischaemia

Impaired oxygen delivery to the gut occurs in shock, and its associated alteration in mesenteric blood flow. During reperfusion, injury occurs and macrophages are acti-vated with release of IL-1, IL-6, TNF-α and free radicals, which further increase intestinal permeability and encourage endotoxin and bacterial translocation.

Reticuloendothelial system

The next barrier to a generalized septic state is the liver and the spleen. Bacteria can be cultured from these organs, the portal circulation and the intestinal lymph nodes after massive physiological insults. If the state of the reticulo-endothelial system in the liver is healthy, it should be effective in neutralizing a moderate bacterial and endotoxin load. If the liver is impaired, Kupfer cell malfunction occurs and endotoxins and bacteria are released into the systemic circulation.

Free radicals

Oxygen free radicals also contribute to MOF by damage to the microvascular circu-lation. They are generated during reperfusion when oxygen reacts with hypo-xanthene, a metabolic product of ATP that accumulates during ischaemia, and is converted into the superoxide anion. The intracellular antioxidants are not capable of neutralizing this massive free radical load with consequent endothelial damage. This attracts neutrophils and encourages them to degranulate with the release of many inflammatory mediators, all of which play a role in the SIRS.

Further reading

D'Amico R, Pifferi S, Leonetti C *et al.* Effectiveness in antibiotic prophylaxis in critically ill adult patients: systematic review of randomized controlled trials. *British Medical Journal,* 1998; **316:** 1275–1285.

Deitch EA. Multiple organ failure. *Advances in Surgery,* 1993; **26:** 333–356.

Friedman G, Silva E, Vicent JL. Has the mortality of septic shock changed with time? *Critical Care Medicine,* 1998; **26:** 2078–2086.

Miller PR, Kincaid EH, Meredith JW, Chang MC. Threshold values of intramucosal pH and mucosal–arterial CO_2 gap during shock resuscitation. *Journal of Trauma,* 1998; **45:** 868–872.

Parrillo JE. Pathogenetic mechanisms of septic shock. *New England Journal of Medicine,* 1993; **328:** 1471–1477.

Related topic of interest

Nutrition in the surgical patient (p. 233).

NON-SPECIFIC ABDOMINAL PAIN

Nick Lagattolla

Fifty per cent of patients initially presenting to hospital with acute abdominal pain do not have a definitive diagnosis. This is still the case in 30% of patients admitted. In the absence of evidence of surgical, gynaecological or medical disease, these patients may be termed as having 'non-specific abdominal pain' (NSAP) or 'abdominal pain of unknown origin'.

Epidemiology

Approximately half of those initially diagnosed with NSAP will leave hospital having been told they have dyspepsia, constipation, dysmenorrhoea, mesenteric adenitis or gastroenteritis. These are not absolute diagnoses, and therefore the percentage of cases of acute abdominal pain that remains 'non-specific' is probably between 40% and 50%. The diagnosis has been entertained at all ages, but the implications may differ.

In up to 30% of children with NSAP, symptoms are recurrent, and many will be submitted to appendicectomy. In eight out of 10 such cases the appendix will be normal. However, in children it is important to rule out acute appendicitis, which is potentially serious if missed, and is eminently treatable as the next most common cause of acute abdominal pain presenting to hospital.

This diagnosis, however, should only be a diagnosis of exclusion in those aged over 50, as over 10% of those presenting (a higher proportion than would be expected) will develop a malignancy within the next 3 years. Additionally, 10% of the over 70s will develop ischaemic heart, abdominal aortic or mesenteric vascular disease over the same time period.

Symptoms and signs

- Acute onset of abdominal pain; may be diffuse but usually in the right iliac fossa.
- Vomiting and anorexia are absent.
- Rarely signs of systemic ill-health such as pyrexia, flushing or tachycardia.
- No signs of peritonism or peritonitis.
- Symptoms usually self-limiting, often disappearing after one night in hospital.

Differential diagnosis

In children and young adults, the chief differential is acute appendicitis. Patients with non-specific abdominal pain more commonly undergo appendicectomy, but have been shown not to have a greater incidence of acute appendicitis.

In those of school age this must be differentiated from the so-called 'functional abdominal pain'. There is often a classical history, and apparently severe pain that thoroughly outweighs any abdominal signs present. This has a basis in psychiatric illness and is very difficult to treat.

Women may have endometriosis, causing abdominal pain in the absence of discrete abdominal signs. A full gynaecological history must be taken, and, if indicated, a thorough pelvic examination must be performed otherwise tubo-ovarian disease may easily be missed.

Though the middle-aged patient with non-specific abdominal pain is at no greater risk of developing peptic ulceration or cholelithiasis, these are common conditions, and it may be advisable to screen for those in this age group.

While an elevated WBC may suggest the presence of a focus of inflammation, a normal count is no guarantee of diagnosis.

Management

A positive diagnosis precludes the need for surgical exploration for treatment or diagnosis. The correct management involves a positive diagnosis of non-specific abdominal pain, reassurance that there is nothing seriously wrong, and discharge from the emergency setting. If a surgical diagnosis cannot be excluded and the patient is admitted, a correct diagnosis may be made upon review the next morning, by which time the symptoms may have resolved. Adults may be given an appointment for a biliary ultrasound scan to exclude gallstones, or an endoscopy to exclude peptic ulceration, and be reviewed in the out-patient clinic. Certainly, if no cause for abdominal pain in a middle-aged patient is apparent after admission to hospital, or a diagnosis of NSAP is made, then some form of follow-up should be offered.

The elderly should not be diagnosed as having non-specific abdominal pain. It is likely that there is some pathology detectable to account for the pain and even if no cause is apparent they should be followed-up in the out-patient clinic.

Further reading

de Dombal FT. Diagnosis and prognosis of patients with non-specific abdominal pain (NSAP). *Current Practice in Surgery*, 1994; **6:** 186–189.

Related topics of interest

Acute appendicitis (p. 4); Assessment of the acute abdomen (p. 41); Irritable bowel syndrome (p. 201).

NUTRITION IN THE SURGICAL PATIENT
Chris Perera

Nutrition plays a vital role in wound healing and collagen maturation, and it boosts the energy reserves of the body. The combination of infection and injury (surgery or trauma) particularly predisposes to malnutrition. These additional stresses inhibit the ketotic response to starvation and encourage the preferential mobilization of muscle protein. The immune response to infection also becomes downregulated and T cell, B cell and macrophage function deteriorates.

Nutritional support

There is evidence of reduction in postoperative complications and length of hospital stay if supplemental sip feeding is started as soon as the patient can take fluid post-operatively. The indications for nutritional support include:

- Protracted post-operative recovery. For example, sepsis.
- Intestinal failure. For example, peritonitis or enterocutaneous fistulae.
- Profound requirements. For example, large burns, major trauma.
- Pre-operative malnutrition. For example, geriatric patients from homes, carcinoma of the oesophagus.
- Unconscious patient. Head-injured patients, ventilated patients in the ICU.

Consequences of surgery

Abdominal operations result in a degree of gut dysfunction, the extent of which depends upon the severity of the disease pathology and on the type and trauma of the surgery. The sequence of intestinal recovery after a laparotomy is often predictable, small bowel recovering first followed by the stomach and then the colon. If enteral nutrition is withheld, functional gut mass reduces, the enterocytes decline in number and the villi flatten. The mucosal barrier then weakens which encourages bacterial translocation into the portal circulation. Endotoxins can be released from these Gram-negative bacteria and lead to endotoxic shock and circulatory failure.

Enteral vs parenteral

The preferred nutritional route is oral or enteral rather than parenteral. Food has a trophic effect on the intestine which is well known for example in the context of the compensatory hyperplasia which occurs in response to intestinal resection and may be mediated by dietary fat. Villous atrophy occurs despite parenteral feeding, perhaps because luminal stimulation is required or because parenteral feeds have lacked glutamine, an important gut fuel.

Enteral feeding

Specialized enteral feeds come in two varieties.

1. *Elemental.* This consists of the L-amino acids and sugars. This diet is non-antigenic and can be as effective as steroids in inducing remission in children with IBD. The main disadvantage is the high osmolarity, which often produces profound diarrhoea.

2. Defined. This is based on milk protein and consists of peptones, medium chain triglycerides and polysaccharides.

There is no need to wait for bowel sounds to commence enteral feeding, which should be started at 10 ml/hour and gradually increased. Six hourly aspiration on the NG tube can ascertain whether the feed is being absorbed.

Percutaneous endoscopic gastrostomy (PEG)

Other methods of feeding should be considered before rushing to parenteral nutrition. The PEG is an ingenious way of placing a gastrostomy. It is achieved by incising over the illuminated tip of the endoscope whilst it is in the stomach and then railroading a feeding tube through the gastric and abdominal puncture hole. Most indications for this procedure are neurological: stroke, motor neurone disease, head injury, bulbar palsy. Complications are few, but can be serious, for example: feeding tube displacement or colonic puncture.

Feeding jejunostomy

A feeding jejunostomy can be positioned at the time of surgery if nutritional support is anticipated post-operatively. Unfortunately, there is no satisfactory indicator of malnutrition pre-operatively. Reduced serum albumin, reduced serum transferrin, triceps skinfold thickness and a diminished absolute lymphocyte count is as good an indicator as clinical judgement.

A purse-string suture is first sewn over a jejunal loop and the feeding tube is then inserted with a trocar into the lumen via a 4-cm submucosal tunnel. The purse-string suture is then carried on to the underside of the abdominal wall in order to keep the jejunum flush with the parietal peritoneum. Unfortunately, these tubes often fall out if not adequately secured. Regular flushing is required to prevent blockage.

Total parenteral nutrition (TPN)

The daily nutritional requirements are 14 g of nitrogen (this must include the essential amino acids), 2000 non-nitrogen calories (including the three essential fatty acids), with added vitamins and minerals (magnesium, selenium, zinc, copper, chromium and manganese are essential trace elements). The essential fatty acids, arachidonic, linoleic and linolenic acid, are required for cell membrane structure and prostaglandin synthesis. This cocktail is usually given by a single 3-l bag into a central vein.

Complications of TPN

TPN, as well as being non-physiological, has a substantial complication rate and occasional mortality.

1. Access. Attempts at subclavian or internal jugular cannulation can produce a pneumothorax, thoracic duct or arterial puncture, or a brachial plexus injury. Advocates of peripheral venous feeding avoid this problem but cannulae need to be changed daily to avoid the irritant nature of a hyperosmolar and low pH solution which readily causes a thrombophlebitis. Long lines from the anticubital fossa to the SVC can avoid this problem. Other complications include central vein thrombosis, air embolism and catheter tip embolism.

2. Infection. Infected lines need to be removed, the tips cultured and the cannulae resited after 24 hours, preferably on the other side. The responsible organisms are usually *Staphylococcus epidermidis or S. aureus* but fungi may also be cultered. Diagnosis is made by inspecting the site, excluding other sources of infection and taking blood cultures through the line itself. Infection risk is minimized by using a tunnelled line (Hickman line), inserting under sterile conditions, avoidance of several side-arm ports and keeping bag changes to a minimum.

3. Metabolic. A multitude of metabolic derangements are common. Daily urea, electrolytes with regular blood glucose monitoring and twice weekly liver function tests are mandatory. Alkaline phophatase and bilirubin levels rise to a plateau after a few days from the cholestasis that TPN produces. Glycosuria, hyperglycaemia and hyperkalaemia indicate glucose intolerance and require the gradual introduction of insulin into the regime.

Glutamine

This dibasic amino acid acts as a shuttle for ammonium from peripheral tissues to the liver and the kidney and its five-carbon skeleton serves as an important fuel for lymphocytes and gastrointestinal mucosal cells, mainly in the small intestine and the colon. Catabolic patients deplete body protein rapidly. Enteral feeds contain 5–8 g of glutamine/100 g protein, but TPN contains none due to stability problems. Glutamine (20 g or more) given parenterally can attenuate the depletion and the gut mucosal atrophy.

A typical regimen for providing enteral or parenteral nutritional support in surgical patients

Fluid/water requirements	25–35 ml/kg/24 h
Protein/nitrogen requirements (1 g nitrogen = 6.25 g protein)	0.15–0.20 g nitrogen/kg/24 h 10–14 g nitrogen/24 h
Energy requirements	25–40 kcal/kg/24 h (rarely >35 kcal/kg/24 h)
Carbohydrate (4 kcal/g) Fat (9 kcal/g)	Usually mixed source with both carbohydrate and fat
Minerals	Calcium 0.11 mmol/kg (± 2.25 mmol) Magnesium 1 mmol/kg (± 2 mmol) Phosphate 2 mmol/kg (± 10 mmol) Zinc 0.3 μmol/kg
Vitamins/trace elements	Fat- and water-soluble vitamins plus additrace

Further reading

Bower RH, Cerra FB, Fershadsky B *et al.* Early enteral administration of formula (IMPACT) supplemented with arginine, nucleotides and fish oil in intensive care patients: results of a multicentre prospective randomised controlled trial. *Critical Care Medicine*, 1997; **23:** 436–449.

Griffiths RD, Jones C, Palmer TE. Six month outcome of critically ill patients given glutamine supplemented parenteral nutrition. *Nutrition*, 1997; **13:** 295–302.

McWhirter JP, Pennington CR. Incidence and recognition of malnutrition in hospital. *British Medical Journal*, 1994; **308:** 945–948.

Spain DA, McClave SA, Sexton LK *et al.* Infusion protocol improves delivery of enteral tube feeding in the critical care unit. *Journal of Parenteral and Enteral Nutrition*, 1999; **23:** 288–292.

Uehara M, Plank LD, Hill GL. Components of energy expenditure in patients with severe sepsis and major trauma: a basis for clinical care. *Critical Care Medicine*, 1999; **27:** 1295–1302.

OESOPHAGEAL CANCER

Simon Gibbs, Christopher Lattimer

The outlook for patients with oesophageal cancer is poor, the overall survival rate at 5 years remaining about 5%. At least 50% of all patients present with inoperable disease. The primary therapeutic aim is prompt and lasting palliation from dysphagia. The condition is twice as common in men, occurring in middle age or the elderly. Northern China has a particularly high incidence of squamous cell carcinoma at 35 per 100 000 (over eight times that seen in Europe and USA), where the disease is seen in younger patients.

Pathology

Worldwide most are squamous cell tumours and associated with poor living conditions. Adenocarcinomas are becoming almost as common now in developed countries. Nearly all cardiac lesions are gastric adenocarcinomas and will be considered under Gastric cancer. Oat cell (small cell undifferentiated) and signet ring types have a particularly poor prognosis. Spread is usually direct along submucosal lymphatics, leading to satellite nodules. Further lymphatic spread is to oesophageal and regional nodes, and haematogenous spread is mainly to the liver and lungs. The length of the tumour, depth of invasion, circumferential and longitudinal resection margins, and node status are the best determinants of survival.

Aetiology

Smoking, heavy alcohol consumption and a diet high in nitrosamines are associated with an increased risk of developing squamous cell carcinoma. The precise cause of the explosion in the incidence of lower oesophageal adenocarcinoma is unknown, although the prolonged use of strong anti-acid therapy is implicated. Duodeno-gastro-oesophageal reflux of bile salts may also be important.

Condition	Increased risk
Achalasia	7×
Barrett's oesophagus	50×
Lye stricture	22×
Post-cricoid web	9×
Peptic stricture	6×

Presentation

The most common presenting symptom is dysphagia. It is relentlessly progressive, starting with solids, then liquids and then the patient's own saliva. Weight loss and wasting are commoner with squamous cell carcinoma. Some adenocarcinomas present with very little weight loss. Unusual presentations include chest pain, cervical lymphadenopathy, left recurrent laryngeal nerve palsy, aspiration pneumonia, jaundice (liver metastasis), preprandial coughing (tracheo-oesophageal fistula) and massive haematemesis (aorto-oesophageal fistula). In Northern China, screening by exfoliative cytology with a net balloon is used to detect early disease.

Examination

Clinical examination consists of a general nutrition assessment (e.g. wasting, cachexia) and the detection of secondary disease (clinical staging), such as a knobbly liver, cervical node or lobar collapse.

Diagnosis

Barium swallow may suggest the diagnosis but the gold standard investigation is upper gastrointestinal endoscopy. The former provides better visualization and a record of the problem with demonstration of the suitability of the stomach for reconstruction. Endoscopy yields material for histology and is better at assessing smaller lesions and lesions of the cardia, unless the lesion is very tight and obstructs passage of the endoscope. The proximal and distal extents of the tumour are measured from the incisor teeth.

Assessment

Once the diagnosis has been made, an attempt to stage the disease is undertaken. If a chest X-ray is clear, a thoracoabdominal CT scan is performed to detect distant metastases if present. Occasionally liver ultrasound may pick up metastases that are missed by CT. If the patient is not fit for surgery, CT is useful prior to any palliative chemo-radiotherapy. If the patient is considered fit for surgery an endoscopic ultrasound scan is arranged. This allows accurate staging of local spread (CT is notoriously unreliable for staging local spread), the tumour being graded between T1–4, N0–1. T1–3 tumours are considered locally operable irrespective of position. Patients with operable adenocarcinomas undergo staging laparoscopy to rule out peritoneal seedling metastases. Patients with operable squamous cell lesions are referred for a staging bronchoscopy to rule out pulmonary invasion. Should the investigations at any point show no chance of complete disease resection, the patient is referred for palliative treatment. If the disease is staged as operable, abstinence from smoking and pre-operative chest physiotherapy all contribute to an improved postoperative recovery. Preoperative pulmonary function tests and echocardiogram allow a much more quantitative assessment of fitness for surgery.

Nutrition

Full nutritional resuscitation with a high-protein liquid diet, supplemented with vitamins and minerals, is advisable. If dysphagia is complete, the obstructing food bolus can occasionally be removed with endoscopy, allowing the placement of a fine-bore feeding tube.

Surgery

There are several surgical approaches.

1. Ivor–Lewis procedure. In this procedure the stomach is mobilized through a midline abdominal incision. The lesion is approached via a right thoracotomy and the anastomosis (usually, jejunal–oesophageal) takes place in the chest. An anastomosis above the azygos vein usually yields better functional results[c].

2. **_McKeown three stage._**   This technique involves the addition of a cervical incision to the last procedure. A cervical anastomosis (usually, gastro–oesophageal) is achieved, and virtually all the oesophagus is removed.

3. **_Ong trans-hiatal dissection._**   In this procedure the thorax is not directly entered. The entire operation is performed via a laparotomy and neck incision. The tumour is dissected free with a hand introduced into the posterior mediastinum, and another passed down behind the manubrium and trachea.

4. **_Abdomino-thoracic oesophago-gastrectomy._**   A laparotomy is performed through an upper abdominal incision parallel to the right costal margin and extending to the left costal margin at the level of the 7th interspace. The stomach is then mobilized and the incision is extended right across the chest to gain access to the tumour. A jejunal loop is anastomosed to the remaining oesophagus. This exposure is only appropriate for lesions of the cardia.

5. **_Trans-thoracic oesophago-gastrectomy._**   As performed by Manson in Swansea, a left thoracotomy is performed and the diaphragm is detached from the chest peripherally, allowing easy exposure of the stomach and the short gastric vessels facilitating their division. This exposure is only appropriate for lesions of the cardia or very lowest part of the oesophagus.

6. **_Extended lymphadenectomy._**   This may be performed in addition to the above procedures to give a more extensive lymph node clearance, and thereby improve survival. Whilst this has been shown to have a significant effect on survival in the Japanese trials[a], no large trials have shown this in Europe to date.

Choice of approach

The advantage of an intrathoracic operation is that direct tumour dissection and lymphatic dissection can be carried out, a necessary requisite for a radical operation. A cervical anastomosis has the obvious advantage that, if it leaks, fatal mediastinitis is less likely. Blunt trans-hiatal dissection can be hazardous if major vessels are inadvertently torn (e.g. the azygous vein). If the integrity of the thorax is preserved, postoperative respiratory complications are reduced. Resection should strive to obtain at least 10 cm of macroscopic clearance if possible.

Continuity

Gastrointestinal continuity is usually restored with stomach after its mobilization on the right gastroepiploic artery. This is achieved by a hand-sewn anastomosis or an EEA staple gun. A pyloromyotomy is usually performed at the end of the operation to encourage early gastric emptying because the vagus nerves have been necessarily divided[c]. Reconstruction with free jejunal transfers or colonic mobilization procedures increases the risk of anastomotic failure[c]. The 30-day operative mortality rate approaches 10%.

Complications

Atelectasis, pneumonia and respiratory failure frequently occur. Specific postoperative complications include left recurrent laryngeal nerve palsy, phrenic nerve injury and chylothorax due to thoracic duct injury. A contrast swallow should be performed at 6–7 days to ascertain anastomotic integrity before oral intake commences[b].

Neoadjuvant treatments

There is now evidence that the pre-operative administration of adjuvant chemotherapy will improve 5-year survival in operable patients[a]. This treatment appears to increase 'operability', and the final decision on operability should be made after this treatment is given[c]. Operating on previously inoperable patients who have been apparently 'downstaged' by this treatment is appropriate but there have been worries about early disease recurrence[c].

Palliation

Non-surgical palliative treatments are divided into radiological and endoscopic techniques to relieve obstruction, chemotherapy, and radiotherapy. Non-surgical procedures are indicated for patients with advanced disease, disabling concomitant medical conditions, and those too infirm by age.

1. Stenting. This is the commonest palliation and has superseded intubation. It can be performed radiologically or endoscopically. The stents are self-expanding, metallic or plastic, covered or non-covered. They treat dysphagia and allow the patient to commence oral nutrition again. Covered stents are the treatment of choice for tracheo-oesophageal fistulae. Obstruction can occur with food bolus, tumour encroachment or migration of the stent. They are used in combination with PPIs which reduce reflux symptoms that often ensue. They are less suitable for upper-third tumours, as they can lead to pharyngeal irritation, intractable pain, and interfere with pharyngeal phase of swallowing.

2. Laser. Polypoid lesions are most suitable for laser therapy, with the neodynium yttrium–aluminium–garnet (YAG) laser, which recanalizes by vaporization[b]. Multiple treatment sessions are necessary, under GA normally. Similar results have been achieved with bipolar diathermy[b]. Endoscopic injection of absolute alcohol is under trial.

3. Radiotherapy. This is used primarily for squamous cell lesions, but can also be given to adenocarcinomas. It is given traditionally by external beam or an intracavity source (brachytherapy). Squamous cell carcinomas are more radiosensitive then adenocarcinomas[c].

4. Chemotherapy. This has some use by itself as a combination of agents though it is usually given in combination with radiotherapy. It is hoped trials of newer agents may yield better results. The palliation provided by combination chemotherapy is brief.

Further reading

Bancewicz J. Palliation in oesophageal neoplasia. *Annals of the Royal College of Surgeons of England*, 1999; **81**: 382–386.

Griffin SM. Surgery for cancer of the oesophagus. In: *Upper Gastrointestinal Surgery – A Companion to Specialist Surgical Practice*, 1997; W.B. Saunders.

Watson A. Operable oesophageal cancer. Current results from the west. *World Journal of Surgery*, 1994; **18**: 361–367.

Related topics of interest

Gastric cancer (p. 135); Nutrition in the surgical patient (p. 233).

OESOPHAGEAL DYSMOTILITY

Simon Gibbs

Oesophageal motility disorders usually present with either dysphagia, chest pain or both. Endoscopy excludes an obstructive cause within the oesophagus and cardiac investigations are normal. Neurological causes such as CVA are ruled out. The dysphagia is characteristically intermittent and worse for liquids than solids. This alerts the investigator that the cause is not likely to be obstructive if dysphagia is progressive and worse for solids first. Pain may occur on swallowing (odynophagia) or be retrosternal and crushing in character.

Classification

Classification is into primary motor disorders, when only the oesophagus is involved, and secondary motor disorders, when the oesophagus is involved as part of a systemic condition.

Primary	Secondary
Cricopharangeal spasm	Amyloidosis
Diffuse oesophageal spasm	Scleroderma
Nutcracker oesophagus	Presbyoesophagus
Achalasia	Diabetes mellitus
Non-specific disorders	Chagas' disease
	GORD

Investigation

Investigation is by barium swallow, endoscopy and oesophageal manometry.

1. Barium swallow. The salient radiological features include barium filling of a cricopharyngeal spasm-related pouch, the corkscrew oesophagus in diffuse oesophageal spasm, the mega-oesophagus in Chagas' disease and achalasia and the 'rat-tail' narrowing at the distal oesophagus in achalasia with 'flocculation' of barium above the food residue. Fluoroscopic screening with barium or barium-coated bread or marshmallow provides a greater visualization of disordered peristalsis[c].

2. Endoscopy. This is helpful in excluding an obstructing lesion, such as carcinoma or stricture, by unhindered passage of the scope into the stomach. It can also provide tissue samples for histology.

3. Manometry. Oesophageal manometry permits assessment of oesophageal motor function and is essential for an accurate diagnosis. In static manometry, pressure transducers are placed 5 cm apart along the oesophagus (25 cm long), and pressures are recorded against time allowing a manometric profile to be generated both at rest and in response to wet swallows. Abnormal features include high resting sphincter pressures, inadequate sphincter relaxation and incoordination of sphincter activity. Non-propagated peristalsis, peristaltic velocity and the normal 'after-contraction' of the lower oesophageal sphincter can also be recorded. The primary peristaltic wave normally travels at 2–4 cm/s, lasts 4 s at any one point and produces an occlusive pressure of 30–120 mmHg. Distension of the lower oesophagus results in a secondary peristaltic wave.

Cricopharyngeal spasm and pharyngeal pouch

Cricopharyngeal spasm presents in the elderly with the feeling of a lump in the throat. Occasionally, external compression from cervical adenopathy or thyroid enlargement may present in this way. The diagnosis is made by manometry when a high resting upper oesophageal sphincter (UOS) pressure, sphincter incoordination and impaired sphincter relaxation may be recorded, in the presence of a normal CT scan. If severe, treatment by cricopharyngeal myotomy should be considered.

A pharyngeal pouch (Zenker's diverticulum) may develop as a result of chronically high UOS pressure. This is a true pulsion diverticulum occurring at the pharyngo-oesophageal junction (Killian's dehiscence). Whilst some studies have clearly shown high UOS pressures in association with these pouches others have shown normal pressures[b] (however, UOS pressure is notoriously difficult to measure). The pouch gradually enlarges until food starts to collect within it and this compresses the upper oesophagus to produce the clinical symptoms of latent regurgitation, nocturnal aspiration and a palpable lump (usually on the left). Squamous carcinoma occurs in 10% of cases[c]. Diagnosis is made by barium swallow because pouch perforation is a recognized complication of endoscopy and manometry is difficult. Treatment is by pouch excision and primary closure through a lateral cervical incision. A cricopharyngeal myotomy over 2–3 cm is then performed.

A more minimally invasive technique for elderly patients with smaller pouches is to introduce an endoscopic GIA stapler through the mouth and fire it whilst grasping the distal portion of the pouch neck (this will by definition cut the underlying cricopharyngeus).

Nutcracker oesophagus

This is the commonest manometric abnormality characterized by propagated very high pressure contractions (at least two standard deviations above normal). It usually causes chest pain (97%) rather than dysphagia (10%) and often progresses eventually to diffuse oesophageal spasm or achalasia[b]. The bouts of chest pain however correlate poorly with the pressure spikes, and manometry may be normal at times with the diagnosis only being proven at a follow up manometry. Treatment is primarily with a calcium channel blocker such as Nifedipine[c]. Dilatation by bougienage has also been effective, although Winters et al. (1984) found that 'placebo bougienage' was just as effective suggesting contact with the doctor was probably more important than the dilatation itself[b]. Long myotomy may be necessary in severe cases.

Diffuse oesophageal spasm

Diffuse oesophageal spasm presents with dysphagia both for liquids and solids, and chest pain and is precipitated by eating and anxiety. In this condition dysphagia rather than chest pain is the dominating symptom. A barium swallow can diagnose extreme cases by demonstrating the characteristic 'corkscrew' oesophageal appearance. Manometry is essential for diagnosis when high-pressure non-propagated contractions are recorded in the presence of other normal contractions. Thus regurgitation is uncommon unlike achalasia. Treatment is with glycerol trinitrate or calcium channel blockers[b]. Oesophageal dilatation or a long myotomy may be necessary in refractory cases.

Achalasia

Achalasia (cardiospasm) is a functional obstruction at the lower oesophageal sphincter characterized manometrically by a high resting sphincter pressure with failure of relaxation and impaired oesophageal body peristalsis. Histologically, there is a reduction in the number of ganglion cells in the myenteric plexus. The condition affects both sexes equally and presents with a long history of intermittent dysphagia. An erect chest radiograph may demonstrate a widened mediastinum, an air/fluid level, aspiration pneumonitis and absence of the gastric air bubble. The 'rat-tail' appearance of the lower oesophagus after a barium swallow is characteristic. Pharmacological treatment with anticholinergics, nitrites or calcium antagonists is mostly unsatisfactory. Endoscopic injection of Botulinum toxin has been used recently with some success but needs repeated procedures[b]. Controlled pneumatic dilatation under radiological screening with a balloon passed over a guidewire is successful in over 75% of patients[b]. Surgery is the most effective management and involves a single anterior myotomy at the cardia (Heller)[b]. The longer the oesophageal myotomy the greater the incidence of postoperative reflux which is why a 'generous' myotomy should be covered with a partial fundoplication[c]. In advanced cases resection may be necessary. Endoscopic surveillance should be carried out every 2 years as the condition is pre-malignant for squamous cell carcinoma[c].

Scleroderma

This systemic disorder causes fibrosis within the smooth muscle portion of the oesophagus. This leads to dysphagia and heartburn (due to acid reflux), and these patients have a high incidence of Barrett's oesophagus[b]. Since the upper third of the oesophagus is largely unaffected, the motility trace is very characteristic showing essentially normal propagated swallows in the upper third with profound hypo-motility of the lower two thirds and decreased LOS pressure. The distal oesophagus may also be grossly dilated. Treatment includes PPIs, bougienage for strictures, and anti-reflux surgery.

Reflux-induced motility disorder

Patients with GORD refractory to PPI treatment, or with endoscopic stigma of GORD, should be referred for pH and manometry prior to a fundoplication procedure. It is often noted that there is a manometric abnormality of the lower oesophagus with low amplitude, disordered contractions, resulting in poor peristalsis. This is classically associated with chronic acid reflux into the oesophagus and will recover to a greater degree after fundoplication is performed. If other manometric abnormalities are discovered then further investigations such as CT and neurological screens should be performed prior to fundoplication, as GORD may not be the cause of the symptoms. In some patients with GORD there is upper oesophageal sphincter spasm leading to dysphagia[c] but this is much more uncommon.

Paraneoplastic syndrome

Rarely patients with lung tumours may present with neuromuscular dysphagia. The tumour, usually oat cell, secretes peptides which have a direct effect on oesophageal motility, promoting disordered contraction. A chest X-ray will often show the tumour, suggesting the diagnosis.

Further reading

Evans DF, Robertson CS. Pathophysiology and investigation of GORD and motility disorders. In: *Upper Gastrointestinal Surgery – A Companion to Specialist Surgical Practice*, 1997; W.B. Saunders.

Griffiths Pearson F *et al. Neuromuscular disorders – Part V: Esophageal Surgery*, 1995; Churchill Livingstone.

Watson A. Oesophageal function and motility disorders. *Recent Advances in Surgery*, 1993; **16:** 63–86.

Related topics of interest

Gastro-oesophageal reflux (p. 146); Oesophageal cancer (p. 237).

ORGAN TRANSPLANTATION: PRINCIPLES

Nick Lagattolla

Before the 1970s the inevitable result of severe renal, hepatic, pulmonary or cardiac failure in children and young adults was an early death. Organ transplantation has dramatically altered the prognosis for many sufferers, particularly renal. More recently, hepatic and pancreatic transplants have offered new promise for terminal liver failure and diabetes mellitus.

Donor origin

All currently undertaken organ transplants are allogeneic in nature, defined as the transplantation of an organ from a different individual of the same species. These include live-related and cadaveric organs, which are termed allografts. A live-related donor may only be a source of a kidney or a hepatic segment, whereas cadaveric organ transplants include renal, hepatic, cardiac, pulmonary, corneal, cutaneous, intestinal, pancreatic or combinations. Xenografts are still totally experimental and are generally porcine in origin.

History

Because of the paired nature of the kidney, human renal allografting was investigated as early as the 1930s, though without success. The first reports of successful transplantation between identical siblings was not until the 1950s. The first successful cadaveric renal transplants were reported in 1963. Heart transplants have been performed since 1967 after Christian Barnard first successfully performed the procedure. Liver, pancreatic and corneal transplantation were also pioneered in the late 1960s.

Major advances in immunology research and immunosuppressant pharmacology occurred in the 1960s resulting in this decade as the dawn of the transplant age. Transplant programmes, most prominantly renal, have been running since this time. Technical improvements, particularly in organ harvesting and storage, improved immunosuppression, and greater public awareness in donation have greatly enhanced the effectiveness of transplantation.

More recently, massive intestinal transplants in children and adult limb transplants have not fared particularly well as yet, though both have been undertaken. Combined heart-lung transplantation is feasible for end-stage pulmonary failure, a procedure that may carry better results than single lung transplantation, and that is technically less demanding than it sounds.

Histocompatability

Cell membrane-bound glycoproteins called human leukocyte antigens (HLA) incorporate the gene product of a complex found on the short arm of chromosome 6. There are two classes of HLA antigens, HLA-I and HLA-II and both confer histocompatability. The term leukocyte in HLA reflects the cell type upon which they were first identified; HLA-I and HLA-II are present on all cell surfaces, and it is these antigens that are responsible for sensitizing T-lymphocytes to foreign proteins.

The HLA-I class gene has A, B and C loci and the HLA-II class gene has three loci termed DP, DQ and DR. Histocompatability matching is undertaken at the HLA-A, HLA-B and HLA-DR loci. Compatability at the last locus carries the greatest significance in terms of achieving a good match.

Rejection and immunosuppression

This is the consequence of the host body reaction to foreign antigens. Rejection can be hyperacute, acute or chronic. Hyperacute rejection follows previous exposure to foreign HLA antigens, as might occur after homologous blood transfusion or previous transplant exposure. Circulating recipient anti-HLA antibodies will instantly identify and bind donor endothelial HLA antigens with ensuing intravascular coagulation and graft failure.

Immediate or very early failure of an organ transplant may not be due to an immunological process. Technical complications such as arterial or venous insufficiency or outflow tract obstruction, or failure of the donor organ to survive ex-vivo are important causes of early failure. Technical failures require instant diagnosis and surgery to restore function if the graft is to survive.

Acute rejection is mostly T-lymphocyte mediated. Recipient T-lymphocytes become sensitized to donor HLA antigens. Stimulated further by recipient macrophage-derived interleukin-1, the T-lymphocytes produce interleukin-2 which induces clonal expansion of the T-lymphocytes, and their transformation into cytotoxic T-cells. Complex cytotoxic interactions supervene, with resultant donor organ damage. Chronic rejection may represent the end result of an attenuated acute rejection process, with supra-added characteristic donor organ fibrosis. Progressive graft failure occurs over months or years.

Without pharmacological means of suppressing these cytotoxic immunological events, all non-related HLA-dissimilar allografts would be rejected. Triple prophylactic therapy using cyclosporine, azathioprine and prednisolone is used to mediate rejection. Cyclosporine is an intracellular calmodulin inhibitor which effectively blocks the clonal expansion of T-lymphocytes. Azathioprine is metabolized to mercaptopurine which has diverse immunosuppressive actions. Systemic immunoglobulins and monoclonal antibodies are alternative strategies.

Further reading

Lafferty K, Prowse S, Simeonovic C, Warren HS. Immunobiology of tissue transplantation. In: Paul WE, Fathman CG, Metzgar PJ, eds. *Annual Review of Immunology*, 1983; 143–173.

Mason DW, Morris PJ. Effector mechanisms in allograft rejection. *Annual Review of Immunology*, 1986; **4:** 119–145.

Serup P, Madsen OD, Mandrup-Poulsen T. Islet and stem cell transplantation for treating diabetes. *British Medical Journal*, 2001; **322:** 29–32.

PANCREATIC CANCER

Nick Lagattolla

Carcinoma of the pancreas is a highly malignant growth of the acinar cells of the exocrine pancreas. It affects about 10/100000 population, and the incidence is rising. Two males are affected for every female. It is rare before the age of 45, and thereafter the incidence rises progressively with age. Aetiological factors include smoking, which approximately doubles the risk, possibly an elevated dietary fat intake and diabetes mellitus.

Pathology

Sixty per cent of pancreatic carcinomas occur in the head of the gland. Spread rapidly occurs to draining lymph nodes and local structures. The common bile duct is frequently invaded and obstructed, causing obstructive jaundice. The pancreatic duct is also invaded, and acute pancreatitis may result. Carcinomas of the head may spare the common bile duct but invade the duodenum and obstruct it, resulting in gastric outlet obstruction. Whether the common bile duct or duodenum is obstructed first, such is the rapid progression of the tumour that obstruction of the other frequently occurs.

Clinical examination

Thirty to sixty per cent of patients present with obstructive jaundice. Pain occurs in 50% and is usually felt in the back. This is usually indicative of a particularly poor prognosis, suggesting that the malignancy has eroded into posteriorly related prevertebral structures. Abdominal pain may, however, be the only presenting feature. Loss of weight is rapid and progressive, and occurs in 80% of cases. Less typical symptoms include: diarrhoea, general malaise, abdominal distension, nausea and vomiting. Trousseau's sign is migrating superficial thrombophlebitis (thrombophlebitis migrans) and this may occur in occult pancreatic carcinoma.

Clinical examination rarely identifies an abdominal mass. However, in the presence of painless jaundice, a palpable gall bladder suggests that the jaundice is not due to gallstones, but rather is due to a malignant obstruction of the common bile duct, usually a pancreatic carcinoma (Courvoisier's law). Transcoelomic spread may occur, resulting in ascites, and spread to the liver may cause hepatomegaly, which may be easily palpable in an emaciated abdomen.

Investigations

- Ultrasound is used to confirm a dilated extrahepatic biliary tree, and may visualize a mass in the head of the pancreas.
- CT scanning should be performed to enable the size of the tumour to be assessed, along with the liver for metastases, and spread to local structures that would affect the resectability of the tumour, such as the portal vein. Tumours in the body or tail of the pancreas can be confirmed by CT scanning.
- A histological diagnosis is essential to guide further management, as occasionally, chronic pancreatitis may present with obstructive jaundice or cause a

localized pancreatic mass. Rarely, tumours in the pancreas may be benign. CT- or ultrasound-guided percutaneous fine-needle aspirate or biopsy usually provides a diagnosis.

- ERCP may be used to obtain samples for cytology from the pancreatic or common bile duct.

Treatment

The aim of the above staging procedures is to assess the tumour with a view to resection, which is the only chance of cure. Tumours greater than 2 cm in diameter and those that have spread to the liver or lymphatics are not curable by surgery. The operation to resect a carcinoma of the pancreas is a radical Whipple's procedure for tumours in the head or body, and distal pancreatectomy with splenectomy for tumours in the tail. If resection is not possible, or if the patient is unfit for major surgery, the prognosis is dismal. Frequently, despite adequate pre-operative investigations, a tumour is found to be unresectable only after an exploratory laparotomy with a trial of dissection of the pancreas. This may be due to invasion of vital local structures, or the presence of hitherto unknown lymphatic involvement. Ultimately, less than 10% of cases are amenable to surgical resection, and a cure may be achieved in less than 1%.

Prognosis

The mean survival after diagnosis is 6 months without resection, with only 10% of patients still alive at 1 year. Following resection, the 5-year survival is 4%, but there is a 10–20% operative mortality rate.

The prognosis is much better if the carcinoma is found to arise from the ampulla of Vater. This presents in an identical fashion to carcinoma of the head of the pancreas, and if treated conservatively has the same appalling prognosis, but if it is resected, the survival rate after 5 years is 15%.

Surgical palliation

Obstructive jaundice is best relieved by stenting the malignant biliary stricture. This can be performed at ERCP, or as a radiological procedure using a percutaneous transhepatic route through dilated biliary radicles, gaining entry into the common bile duct from above. Self-expanding stents offer excellent palliation in the short term, but may become blocked, and may migrate. They can, however, be replaced. The procedures used to place them are performed under local anaesthesia under sedation. They may be used as a temporary measure to relieve a patient of severe jaundice while surgery is planned. Transhepatic stenting offers an advantage in that an external biliary drain may be left in situ to decompress the biliary tree, and this may be useful should oedema occur at the stented site inhibiting free drainage, or as access for cholangiography or for further procedures.

Open surgery has a role in the palliation of symptoms should minimally invasive procedures fail. Jaundice is relieved by means of a biliary bypass, best achieved using a loop cholecystojejunostomy or a choledochojejunostomy fashioned as a Roux-en-Y. As many patients later additionally develop duodenal obstruction, the stomach is bypassed prophylactically by means of an antecolic gastrojejunostomy. The afferent and efferent limbs of the loop of jejunum used in the biliary bypass may be anastomosed to avoid small bowel contents passing to the biliary tree.

Endocrine pancreatic tumours

Tumours derived from endocrine cells and which are therefore active endocrinologically are insulinoma, glucagonoma, VIPoma (vasoactive intestinal polypeptide) and gastrinoma. Rarer tumours derived from exocrine portions are cystadenoma and its malignant form cystadenocarcinoma. Tumours of the ampulla of Vater are usually malignant, however, rarely, benign adenomyomas are encountered.

1. Insulinoma. These produce insulin and present with features of hyperinsulinaemia often referred to as Whipple's Triad. This comprises syncopal episodes during which there is proven hypoglycaemia, the episodes being reversed by the administration of glucose, and the reproduction of the same syncope by fasting. Though most insulinomas are benign, there is a malignant potential, and these tumours are best treated surgically. In some cases, a malignant insulinoma may already have metastasized at presentation, or possibly no tumour can be localized at all. Then surgery has little to offer, and medical treatment with diazoxide is started.

2. Glucagonoma. These are usually benign and present with diabetes mellitus and weight loss due to the overproduction of glucagon. They also produce a peculiar but typical circular erythematous truncal skin rash. Symptoms may be controlled with insulin.

3. Vipoma. These produce vasoactive intestinal polypeptide, and present with profuse, watery diarrhoea. The inhibitory intestinal peptide somatostatin, or its synthetic analogue octreotide can be used to control the diarrhoea, or the tumour can be localized and resected.

4. Gastrinoma. These present with recurrent peptic ulceration. Sixty per cent of these are malignant, and they are best resected. However, up to 30% of gastrinomas lie outside the pancreas, and localization may prove very difficult.

Further reading

Glazer G, Coulter C, Croyton ME. Controversial issues in the management of pancreatic cancer. *Annals of the Royal College of Surgeons*, 1995; **77**: 111–122, 174–180.
Rothmund M. Localization of endocrine pancreatic tumours. *British Journal of Surgery*, 1994; **81**: 164–166.
Watanapa P, Williamson RCN. Surgical palliation for pancreatic carcinoma. *British Journal of Surgery*, 1992; **79**: 8–20.

Related topic of interest

Jaundice – investigation (p. 203).

PENILE CONDITIONS AND SCROTAL SWELLINGS

Christopher Lattimer, Omar Faiz

Penile conditions

Phimosis

This condition arises due to a narrow preputal meatus. The foreskin cannot usually be retracted until 3 years of age. In children phimosis presents with recurrent balanitis, ballooning on micturition and UTIs. In adults this condition is acquired and occurs secondary to chronic balanitis. Occasionally, the opening in the foreskin is so small that urinary outflow obstruction ensues. Foreskin fissuring and pain is common during sexual intercourse. These patients are best treated with circumcision.

Paraphimosis

This condition occurs when a tight foreskin is retracted behind the glans penis resulting in progressive glandular engorgement. It may follow masturbation, intercourse or retraction during urination. A tight foreskin predisposes towards the development of this condition. Emergency treatment involves manual reduction; however, if this fails, a dorsal split procedure followed by an elective circumcision is required.

Balanitis xerotica obliterans

This condition is equivalent to lichen sclerosis et atrophicus in the female. It presents as chronic balanitis which often involves the urethral meatus and is characterized by a fibrous plaque which welds the foreskin to the glans.

Circumcision

The medical indications for circumcision are phimosis, paraphimosis, chronic balanitis and vesico-ureteric reflux. There is no medical indication for neonatal circumcision, but it can be performed for religious reasons. The contraindications to circumcision include hypospadias and other conditions, such as urethral stricture, where the foreskin may be necessary for the formation of a urinary conduit. The procedure involves separation of the foreskin from the glans and then removal of the foreskin by direct dissection leaving an adequate cuff of 'mucosa' which is then sutured to the skin. Bipolar diathermy should be used as the inadvertent use of monopolar diathermy can result in penile necrosis. In neonatal circumcision a plastibell dome is placed between the separated glans and the foreskin. A ligature is then tightened around the foreskin at its base. After 7–10 days a natural separation occurs.

Carcinoma

Squamous cell carcinoma of the penis occurs more commonly in uncircumcised men often in association with a poor standard of hygiene. Circumcised males rarely develop the disease. It is predominantly locally invasive but can spread to inguinal lymph nodes. Distant metastases are extremely rare. Presentation occurs late as the lesions lie beneath the foreskin. Primary treatment for small lesions is by external beam radiotherapy or laser therapy[b], however recurrences require excision. Occasionally radical excision is indicated with complete genito-scrotal clearance leaving a permanent perineal urostomy. Trials have commenced to determine whether primary chemotherapy can downstage advanced carcinomas thereby making them amenable to surgery[b].

Erythroplasia of Queryat

This condition presents as a deep red lesion over the whole surface of the glans. Histology reveals a carcinoma-in-situ. Treatment with topical 5-fluorouracil is usually curative.

Penile warts

Penile warts (condylomata lata) are sexually transmitted. They are caused by human papillomaviruses (HPV). Glandular or foreskin warts can be treated topically with 5-fluorouracil cream, podophyllin or scissor excision. Urethral warts require urethroscopic excision or diathermy.

Impotence

Impotence may be caused by vascular, neurological, psychological, post-surgical, pharmacological or endocrine factors. The preservation of early morning tumescence is suggestive of a psychological cause. Intracorporeal prostaglandin and papaverine injections or inflatable prostheses are of benefit in a minority of patients. Recently however Sildenafil (Viagra), an agent taken orally that increases penile blood flow, has become available. Viagra can only be prescribed on the NHS under circumstances where the impact of impotence is marked on the patient's social activities, mood or interpersonal relationships.

Priapism

This condition is associated with sickle cell anaemia, leukaemia, spinal cord injury and pelvic malignancy. Typically the corpora cavernosa are erect whilst the glans and corpus spongiosum remain flaccid. Initial detumescence therapy is achieved by trans-glandular corpus cavernosal aspiration. In resistant cases, a corpora-saphenous shunt is required. This procedure is usually successful and 50% of patients retain potency[c].

Peyronie's disease

In this condition a fibrous plaque is responsible for producing either dorsal or lateral curvature of the penis when erect. This condition is associated with penile trauma, retroperitoneal fibrosis, desmoid tumours, Dupytren's contracture and Reidel's thyroiditis. The diagnosis is best established by a Polaroid photograph but clinically the scarred corpora can usually be palpated. The efficacy of medical treatment including Vitamin E and aminobenzoic acid has not been clearly established[b]. Surgical treatment involves producing an artificial erection by intracorporeal injection of saline and either excising the plaque or plicating the opposite side with reefing sutures (Nesbit's procedure).

Scrotal swellings

Hydrocele

Hydroceles are classified into four types.

*1. **Vaginal hydrocele.*** This is the commonest type of hydrocele. It arises as a serous fluid collection within the tunica vaginalis. Vaginal hydroceles occur most commonly as a primary condition, however, it can also arise secondary to other scrotal pathology such as: tumours, orchitis, torsion or following hernia repair. Aspiration therapy is simple, and although recurrence is inevitable, this can be used for patients who are elderly and unfit for general anaesthesia. Differing approaches have been described for definitive surgical treatment. The commonly utilized procedures include: hydrocele excision, Jaboulay's sac eversion technique, the bloodless operation of Lord involving sac plication, and Wilkinson's operation where the testis is placed outside the tunica.

*2. **Congenital hydrocele.*** In this condition fluid collects within a patent processus vaginalis. The hydrocele connects with the general peritoneal cavity and, consequently, increases in intra-abdominal pressure are transmitted to the hydrocele. Although the connection is usually too small for intra-abdominal contents to pass through, this type of hydrocele is best considered as a hernia presenting in infancy or early childhood with only fluid filling of the sac.

*3. **Infantile hydrocele.*** In this type of hydrocele the processus vaginalis is obliterated at the deep ring leaving a fluid collection anterior to the testis and cord.

*4. **Hydrocele of the cord.*** This occurs when part of the processus vaginalis separates leaving a discrete fluid collection at that site. On clinical examination the hydrocele can be palpated along the spermatic cord. Specifically, the swelling is separate from the testicle, one can get above it and it descends with downwards testicular traction.

Epididymal cysts

These are often multiple and can be palpated separately from the testis. They usually contain clear fluid, however when the contents are cloudy they are termed spermatoceles. A spermatocele is a retention cyst of the epididymis whereas the more usual epididymal cyst results from focal epididymal degeneration. Large size and local pain are the usual indications for cyst removal.

Torsion

This condition peaks in incidence during the teens and is rare after 35 years of age when epididymitis becomes the commoner cause of scrotal pain. Torsion occurs more commonly in undescended testes, as normal descent is usually associated with a secure, non-rotating testis in the scrotum. Three anatomical factors predispose towards torsion. These include: *testicular inversion,* where the testis lies transversely or upside down; *high investment of the tunica vaginalis,* which results in the testis hanging like a clapper in a bell and; *true torsion* which results from separation of the epididymis from the testis permitting twisting between these two structures. Patients present with sudden pain, often with similar previous episodes, and an extremely tender testicle. Colour Duplex sonography and technetium scanning can confirm the diagnosis[b] but delay for these investigations to be performed is unacceptable and emergency exploration is required for all suspected torsions. Controversial evidence suggests that an immune reaction may be lodged in response to the infarcted testicle with immunological sensitization to sperm leading to infertility in some cases[b]. A midline incision confirms the diagnosis and allows fixation of the opposite testis (orchidopexy). Gangrenous testes should be removed but those of dubious viability should be left in situ.

Varicocele

This is a varicose dilatation of the pampiniform plexus, or cremasteric veins which surround the lower spermatic cord. Nearly all varicoceles (95%) arise on the left side. This may be due to an absent valve in the terminal testicular vein where it drains into the left renal vein. Examination of the patient reveals a scrotal swelling which is likened to a 'bag of worms'. Varicocele may cause infertility in some men[b]. Definitive treatment is either by surgery or selective testicular vein embolization. The former involves exposure of the testicular artery by the high retroperitoneal approach and ligation of its surrounding veins (Palomo procedure).

Further reading

Cuckow PM, Frank JD. Torsion of the testis. *BJU International*, 2000; **86**(3): 349–353.
Demas BE, Hricak H *et al.* Varicoceles. Radiological diagnosis and treatment. *Radiology Clinics of North America*, 1991; **29**(3): 619–627.
Pizzocaro G, Piva L *et al.* Up-to-date management of carcinoma of the penis. *European Urology*, 1997; **32**(1): 5–15.

Related topics of interest

Common paediatric conditions (p. 96); Inguinal hernia (p. 179); Testicular tumours (p. 319).

PEPTIC ULCERATION

Simon Gibbs, Christopher Lattimer

A peptic ulcer is the final morphological result of the interplay between the aggressive acid-peptic forces and the mucosal resistance to ulceration. Whilst acid attack is a marked feature of duodenal ulcer (DU), impaired mucosal resistance appears to be more important for gastric ulcer (GU). The discovery of *Helicobacter pylori* (HP), and the introduction of H_2 receptor antagonists, and more lately proton pump inhibitors (PPIs), has resulted in a dramatic decrease in the need for surgical intervention.

Duodenal ulcer (DU)

Epidemiology

DU disease has declined in prevalence over the past 30 years and is now occurring in a progressively older population. Previously, half of all operations performed for DU were done for pain, but now over 98% are performed as an urgent intervention for complications: perforation, haemorrhage or obstruction. Mortality rates for emergency surgery have changed little for 20 years despite an increase in the overall age of the patient at emergency operation. *H. pylori* (HP) infection is common and associated with low social class and poor living conditions.

Risk factors

Cigarette smoking, stress, NSAIDs, corticosteroids and infection with HP are risk factors for DU development. NSAIDs deplete endogenous mucosal prostaglandin making the mucosa more susceptible to ulceration. Smoking impairs ulcer healing, accelerates gastric emptying, increases acid secretion and decreases pancreatic bicarbonate secretion. HP is postulated to induce areas of chronic inflammation and metaplasia that are much more susceptible to acid attack. About 90–95% of patients with a DU are HP positive on urease testing and thus any patient that presents with a DU should have a course of eradication therapy[b]. Most people with HP infection however, do not develop ulcers. The continued presence of HP can be detected by a hydrogen breath test.

Physiology

Duodenal ulceration is associated with higher mean basal acid and maximal acid outputs often with reduced bicarbonate secretion by the duodenal mucosa. Gastric emptying is usually rapid and the total parietal cell mass is enlarged. The presence of multiple ulcers in the first and second part of the duodenum should raise the possibility of Zollinger-Ellison syndrome (hypergastrinaemia secondary to a gastrinoma).

Medical treatment

Cessation of smoking and the intake of NSAIDs and alcohol, a change to a less stressful lifestyle, and a period of bed rest are general measures proven to be effective for helping to heal ulcers[c]. The profound acid suppression induced by therapy with H_2 antagonists or PPIs has largely obviated the need for elective operations for ulcer pain such as proximal gastric vagotomy (parietal cell vagotomy, highly selective vagotomy). It is now established beyond reasonable doubt that duodenal ulceration is almost always associated with HP infection. HP may also play a lesser role in gastric ulceration. Eradication of this organism with triple therapy (amoxycillin 1000 mg b.d., clarithromycin 500 mg b.d., omeprazole 20 mg b.d.) heals the ulcer with rates better than those of H_2 antagonists alone and considerably reduces recurrence[a]. Re-infection does appear to occur but the mechanism of this is as yet unknown.

Elective surgical treatment

Elective duodenal ulcer surgery is now uncommon. It is indicated in patients with resistant ulcers despite eradication therapy, or who are non-compliant with medical therapy, or who are chronically dependent on NSAIDs. Truncal vagotomy is the most commonly performed operation although very few are actually undertaken. The vagotomy must be high enough to get all nerves to the stomach including the 'criminal nerves of grassi' which come off the main vagal trunks very early. Truncal vagotomy results in extensive parasympathetic denervation of the gastrointestinal tract and may produce long-term problems such as gallstones and diarrhoea. A truncal vagotomy requires a gastric drainage procedure (gastroenterotomy or pyloroplasty) which in itself may promote bilious vomiting, chronic gastritis, stomal ulceration and an increased risk of gastric adenocarcinoma. Increased gastric emptying may also predispose to diarrhoea and the early (osmotic) and late (hypoglycaemic) dumping syndromes. Some of these complications can be avoided by employing a selective vagotomy (which preserves the coeliac and hepatic branches, but still requires a drainage procedure). A highly selective vagotomy (which also preserves the terminal branches of the gastric nerves which are relaxant to the pylorus, thereby avoiding the need for a drainage procedure) may also reduce complications. The mortality from vagotomy is low (0.1–0.3%)[b], and all these operations can now be performed laparoscopically by experts.

Surgery for complications

1. Perforation. Sudden onset of pain with peritonitis is the usual emergency presentation but these symptoms are masked in the elderly or patients on steroids or immunosuppressives. Sub-diaphragmatic air is present on an erect chest radiograph in 70% of patients[b]. Maintenance of the upright position 10 min prior to taking the film further increases the detection rate of a perforation. A right lateral decubitus film or a water-soluble contrast swallow may also aid diagnosis. Management involves fluid resuscitation, antibiotics and surgery if the patient is fit enough. Direct ulcer suture, omental patch placement and a thorough abdominal lavage with tube drainage of the right upper quadrant is the commonest procedure. A partial gastrectomy is required if the ulcer is huge and closure would result in duodenal stenosis. Patients who are unfit for surgery can be managed conservatively. All patients should be given a course of triple therapy against HP. Patients with a definitive aetiology (NSAIDs) or those not previously taking H_2 antagonists or PPIs, should have appropriate postoperative anti-ulcer advice (such as advice against smoking, alcohol, stress, and avoiding further NSAID ingestion etc.). Follow up endoscopy is only required if symptoms recur after cessation of medical therapy.

2. Obstruction. DUs may cause outlet obstruction by scarring, oedema or impaired gastric motility. Barium meal often helps in the diagnosis, by demonstrating an ulcer and showing an enlarged stomach. Clinically a 'succussion splash' may be present. Endoscopy confirms a 'stomach lake' and a tight pylorus. Initial management should involve PPI therapy and nasogastric decompression for 3–5 days to allow any oedema to settle. Failure to re-establish motility and the presentation of a severely malnourished patient are indications for surgery. A gastroenterostomy is usually required.

3. Haemorrhage. This is discussed elsewhere (see Upper gastrointestinal haemorrhage).

Gastric ulcer

Epidemiology

Gastric ulcers (GUs) were commoner in young women before the 1970s and presented with perforation. Now they are relatively uncommon and present in the elderly with bleeding. The role of surgery is almost exclusively limited to the complications of the disease.

Risk factors

These include tobacco, alcohol, cocaine and HP infection. Approximately 10% of people taking NSAIDs have an acute gastric ulcer (H_2 receptor antagonists or PPIs should be taken concomitantly with NSAIDs). GUs frequently develop in inflamed, atrophic or metaplastic gastric mucosa. They are most frequently found near the incisura on the lesser curve in close approximation to an atherosclerotic left gastric artery. Pre-pyloric ulcers behave like DUs but are ineffectively treated by operations for DU. Differentiation from a malignant ulcer is essential. At endoscopy all such ulcers require four-quadrant biopsy.

Barium meal

This may be useful in aiding diagnosis particularly prior to endoscopy. It may show classic 'hour-glass' cicatrization or 'kissing ulcers' on either side of the stomach.

Complications

1. Perforation. Perforated GUs usually require operative intervention. Ulcer excision, either locally or by partial gastrectomy is recommended, except for small benign pre-pyloric ulcers which may be treated by oversewing like a perforated DU. The lesser sac should always be explored in patients where no site for peritonitis is discovered because posterior GUs can be missed. Excision is difficult with large or high posterior ulcers and a partial gastrectomy may be necessary [c].

2. Obstruction. GUs obstruct by producing gastric atony [c]. They also cause severe malnutrition, general ill health and anaemia. They are often large and heal slowly.

Antrectomy with inclusion of the ulcer is the preferred operation for obstruction[c]. Reconstruction is achieved with a roux-en-Y anastomosis.

3. Haemorrhage. This is discussed elsewhere (see Upper gastrointestinal haemorrhage).

Further reading

Johnson AG. Management of peptic ulcer. *British Journal of Surgery*, 1994; **81:** 161–163.
Stabile BE, Passaro E. Surgery for duodenal and gastric ulcer disease. *Advances in Surgery*, 1993; **26:** 275–306.

Related topics of interest

Meckel's diverticulum (p. 218); Upper gastrointestinal haemorrhage (p. 338).

PILONIDAL SINUS DISEASE

Christopher Lattimer, Nitin Gureja

Pilonidal disease (lit. nest of hairs) is a chronic inflammatory condition associated with unwanted hair. The breech of the dermis by the hair allows influx of bacteria to the deeper tissues. It is common in males (4:1), in the 20–40 age group, and most frequently occurs in the natal cleft, although it may occur in the umbilicus, axilla and in the web spaces of the fingers of hairdressers.

Aetiology

There are two main theories as to the possible aetiology of pilonidal sinus disease.

1. Congenital. Less accepted, suggests the presence of a squamous-lined epithelial tract present from birth, in the midline of the natal cleft. The origin of the tract is thought to be either a caudal remnant of the medullary canal, a traction dermoid, or an inclusion dermoid.

2. Acquired. Widely accepted, suggests that a shed hair introduced into a small epithelial pit 'drills' its way into the subcutaneous tissue by mechanical movement of the buttocks. Midline sweat glands or hair follicle orifices may enlarge from the shearing forces imposed upon them and form a pit.

Pathology

Pilonidal sinus consists of a midline pit in the natal cleft with lateral secondary tracks emerging cephalad from it. The primary tract orifice is epithelially lined, whilst the track which may end in a blind cavity or orifice is lined by granulation tissue.

Secondary tracks develop laterally from the primary track, due to an inability for infection to penetrate the fibrous bands overlying the sacrum.

Human capital hair and animal hair have been identified within sinuses as well as buttock hairs.

Clinical presentation

Common in young men, who as described by Frankowiak tend to be 'robust, fat, plethoric type males with narrow pelvis, deep sulcus between folds of thick buttocks, an excessive glandular activity and susceptibility to staphylococcus infection'.

In one study ~11% of patients with pilonidal sinus disease were asymptomatic. However it more commonly presents with features of chronic sepsis; i.e. intermittent discharge, pain and repeated episodes of acute sepsis requiring drainage. In chronic sepsis anaerobes are often the incriminating organism, whilst in the acute situation *Staphylococcus aureus* is often isolated.

Natural history

Pilonidal sinus disease, like acne, is a self-limiting disease. It is characterized by episodes of remission and relapse, most common in the second decade. Patients over the age of 30 years treated by incision and drainage of an abscess, often have no further symptoms[b].

Treatment

Present in the literature is an abundance of reports recommending the ideal treatment for pilonidal disease. Unfortunately the less radical methods are usually associated with high recurrence rates, and vice versa. It is generally accepted that asymptomatic sinus disease should not be treated and managed conservatively. General advice regarding weight loss, improvement in personal hygiene and shaving the sacrococcygeal area should be given to all patients.

*1. **Acute abscess.*** In the acute situation; treatment of incision and drainage of the abscess should be undertaken with packing of the cavity, under local, regional or general anaesthesia. This will achieve healing in ~58% of patients.

Twenty seven per cent of patients will require definitive surgery. This should not be undertaken for at least 10 weeks after drainage.

*2. **Chronic disease.*** Of the various methods described, they can be broadly divided into conservative and radical procedures.

● **Conservative**
1. *Excision of midline pits and clearing of tracts.* In this method pits are excised and the lateral tracts are cleaned with nylon brushes. Secondary openings are also locally debrided. Close attention is given postoperatively to skin cleanliness; with regular shaving of the natal cleft until the wounds have healed.
2. *Laying open of tracts.* The tracts are identified using a probe or using dilute methylene blue and layed open. The granulation tissue lining the tracts is curettaged. This method is associated with a high recurrence rate.

● **Radical excision**
1. *Excision and healing by granulation tissue.* The sinus complex is excised and allowed to heal by 2° intention. This has the disadvantage of prolonged recovery time. Alternatively the excised cavity can be covered with elastomer foam, which is removed on a daily basis to allow cleansing of the wound, and is changed weekly to accommodate for the decreasing size. The reported recurrence rate is between 0–22%.
2. *Excision and marsupialization.* Once the sinus complex has been excised the skin edges are sutured to the pre-sacral fascia. This has a reported recurrence rate of <7%.
3. *Excision and primary closure.* The main problem with this technique is that unless the cavity is completely obliterated, there is a high incidence of wound breakdown. Recurrence rates of between 1–38% have been reported.
4. *Karyadakis' operation.* This is essentially an excision procedure with a lateral–medial advancement flap.
5. *Excision and asymmetric closure.* As (3) above, but the oblique closure disrupts the natal cleft, and discourages the accumulation of hairs in this area. Recurrence rates are very low if primary healing is achieved. Recurrence rates of <5% have been reported, but often involve use of complex procedures like Z plasty

and rhomboid and gluteal flaps. However these radical procedures are often used for recurrent disease.

Further reading

Allen-Mersh TG. Pilonidal sinus: finding the right track for treatment. *British Journal of Surgery*, 1990; **77**: 123–132.

Jensen SL, Harling H. Prognosis after simple incision and drainage for a first-episode acute pilonidal abscess. *British Journal of Surgery*, 1988; **75**: 60.

Karyadakis G. Easy and successful treatment of pilonidal sinus after explanation of its causative process. *Australian and New Zealand Journal of Surgery*, 1992; **62**: 385.

PORTAL HYPERTENSION

Nick Lagattolla

Pathology

Chronic hepatic disease may lead to obstruction of the intrahepatic veins, raising the portal venous pressure above its usual limit of 10 mmHg. Common causes include alcoholic liver disease and chronic viral (B, C or D) hepatitis. Increased portal venous pressure results in the distension of existent, usually microscopic, portasystemic venous anastomoses. These occur at numerous sites, most importantly in the wall of the lower oesophagus where the left gastric (portal) and azygous (systemic) veins communicate. These become oesophageal varices, and they frequently cause life-threatening haemorrhage.

The severity of the causative hepatic disease is classified according to Child's classification, or its modification as proposed by Pugh, according to five parameters: serum bilirubin, albumin, the presence of ascites, encephalopathy and the nutritional state (Child) or prothrombin time (Pugh). The patient is graded into one of three classes, A, B or C. These are commonly used in the assessment of prognosis, fitness for anaesthesia or requirement for surgery.

Clinical features

Portal hypertension may carry the stigmata of chronic liver disease, with clubbing of the nails, liver palms, spider naevi, ascites, peripheral (hypoproteinaemic) oedema, leuconychia, and wasting of the muscles, particularly if the cause is alcohol. An enlarged liver may be present, although the spleen is more likely to be enlarged. Cutaneous portasystemic anastomoses may be evident, such as the 'caput medusae' around the umbilicus (which is usually not completely circumferential), or around abdominal scars or stomas. Jaundice, liver flap and encephalopathy may be features of acute hepatic failure.

Variceal haemorrhage

Oesophageal varices bleed torrentially and result in 50% of deaths from gastrointestinal bleeding. Occasionally, gastric varices bleed. The diagnosis may be considered on the history of liver disease or alcohol abuse, or may be detected clinically through the above-mentioned signs. However, the diagnosis should be confirmed by gastroscopy, particularly as varices are best treated endoscopically in the first instance.

1. Endoscopic treatment. This involves the intravariceal injection of a vascular sclerosant, usually ethanolamine. Alternative materials are cyanoacrylate glue or thrombin, which works best on bleeding gastric fundal varices. Repeated injections may be necessary, but cannot be repeated more than twice on successive days. Although the immediate success is of the order of 90%, recurrent bleeding is common, with about 40% of patients requiring emergency treatment in the future.

2. Drug treatment. If an emergency endoscopy service is not available, the patient may be treated with drugs. Intravenous vasopressin causes generalized and splanchnic vasoconstriction. Systemic vasoconstriction is less with terlipressin. Intravenous octreotide also reduces portal flow. Drug treatment is not as effective as variceal injection. Twenty five per cent will require further treatment, and vasoconstrictors should be used is as a temporary measure whilst a patient is transferred to a specialist unit.

3. Balloon tamponade. Oesophageal intubation for balloon tamponade is more effective than medical treatment. This is achieved using a Sengstaken–Blakemore tube. This is a wide-bore tube with four external ports: two to allow inflation or deflation of oesophageal and gastric balloons, and two ports for oesophageal and gastric suction. The Minnesota tube is a similar device that lacks the oesophageal balloon. The tube is passed via the nose into the stomach and 300 ml of air is used to inflate the gastric balloon. The tube is withdrawn until the balloon impinges on the gastric cardia, and tension is kept on the tube to maintain pressure on the cardia. This effectively prohibits portal blood from filling the oesophageal varices. Inflation of the oesophageal balloon is not always required. Suction is necessary to prevent aspiration from the oesophagus, and absorption of an excessive protein load from gastric luminal blood which may precipitate encephalopathy.

4. Surgery. If conservative measures do not arrest haemorrhage, emergency oesophageal transection and gastric devascularization must be undertaken. Emergency portacaval bypass may help, but this is risky and may precipitate encephalopathy.

Long-term treatment of portal hypertension

1. Medical management. Spironolactone, the aldosterone antagonist potassium-sparing diuretic, may be prescribed to reduce ascites, which is at least in part due to secondary hyperaldosteronism in chronic liver disease. The beta-blocker propranolol may be given to reduce portal venous pressure. Alcohol is prohibited, whether or not the underlying cause is alcoholism.

2. Shunting of ascites. Gross and debilitating ascites may be shunted into the venous system by means of a peritoneal–jugular shunt. These tubular shunts are tunnelled subcutaneously from the peritoneal cavity to the internal jugular vein. Two devices are in common use, the LeVeen and Denver shunts, the former incorporating a one-way valve. These frequently become blocked by fibrinous deposits at their peritoneal end and their use in hepatic ascites is limited.

3. Repeated endoscopic sclerotherapy and banding. Oesophageal varices may be endoscopically banded. This is not as effective as injection sclerotherapy for bleeding varices, but may be a better elective treatment. Repeated treatments are usually necessary.

4. Portasystemic shunting. Many patients relapse after initial or repeated successful conservative management. Surgery may be effective in reducing portal venous pressure by means of a portocaval bypass. In those unfit for surgery, TIPS, as outlined below, may be of use. If the patient is fit for anaesthesia, a distal lienorenal shunt or a portacaval shunt may be performed. Rarely, portal hypertension may be due to thrombosis of the splenic vein, causing left-sided or sectorial portal hypertension. This may be treated by splenectomy.

5. Liver transplantation. The non-alcoholic patient with severe chronic liver disease may be suitable for hepatic transplantation, though this is not a therapeutic option in the emergency treatment of variceal haemorrhage.

Transjugular intrahepatic portasystemic anastomosis (TIPS)

Portal hypertension may be relieved by the formation of an intrahepatic anastomosis between branches of the hepatic and portal veins. This is performed under radiological control via the right internal jugular vein, and is known as transjugular intrahepatic portasystemic anastomosis (TIPS). A catheter is passed into and through the wall of a hepatic vein until a wire can be passed into a branch of the intrahepatic portal vein. The resultant fistulous tract is dilated and self-expanding vascular stents are positioned within the fistula to maintain patency. The procedure is complicated by shunt stenosis or thrombosis, and may precipitate encephalopathy. This may be a useful minimally invasive procedure to reduce portal venous pressure in the short term, mainly in those too unfit for portocaval bypass surgery, or in those awaiting hepatic transplantation. TIPS is being evaluated in acute variceal haemorrhage.

Further reading

Copeland G, Sheilds R. Portal hypertension and oesophageal varices. *Surgery*, 1991; **98**: 2342–2347.

Jalan R, Redhead DN, Hayes PC. Transjugular intrahepatic portasystemic stent. *British Journal of Surgery*, 1995; **85**: 1158–1164.

Sarin SK, Lamba GS, Kumar M *et al.* Comparison of endoscopic ligation and propranolol for the primary prevention of variceal bleeding. *New England Journal of Medicine*, 1999; **340**: 988–993.

Related topics of interest

Jaundice – investigation (p. 203); Upper gastrointestinal haemorrhage (p. 338).

POSTOPERATIVE CARE AND COMPLICATIONS

Nick Lagattolla

Immediate care

Immediately following surgery the patient is placed on the recovery ward in the theatre suite, where vital signs are measured by a specialist nurse with anaesthetists in close attendance. Problems arising as a direct consequence of the surgery will be evident, and the patient's proximity to the operating theatre makes immediate re-exploration feasible.

Ward care

Patients are monitored for adequate pain relief and the development of postoperative complications. Drainage from wound drains and nasogastric tubes needs to be monitored. Intravenous infusions, for both fluids and medication such as analgesic infusions, are very carefully controlled and charted. Whilst the above is mostly the province of the nursing staff, overall care is shared, and the surgical team must assume equal responsibility.

Pain relief

Adequate analgesia is necessary to allow patients to breathe deeply and cough without undue pain. Continuous analgesic regimens provide excellent pain relief. Low-dose opiates (usually morphine) may be continually infused through an epidural catheter or intravenously. Patient-controlled analgesia (PCA) is safe and effective but requires close surveillance. Opiates may also be infused continuously subcutaneously.

Blood tests

FBC and U&E should be requested on the morning following major surgery. A fall in haemoglobin may require a blood transfusion. Electrolyte imbalances may be addressed by modifying the intravenous fluid regimen. A rising urea and creatinine may signify impending prerenal failure, and intravenous fluids may need to be increased.

Nasogastric tubes and drains

Nasogastric tubes may cause difficulty in breathing and are best removed at the earliest convenience. Occasionally, the stomach becomes atonic, and there is a copious nasogastric aspirate. If this occurs, the tube should be left in place on free drainage. Drains should be removed at the earliest opportunity, usually if drainage has been minimal for 2 days, and certainly when they cease to drain anything.

Intravenous fluid requirement

The normal daily intake is between 2.5 and 3.0 litres of fluid, with approximately 100 mmol sodium and 60 mmol potassium per day. The postoperative patient is not a normal situation, however. Fluid requirement may be less over the initial day, due to the metabolic response to trauma, however, there will have been fluid losses incurred during surgery. A standard intravenous regimen is thus 2 litres of 5% dextrose and 1 litre of 0.9% saline per day, each litre containing 20 mmol potassium. It is important to note excess fluid losses from drains, tubes, stomas or fistulae and replace these amounts with potassium supplemented 0.9% saline. Patients may rapidly become dehydrated with large nasogastric aspirates or high-output fistulae or stomas.

Oral fluids and feeding

If a patient has a nasogastric tube, there is no harm in allowing sips of fluid. Following abdominal surgery, a safe rule is that if bowel sounds are present, oral fluids may be started. When patients have passed flatus or faeces, they may take a light diet.

Post-operative complications

These are classified into early, intermediate and late. Late complications are specific to the condition being treated. These occur after some months have elapsed, and are considered during follow-up. Complications arising on the ward occur early (days) and intermediate (weeks) after surgery.

Pulmonary collapse

This is a common cause of an early postoperative pyrexia which disappears as the patient coughs up mucus which has been plugging a subsegmental bronchus. However, patients with poor respiratory function with major bronchial plugging may develop respiratory distress, and arterial blood gases must be performed. The patient is put on oxygen and a chest X-ray is requested. Treatment options include chest physiotherapy, bronchoscopy and suction, and, if there is respiratory failure, admission to the ICU for ventilation.

Chest infection

Minor infections are common in smokers or those with chronic lung disease, and are often the cause of a persistent postoperative pyrexia. The patient will be coughing sputum which should be sent for culture. A frank pneumonia is unusual but may cause respiratory failure necessitating intensive care. Infections usually occur in collapsed pulmonary segments, and postoperative chest physiotherapy does much to clear the airways and avoid infection.

Aspiration pneumonia

Gastric contents may be aspirated into the right lower lobe where it may cause a severe pneumonitis and consolidation. This is a potentially serious complication that usually arises on induction or recovery from anaesthesia. It may be avoided on the ward by nasogastric intubation in those with an ileus or gastric stasis. However, early removal of unnecessary nasogastric tubes may actually prevent aspiration by facilitating coughing.

Deep venous thrombosis

This causes a painful swollen leg. Clinically there is calf tenderness. If suspected, the patient should have ascending phlebography. A duplex scan may be sufficient to diagnose femoral or popliteal thrombosis, but may miss calf thrombosis. The patient is heparinized, and this is monitored by daily activated partial thromboplastin times. Warfarin is started simultaneously, and the heparin is stopped as soon as the pro-thrombin time is under control. If the patient cannot be anticoagulated and has a proximal thrombosis, or if there is a large free iliofemoral thrombus, a caval filter may be necessary to prevent pulmonary embolism.

Pulmonary embolism

This is responsible for 3% of all hospital deaths, despite routine prophylaxis with anticoagulants. A total of 2.5% of pulmonary emboli are fatal, and recurrent emboli occur in 30% if untreated. It may result in sudden death, or present with pleuritic chest pain, haemoptysis and shortness of breath. Signs include elevation of the jugular venous pulse, tachycardia, hypotension, a pleural rub, and hypoxia on blood gas estimation. There may be no signs of a deep venous thrombosis. This is treated on suspicion with full heparinization. Despite this, recurrent emboli occur in up to 10% of cases. Pulmonary embolism may be confirmed with ventilation/perfusion lung scanning. Major pulmonary emboli causing severe cardiorespiratory effects may require intensive care, pulmonary thrombectomy or thrombolysis.

Haemorrhage

Primary haemorrhage occurs at the time of surgery. Reactionary haemorrhage occurs within hours of surgery from vessels that initially constrict but later bleed, or as a result of a slipped ligature. Secondary haemorrhage usually results from localized infection, ulceration or malignancy causing erosion of a vessel wall. It occurs 1 or 2 weeks after surgery, and may be torrential and life-threatening.

Anastomotic leak

A gastrointestinal anastomosis may break down giving rise to serious complications. Factors that contribute to anastomotic leaks or dehiscence include ischaemia or tension of the bowel ends, or local contamination at the time the anastomosis was fashioned. The leak must be drained, and the bowel ends exteriorized if possible, or a proximal diverting stoma may be created.

Wound dehiscence

The oozing of haemoserous fluid from an abdominal wound is an ominous sign. This may occur at around one week, and it indicates that the wound is coming apart or dehiscing. Localized dehiscence may result in strangulation of a knuckle of bowel. Full-length dehiscence may result in evisceration. These constitute surgical emergencies, and resuturing is mandatory. Dehiscence may occur as a result of weak abdominal musculature from previous surgery, but more often as a result of suture line tension and resulting tissue strangulation and ischaemia. Wounds should be sutured to be approximated not strangulated (opposed not necrosed).

Wound infection

This is common after contaminated operations. Up to 20% of all wounds may become infected. A persistent, postoperative pyrexia must prompt examination of the wound. Infecting organisms are often Gram-negative following bowel surgery. Wounds from clean operations that become infected usually harbour staphylococci. Minor infections respond to antibiotics. Small superficial collections usually drain satisfactorily after removal of two or three sutures. If a wound abscess results, formal drainage is necessary, and the wound is left open to heal by secondary intention.

Cardiac

Myocardial infarction and left ventricular failure with acute pulmonary oedema may occur in the postoperative period. An ECG and chest X-ray must be performed on patients who have chest pain or become short of breath. Acute pulmonary oedema responds well to intravenous diuretics.

Acute renal failure

Hypovolaemia or hypotension results in reduced renal perfusion. The urinary output may fall below the accepted lower limit of the acceptable range, which is 30 ml/hour. This should initially be managed by administration of intravenous crystalloid fluid. If the patient is adequately hydrated and still producing insufficient urine, a bolus dose or continuous infusion of frusemide is given. If this state of prerenal failure and oliguria is allowed to continue, acute renal tubular necrosis will ensue. This will result in an aneuric phase which may last for 2 days, representing tubular necrosis. The urea and creatinine rise, and there will be a metabolic acidosis. Following this there is a phase of polyuria as the kidney recovers. Both these phases need to be treated by careful fluid management. If the urea fails to fall or approaches 35 mmol/l, or if there is hyperkalaemia, haemofiltration or dialysis may be indicated.

Acute retention of urine

This is common in men after abdominal or bilateral inguinal hernia surgery. There is usually a history of bladder outflow obstruction. Urethral or suprapubic catheterization is required. The patient is referred to the urologists for cystoscopy and a TURP. This may, rarely, occur in a woman. There may be an underlying urethral stenosis, or a neurological cause, possibly multiple sclerosis.

Psychiatric

Acute confusional states are common in the elderly or alcoholics. The diagnosis in the latter is likely to be acute alcohol withdrawal, and is treated with intravenous or oral chlormethiazole. Vitamin B complex should also be administered. In the elderly, confusion may signify an underlying infection, anaemia, hypoxia or metabolic derangement. It is highly non-specific, and the patient must be fully investigated.

Paralytic ileus

This represents atonic small intestine, and some degree is common after any abdominal operation. The small bowel usually recovers within 24 hours, but occasionally this is prolonged, and the term paralytic ileus then applies. The patient remains distended, and there will be few bowel sounds. Vomiting may occur. Electrolyte imbalance, particularly potassium, predisposes to this. It is managed by continued nasogastric suction if there is vomiting, correction of electrolyte disturbances, and prohibition of oral intake.

Gastric stasis

The stomach may become atonic after abdominal surgery, and may take days to recover its function. This may require nasogastric suction, and prohibition of fluids. Acute gastric dilatation, which probably simply represents extreme gastric stasis, carries a high risk of aspiration and mortality. It may occur following any abdominal surgical procedure, causing discomfort, effortless vomiting, hiccoughs, and abdominal bloating. It is remedied by insertion of a wide nasogastric tube. Contributory electrolyte imbalances, particularly hypokalaemia, must be corrected.

Further reading

Smith JAR. *Complications of Surgery in General.* Oxford: Baillière Tindall, 1984.

Related topics of interest

Blood transfusion (p. 53); Fluid replacement (p. 127); Intestinal pseudo-obstruction and ileus (p. 198); Postoperative pain relief (p. 270).

POSTOPERATIVE PAIN RELIEF

Chris Perera

Postoperative pain is generally inadequately recognized, inadequately monitored and inadequately treated. The introduction of minimally invasive surgery as a substitute for open surgery has resulted in a major decrease in the amount of postoperative pain and consequent prolonged admission for pain control. The establishment of an 'acute pain team' of trained clinicians may be an effective measure to minimize postoperative surgical pain.

Consequences of pain

Postoperative pain increases morbidity and mortality, delays mobilization and prolongs hospital stay. After thoracic or upper abdominal surgery, deep breathing and coughing are inhibited, functional residual capacity decreases and small airways close. Sputum retention leads to resorption collapse of alveoli (atelectasis) especially in dependent lung regions. Myocardial ischaemia in patients with ischaemic heart disease is increased in the presence of pain. Pain also increases the metabolic rate and oxygen demand.

Consequences of pain relief

Postoperative pain relief too has its problems. Opioids, such as morphine, decrease tidal volume and ventilation rate, and make breathing irregular. Carbon dioxide retention is encouraged with an increase in the number and severity of episodes of sleep apnoea. Morphine intoxication should be considered in any drowsy or unresponsive patient following major abdominal surgery. Treatment with 0.1 mg of Naloxone is rapid and effective but may need to be repeated since its half-life is much shorter than most opioids. Opioids suppress rapid eye movement sleep and encourage nausea with vomiting. Subsequent aspiration may be fatal. All patients should avoid smoking the week leading to surgery to improve baseline respiratory function. The pre-admission clinic is an ideal time to give this advice.

Methods

1. *Drug treatment includes:*
- Opioids.
- Non-steroidal anti-inflammatory drugs.
- Paracetamol and combinations (e.g. paracetamol and codeine).

2. *Regional anaesthetic techniques include:*
- Central neuraxial blocks: epidural, caudal and spinal.
- Peripheral nerve blocks (e.g. femoral nerve block).
- Local infiltration.

3. *Psychological methods:*
- Relaxation.
- Hypnosis.
- Psychoprophylaxis.

Routes of administration

1. **Parenteral:**
- Intramuscular bolus on demand.
- Intravenous bolus.
- Continuous infusion.
- Patient-controlled (or nurse-controlled in small children) analgesia (i.v., s.c. or epidural).

2. **Non-parenteral:**
- Oral.
- Buccal/sublingual.
- Rectal.
- Spinal and epidural.
- Intra-articular.
- Transdermal.
- Inhalation.

Advances

The main advances in postoperative pain relief have been the increased appreciation of patient-controlled analgesia and the administration of spinally applied opioids. The concepts of pre-emptive analgesia and psychoprophylaxis are now widely accepted and should be frequently applied.

1. **Patient-controlled analgesia.** Differing individual analgesic requirements at different times for different operations led to the development of patient-controlled analgesia (PCA). Two thirds of patients wait until severe pain develops before requesting analgesia and one third of nurses will not administer analgesics until a request is made by the patient. Once the patient is in control of the pain, anxiety is reduced and pain tolerance is increased. The system requires a rapid response if the patient is to feel in control of the pain. Directly a bolus of analgesia is delivered a 'lock-out' interval ensues to ensure the drug is appreciated before further demands are met. The usual regime is an intravenous 1 mg morphine bolus with a lock-out interval of 5 min. Before taking sole control of the intravenous or epidural delivery of analgesia the patient should be comfortable and told to titrate the drug to a level of tolerable discomfort rather than to total analgesia.

2. **Spinally applied opiates.** These can be given by the epidural or subarachnoid route, and produce a very effective and prolonged analgesia by acting upon the rich concentration of opiate receptors clustered in the dorsal horn of the spinal cord. Morphine is the most widely used drug, but almost all the available drugs have been used. It is relatively lipid insoluble, being distributed in the CSF rather than to the cord, which is unfortunate because its effects are subjected to CSF movements. Any sudden change in position or straining can thereby induce respiratory depression. Consequently, such patients should be monitored with pulse oximetry in a high dependency area. The risk is further reduced by delivery with a slow infusion into the lumbar, rather than the thoracic, spine using a large volume of solvent. The

combination of local anaesthetic and opioid enhances the effect and duration of both agents. Nausea and vomiting, itching, urinary retention and somnolence are the other main drawbacks of its use, but have now been minimized by using very dilute solutions.

3. Other drugs. Clonidine, a selective alpha-2 adrenergic receptor agonist and ketamine, an NMDA receptor antagonist have been added to local anaesthetics given epidurally and caudally to prolong its duration of action.

4. Pre-emptive analgesia. Pre-emptive treatment of pain with opiates, NSAIDs and paracetamol reduces pain for much longer than the expected action of the drug. This is achieved by inhibition of the increase in sensitivity at the post-synaptic spinal cord neurone which painful stimuli produce. Phantom limb pain can be eliminated in this way by ensuring a pain-free interval prior to amputation. Local anaesthetics prolong the pre-emptive effects of opiates. NSAIDS reduce the need for opiates. They are particularly useful in day case surgery and are often given as a suppository following the induction of anaesthesia.

5. Psychoprophylaxis. The ability to cope with pain depends upon individual personality, the perceived support from relatives, the level of distraction, the individual pain threshold and fear of the unknown. A pre-operative anaesthetic visit and an explanation of the surgical procedure both reduce anxiety, although a concise explanation is just as effective as a detailed explanation. Benzodiazepines, given as premedication, help to alleviate anxiety.

Local anaesthesia

Wound infiltration by local anaesthetic at the end of an operation successfully reduces the opiate requirements for most operations including inguinal herniorrhaphy and open cholecystectomy. Topical lignocaine gel can be applied to mucous membranes, split skin grafts or to the suture line following a circumcision. Local anaesthetic application by intercostal, paravertebral, rectus sheath, brachial or femoral cannulation alongside the appropriate nerve can provide long-lasting postoperative pain relief.

Further reading

Ballantyne JC, Carr DB, deFerranti S *et al*. The comparative effects of postoperative analgesic therapies on pulmonary outcome: cumulative meta-analyses of randomized, controlled trials. *Anesthesia and Analgesia*, 1998; **86:** 598–612.

Gould TH, Crosby DL, Harmer M *et al*. Policy for controlling pain after surgery: effect of sequential changes in management. *British Medical Journal*, 1992; **305:** 1187–1193.

Liu SS, Carpenter RL, Mackey DC *et al*. Effects of perioperative analgesic technique on rate of recovery after colon surgery. *Anesthesiology*, 1995; **83:** 757–765.

McQuay HJ. Post-operative analgesia. *Baillière's Clinical Anaesthesiology*, 1999; **13:** 465–476.

McQuay HJ, Moore RA. *An Evidence-based Resource for Pain Relief*. Oxford: Oxford University Press, 1998.

Yeager M, Glass D, Neff R, Brinck-Johnson T. Epidural anaesthesia and analgesia in high risk surgical patients. *Anesthesiology*, 1987; **66:** 729–736.

Related topics of interest

Minimal access surgery (p. 224); Postoperative care and complications (p. 265).

PRE-OPERATIVE ASSESSMENT

Nick Lagattolla

Clinical examination

A full current and past medical history will alert the houseman to possible problems that may need special attention, particularly for the anaesthetist (respiratory or cardiac disorders, glaucoma, epilepsy, cervical arthritis, drug sensitivity), but also for the surgeon (previous surgery) and for the postoperative period (past venous thromboembolism, prostatism, diabetes). The examination should be geared to assessing disorders picked up on the history, but also to detecting unknown disease, for example in the cardiovascular system, hypertension, cardiac murmurs, cardiac failure, arrhythmias, peripheral vascular disease.

Anaesthetic assessment

This will be performed by the anaesthetist, who should have been alerted to potential problems. The patient's fitness for anaesthesia is assessed and graded according to the American Society of Anesthesiology (ASA) scale of 1 to 5. ASA 1 amounts to a fit and healthy individual, and ASA 5 is a moribund patient who is not expected to survive and is undergoing surgery as a last resort.

Blood tests

FBC and estimation of U&E are recommended in all patients. The haemoglobin and potassium levels are important considerations for the anaesthetic, and all the results will provide a baseline should postoperative problems occur. Severely unwell patients with metabolic complications should have arterial blood gases performed, as acidosis reduces cardiac function, and co-existing hyperkalaemia can cause arrhythmias. Patients from the West Indies and Africa must have a sickle-cell screen. Patients undergoing major bowel or arterial operations will need blood cross-matched according to the surgeon's requirement. It is prudent if serum is sent for a group-and-save from all patients having major surgery.

Cardiac

For anaesthetic purposes, an ECG is usually requisite in all patients over the age of 50. If patients are currently symptomatic, either with angina or heart failure, or if they have a history of severe cardiac illness, then the opinion of a cardiologist should be sought prior to a general anaesthetic as measurement of the left ventricular contractility or ejection fraction or an exercise ECG may be indicated. If hitherto unknown murmurs or arrhythmias are detected pre-operatively, these must be investigated first. Patients at risk of bacterial endocarditis should receive prophylactic antibiotics.

Pulmonary

Patients with current symptoms or signs, or a history of chest disease, and the elderly should have a routine pre-operative chest X-ray. Those with chronic airways disease must have simple spirometry and peak flow velocities measured as part of their work-up, and nebulized bronchodilators should be prescribed perioperatively. For surgery involving the thorax, including oesophageal or pulmonary resections, formal pulmonary function tests should be performed.

Nutritional

Chronically debilitating disorders, for example, in the gastrointestinal tract ulcerative colitis, high-output gastrointestinal fistula, or gastro-oesophageal malignancies, result in hypoproteinaemia and electrolyte imbalances. These must be assessed by serum albumin, transferrin, haemoglobin and electrolytes, and potential problems must be addressed pre-operatively. Supplemental enteric or parenteral feeding may be required. Unfortunately, nutritional status is often only considered after its ill effects have become evident with cachexia, gross hypoproteinaemic oedema or poor healing.

Risk of venous thromboembolism

Factors with an increased risk of DVT include advanced age, obesity, cardiac failure, trauma, previous episodes of venous thromboembolism, malignant disease, and major abdominal or pelvic surgery. The last three constitute particularly high risks. Patients may be graded according to their risk of DVT. Patients with no risk factors having minor surgery with early ambulation may not require prophylactic anticoagulation, but ought to wear compression stockings perioperatively. However, all other patients should have prophylactic anticoagulation with either twice daily 5000 IU of heparin or once daily low-molecular-weight heparin subcutaneously. Consideration for full anticoagulation or prophylactic caval filtration should be given to those at very high risk.

Patients on steroids

Long treatment with steroids necessitates intravenous hydrocortisone 100 mg qds to avoid an Addisonian crisis from adrenal suppression.

Day-case surgery

Patients for minor surgery under local anaesthetic need not be screened. Patients for general anaesthesia, and those for intermediate procedures under local anaesthesia, will need to be screened for medical conditions and social factors that are contra-indications to day-case surgery. Initial screening must take place in the outpatient clinic. Clearly those with a history of ischaemic heart disease or chronic lung disease or other medical conditions that may cause intra- or immediate postoperative complications will be unsuitable. Social considerations are also very important. Patients living alone, the elderly or those without a GP may not be suitable.

Further more detailed screening is performed in a pre-admission outpatient clinic. This is best undertaken by the trained nursing staff of the day-case unit who will screen the patient's hospital records, if available, and take a history and perform a clinical appraisal according to a clerking pro forma. Absolute and relative contra-indications to day case surgery will become evident, these having been previously agreed by the anaesthetists responsible for the day case list.

Further reading

Cuschieri A. Preoperative, operative and postoperative cares. In: Cuschieri A, Giles GR, Moosa AR (eds) *Essential Surgical Practice*. London: Wright, 1988.

Powell M. Cardiopulmonary assessment of the surgical patient. *Surgery*, 1993; **11:** 361–367.

Reilly CS. Cardiac risk and its relevance to the preoperative assessment. *Surgery*, 1991; **97:** 2308–2310.

Related topic of interest

Day case surgery (p. 110).

RENAL ACCESS SURGERY

Nick Lagattolla

Progressive chronic renal failure requires treatment with haemodialysis. The creation of arterio-venous fistulas for dialysis and positioning of peritoneal and vascular access catheters is usually the province of the transplant or vascular surgeon, though some nephrologists undertake some of these procedures.

Great advances in the field of transplantation occurred in the 1960s which enabled not only improved survival of patients with renal failure, but fitter patients for transplantation. Hand in hand with improvements in transplant immunology and pharmacology, improved renal access techniques aided the initiation of transplant programmes. The general surgeon should be conversant with not only obtaining access for the purpose of haemodialysis, but with the specific complications of these common and important procedures.

Continuous ambulatory peritoneal dialysis

The peritoneal surface is the barrier across which dialysis occurs in CAPD. The technique allows for dialysis in the home setting undertaken by the patient him- or herself. CAPD is achieved by the instillation of dialysate fluid into the peritoneal cavity through an indwelling intra-peritoneal Tenckoff catheter. This is a silicon tube with multiple perforations in a pig-tailed inner end. The pig-tailed end must be positioned in the lowermost recess of the pelvis for optimal function.

CAPD catheter insertion

It is inserted either as a closed procedure under local anaesthetic, or as a minimally invasive semi-open procedure under a brief general anaesthetic. Under local, a specific introducer is used to guide the catheter into the pelvis. Under a general anaesthetic, a short infra-umbilical incision is made through all layers of the abdominal wall, and using a sponge-holding forceps (Rampley), the catheter is delivered directly into the pelvis. An inner teflon cuff is positioned at the level of the peritoneum. The cuff is incorporated in the peritoneal suture, taking care not to leave too much cuff poking into the peritoneal cavity as adhesions to this may occur.

A trochar is placed on the outer end of the Tenckoff catheter, and the catheter is guided through the rectus sheath such that the outer teflon cuff lies between the outer rectus sheath and the exit site which is usually about 10–15 cm inferolateral to the umbilicus. A titanium connector is placed on the outer end, and the catheter is checked by instilling 500 ml of saline which should then be drained to ensure two-way flow. The incision is carefully closed with interrupted PDS or nylon suture to restore the midline, followed by careful closure of the skin.

CAPD complications

The catheter may block. Early failure is usually technical, the catheter tip usually not lying in the pelvis and ending up wrapped in omentum. Late failures may occur secondary to build up of fibrinous material blocking the catheter tip perforations. Such blocked catheters will need to be removed and replaced.

Incisional hernia is common at the site of CAPD catheter insertion, due to a combination of poor wound healing and peritoneal distension.

Two forms of peritonitis may ensue. Typically, a chronic sclerosing peritonitis occurs, identified by a general pallid thickening of the visceral peritoneum, arising from the constant low-grade irritation of the dialysis catheter and fluid. This is likely to be asymptomatic, but will be encountered should abdominal surgery be undertaken.

Acute peritonitis is common, the patient presenting generally unwell, with abdominal pain and a turbid dialysate. This must be cultured, and the organisms grown are scrutinized as to whether they originate as skin commensals or as intestinal flora. Growth of a skin commensal suggests the cause is infection tracking along the CAPD catheter. Bowel-related organisms suggest that the source is likely to be a co-existing intraperitoneal inflammatory or infective condition.

Antibiotics to which the infecting organisms are sensitive may be given systemically and instilled through the CAPD catheter. This may control the infection, particularly if it is a skin commensal, though in the presence of a foreign body such as the CAPD catheter, this is unlikely. If the infective source is intra-abdominal sepsis, antibiotics alone will not succeed (vide infra).

Catheter removal

This is performed under a general anaesthetic. If a skin-related organism is cultured, removal alone may be sufficient. This is achieved by cutting down along the catheter until the external teflon cuff is encountered. This is freed from adhesions. The catheter beyond the cuff is grasped, pulled and retrieved, leaving the inner cuff in situ. This will do no harm, though its presence should be noted lest complications occur. If the catheter is retrieved incomplete, or it can not be delivered, then the infra-umbilical incision is re-opened, and the inner cuff is freed and delivered and the catheter may be easily withdrawn. The wound is sutured carefully using non-absorbable material.

In the presence of anaerobes or Gram-negative intestinal-type organisms, the underlying peritonitis is likely to be unrelated to the CAPD catheter, and simple removal is insufficient. The patient must be prepared for a laparotomy, the underlying condition is dealt with and the CAPD catheter is removed as a matter of course.

Central venous lines

Internal jugular catheters, frequently with two or even three channels, may be used for vascular access for haemofiltration or haemodialysis. These are inserted percutaneously under a local anaesthetic using a sterile technique. They do not require tunnelling as they are usually a temporary measure, and their diameter and relative inflexibility would render this difficult.

Complications from longer-term indwelling central venous lines include line sepsis, and central venous stenosis or thrombosis. Sepsis is treated by removal of the line. Stenosis may be amenable to angioplasty if symptomatic. Thrombosis may result in venous engorgement of the drainage area, and will usually respond to catheter directed thrombolysis delivered through the access line itself, if carefully repositioned. Following lysis, the catheter is removed, and any underlying stenosis may then be angioplastied.

Arterio-venous fistulae

The anastomosis of a peripheral artery with a neighbouring vein creates high venous flow and pressure in a dilated vein. These arteriolized veins are easy to cannulate, and the pressure and flow are enough to sustain flow through a dialysis machine. Fistulae are usually first created at the wrist, by means of end-to-side cephalic vein–radial artery anastomosis, the Cimino fistula. Complications are rare, apart from occlusion, which is usually due to venous outflow stenosis or occlusion.

Failure necessitates creation of the same on the other wrist, or the formation of a brachiocephalic fistula in the antecubital fossa. This may also be complicated by stenosis or occlusion, but as the arterial flow is higher at this level, a vascular steal phenomenon may occur in the forearm and hand, even resulting in focal necrosis, a situation that requires closure of the fistula. A Warren–Schreibner shunt is a fistula created between the posterior tibial artery and the nearby long saphenous vein.

PTFE vascular access grafts

These are also arteriovenous fistulae, though the connection is established via a length of subcutaneous non-supported non-expanded polytetrafluoroethylene. This is created either as straight graft usually running from the brachial artery in the antecubital fossa up the lateral aspect of the arm to a brachial vein, or as a loop running down the arm from the brachial artery near the axilla and back up to a brachial vein. Loops may also be located in the thigh running from the femoral artery to the femoral or long saphenous vein.

Complications usually involve low graft flow or graft occlusion. Low flow and occlusion are usually due to venous outflow stenosis. Occlusion may supervene on stenosis, and may be cleared using locally instilled thrombolysis followed with graft revision, or by open graft thrombectomy and revision. Because these grafts are located more proximally in the limb, and the PTFE diameter is usually 6 mm, high graft flow can create a distal steal phenomenon, a situation that requires graft removal to remedy.

Further reading

Bell PRF, Wood RFM. *Surgical Aspects of Haemodialysis,* 2nd edn. Edinburgh, Churchill Livingstone, 1983.
Bengmark S, ed. *The Peritoneum and Peritoneal Access for Dialysis.* London, Wright, 1989.

RENAL TUMOURS

Christopher Lattimer, Adrian Simoes

The conditions, which may give rise to renal mass, are as follows:

Benign	Malignant
Simple/multiple cyst	Renal cell carcinoma
Polycystic kidney	Transitional cell carcinoma
Tubular ectasia	Squamous cell carcinoma
Dermoid	Nephroblastoma
Lipoma, angioma, leiomyoma	Sarcoma
Angiomyolipoma	Metastatic (lung, breast)
Oncocytoma	
Tuberculosis	

Polycystic kidney disease

Adult polycystic kidney disease is autosomal dominant and almost always affects both kidneys. On the other hand the infantile type is autosomal recessive with a short life expectancy. The developmental failure of joining of the uriniferous tubules and the collecting tubules lead to the formation of cysts. As the cysts enlarge there occurs progressive impairment in renal function. Symptoms rarely appear before the age of 40. Pain occurs due to the drag on the renal pedicle by the enlarged heavy kidney or from obstruction, infection and haemorrhage into a cyst. Clinic-ally an abdominal mass may be apparent. Depending on the extent of renal deterioration, symptoms of uraemia may be present. Hypertension is found in over half the patients. The diagnosis is ascertained by ultrasonography and CT scanning. Complications include pyelonephritis, calyceal or ureteric obstruction, infection of the cyst, haem-orrhage into a cyst, haematuria and renal failure. The treatment is conservative and supportive with surgery having hardly any role except to relieve pressure effects by excision or de-roofing the offending cyst. This may be also effectively achieved by percutaneous aspiration. As renal function worsens dialysis or renal transplantation will be necessary.

Angiomyolipoma

As the name suggests this is a renal hamartoma comprising of mature fat cells, smooth muscle and blood vessels. Up to 80% of the patients show features of tuberous sclerosis. Typically the lesions are unencapsulated, multiple and bilateral. In the majority of cases they are asymptom-atic. As many as 25% of the patients may present with sudden loin pain, hypotension and massive retroperitoneal haemor-rhage due to spontaneous rupture of the lesion and accompanying haemorrhage. Due to their high fat content they are easily diagnosed on imaging. On ultrasound they appear as very high intensity echoes and on CT scan they have negative density ranging from –20 to –80 Hounsfield units which is pathognomonic. Asymptomatic lesions less than 4 cm need regular follow-up with imaging. Symptomatic lesions or those more than 4 cm need treatment either in the form of renal sparing surgery or embolization.

Renal cell carcinoma (RCC)

Renal cell carcinoma (clear cell, hypernephroma, Grawitz, adenocarcinoma) arises from renal tubular epithelium and comprises 85% of all primary malignant adult renal tumours. It is twice as common in men than women and peaks in incidence between the 6th and 8th decade. The incidence is increasing in both sexes.

1. ***Risk factors.*** Smoking, obesity, coffee, analgesic abuse, phenacetin, cadmium, petroleum products, exogenous estrogens and those working in the shoe and leather industry are all considered to increase the risk. Polycystic disease and acquired cystic disease of the kidney (in patients with chronic renal failure on dialysis) both are reported to increase the incidence too. A familial tendency is present in von Hippel-Lindau syndrome, which comprises RCC, cerebellar and spinal haemangio-blastoma, retinal angioma, phaeochromocytoma with cysts in the pancreas and epididymus. Structural changes are noted in chromosome 3 in both sporadic as well as hereditary RCC.

2. ***Pathology.*** Grossly the tumour is yellow to orange in colour due to the abundance of lipids. They may be associated with haemorrhage, necrosis, secondary cystic changes and calcification. Microscopically the carcinoma may contain clear cells, granular cells and occasionally spindle cells.

3. ***Presentation.*** The classical triad of loin pain, gross haematuria and a palpable mass occurs in only 10% of patients. However, most of these tumours are now detected incidentally on abdominal ultrasound. Other features may be weight loss, anaemia, sudden onset of a varicocele, caval obstruction and symptoms due to distant metastases. RCC may also present as one of the paraneoplastic syndromes:

Hormone	Effect
Endopyrogen	fever
PTH like peptide	hypercalcemia
Erythropoietin	polycythaemia
Insulin	abnormal glucose metabolism
ACTH	Cushing's syndrome
HCG	gynaecomastia
Prolactin	galactorrhea
Enteroglucagon	protein enteropathy

4. ***Investigations.*** Routine blood and urine for microscopy will reveal anaemia and heamaturia. Ultrasonography with Doppler or transoesophageal scanning give more information of IVC involvement. Contrast CT scanning is more sensitive and apart from confirming the diagnosis also helps stage the disease. An MRI will

give added information only in certain cases where CT suggests visceral involvement and also to further evaluate IVC thrombus. Chest CT or X-ray is needed for staging and a bone scan is indicated for bone pain or raised serum alkaline phosphatase. Selective angiography is necessary for nephron sparing surgery or to embolize a bleeding tumour.

5. Staging.

TNM classification

T1	7 cm or less and limited to kidney
T2	more than 7 cm and limited to kidney
T3a	invades adrenal, perinephric tissue but not beyond Gerota's fascia
T3b	tumour thrombus in renal vein or IVC below the diaphragm
T3c	tumour thrombus in supradiaphragmatic IVC
T4	tumour beyond Gerota's fascia
N0	No regional lymph node metastasis
N1	Metastasis in single regional lymph node
N2	Metastasis in more than one regional lymph node
M0	No distant metastasis
M1	Distant metastasis

6. Biopsy. Renal cell carcinoma is one of those few tumours where radical surgery is undertaken without preoperative histological diagnosis[b]. The indications for fine-needle or Trucut biopsy are to differentiate a chronic abscess from a cystic carcinoma, to achieve a histological diagnosis if required in case of metastatic disease and to differentiate a primary renal tumour from a secondary.

7. Management. Radical nephrectomy is indicated for localized disease whereby the kidney with the proximal half of ureter along with the adrenal, perinephric fat and Gerota's fascia are removed with regional infradiaphragmatic lymph nodes up to the aortic bifurcation. For suprahepatic or hepatic IVC involvement, veno-venous bypass or cardio-pulmonary bypass is usually required. Recent advances include laparoscopic radical nephrectomy and nephron-sparing surgery. For advanced and metastatic disease other modalities of treatment available are radiotherapy, hormonal therapy, chemotherapy and immunotherapy. Immunotherapy alone or in combination with chemotherapy have been reported to provide varying response rates. Commonly used agents are interferon alpha and interleukin-2. Some indications for palliative nephrectomy include elimination of paraneoplastic potential, better response rates than with other modalities[c], spontaneous regression of metastases (less than 1%) and the fact that some tumours make hormones (TGF-β) that suppress the immune response.

8. Follow up (post-radical nephrectomy).

Examination	1 mth	6 mthly for 2 yrs	Yearly for 3 yrs
Physical	+	+	+
Laboratory	+	+	+
X-ray chest		+	+
CT abdomen		+	+

Transitional cell carcinoma of the renal pelvis and ureter

Urothelial cancers of the renal pelvis and ureter are rare and account for only 4%. The aetio-logical factors are the same as that for bladder cancer. A majority of patients present with gross haematuria. The other presenting symptoms are flank pain, clot colic and infection. The diagnosis is arrived at by urinary cytology, ultrasonography, IVU, retrograde pyelography, CT scan and MRI. Ureteropyeloscopy offers visualization, biopsy and occasional tumour resection. The definitive treatment is radical nephroureterectomy which involves the removal of the kidney and the entire ureter along with a cuff of the bladder.

Nephroblastoma (Wilms' tumour)

Wilms' tumour is the commonest solid renal tumour in children. It arises from metanephric blastema. The loss of tumour suppressor genes on the short arm of chromosome 11 is associated with both familial and sporadic forms of Wilms' tumour. In the familial variant the patients are typically younger and the tumours are multicentric and bilateral. This tumour is also associated with congenital anomalies such as cryptorchidism, hypospadiasis, aniridia and hemihypertrophy. The presentation is in the form of an abdominal mass and abdominal distension. Gross haematuria is uncommon while hypertension is not. Ultrasound, CT scan and MRI help in the diagnosis, the staging and evaluation of the contralateral kidney. The treatment involves radical nephrectomy, chemotherapy and radiotherapy.

Further reading

Dhote R, Pellicer-Coeuret M, Thiounn N, Debre B, Vidal-Trecan G. Risk factors for adult renal cell carcinoma: a systematic review and implications for prevention. *BJU International*, 2000; **86:** 20–27.

Motzer RJ, Bander NH, Nanus DM. Renal cell carcinoma. *New England Journal of Medicine*, 1996; **335:** 865–872.

Sufrin G, Chasan S, Golio A, Murphy GP. Paraneoplastic and serologic syndromes of renal adenocarcinoma. *Seminars in Urology*, 1989; **7:** 158–171.

RENOVASCULAR SURGERY

Nick Lagattolla

Renal artery stenosis is the most important renal vascular disorder that is amenable to surgical correction. Other rarer disorders include renal artery aneurysm, congenital arterial anomalies, and acute renal artery occlusion.

Renal artery stenosis

Pathology

Seventy per cent of cases are due to atherosclerosis and 30% to fibromuscular dysplasia. The latter occurs mostly in younger patients and is commoner in women. Stenosis of a single renal artery can result in hypertension from stimulation of the renin–angiotensin system of that kidney. Angiotensin is a very potent systemic hypertensive hormone. As a result of the stenosis, the function of the affected kidney reduces and the kidney eventually becomes smaller. If both renal arteries are involved, then hypertension will certainly result, as will progressive renal failure.

Clinical presentation

Systemic hypertension, particularly medication-resistant or the so-called malignant variety, is the most significant result of renal artery stenosis. Hypertension in a general arteriopath with typical symptoms such as headache and epistaxis, may be caused in part by renovascular disease. Males are most often affected. Approximately 2–5% of hypertensives have some degree of renal artery disease, but whether this is cause or effect is very difficult to prove, as addressing the renal artery stenosis may not benefit the hypertension, particularly in atherosclerotics. Flash pulmonary oedema, hypokalaemia with hyponatremia (from secondary hyperaldosteronism) and established renal failure are less common presentations.

Diagnosis

Intravenous digital subtraction arteriography may identify renal artery stenosis; however, this requires a large bolus of intravenous contrast which is nephrotoxic and may precipitate acute renal failure if both kidneys are involved and there is established renal impairment. Selective arteriography utilizes less contrast, and provides better quality films, although it requires a direct arterial puncture. Arteriography is the current gold standard, but is invasive.

The assessment of renal vein renin levels after selective catheterization is an alternative means of establishing diagnosis if doubt remains after the above tests. The changes seen on an intravenous urogram are typical if one side only is affected. The kidney appears smaller, and there is delayed excretion of contrast compared to the normal side. Similar changes are seen on isotope renography. Duplex scanning of the renal arteries is difficult, but if views are obtained, the diagnosis may be established with confidence. CT reconstructions and magnetic resonance arteriography (MRA) are non-invasive, and will detect renal artery stenosis.

Treatment

1. Conservative. In the elderly, medical treatment for hypertension is the optimal treatment. The majority of middle-aged or younger patients can also be controlled by antihypertensives alone, though invasive procedures may be indicated.

2. Minimally invasive. Percutaneous transluminal angioplasty is the usual first-line invasive procedure. This is optimal for all fibromuscular stenoses, and for stenoses of either aetiology in the main part of the renal artery. Ostial stenoses are usually atherosclerotic, and though angioplasty alone is the treatment usually initially offered, primary stenting after angioplasty may carry a better initial patency rate and lower rate of restenosis.

3. Surgical. Ostial stenoses in particular are also treated at open surgery by endarterectomy and patching, or by autologous vein or polytetrafluoroethylene bypass grafting from the aorta to the post-stenotic portion of the renal artery. A very long stenosis from the ostium to the renal hilum may require a nephrectomy, extensive patching of the stenotic segment, and reimplantation on the iliac artery.

All these procedures will reduce systemic blood pressure but will not result in the recovery of lost renal function. Generally, results for both first-time angioplasty and bypass are better for fibromuscular hyperplasia than for atheromatous stenoses. However, about half the patients having angioplasty will need further treatment within two years. The benefit of angioplasty over surgery is that it is far easier to repeat should this be required.

Other renal vascular disease

Renal artery aneurysm

These are rare. They are usually small and saccular, are more commonly seen in association with hypertension, and occur at bifurcations in the artery. The aetiology of these is usually atherosclerosis or medial necrosis. They are usually found by chance on an arteriogram performed for another reason, and they are best left alone as they rarely rupture.

Acute renal artery occlusion

This is rare but is an occasional cause of flank pain of sudden onset. Sudden occlusion of the renal artery is usually embolic, and a source for the embolism should be sought. This is not amenable to surgery. Iatrogenic causes include thrombosis during renal artery angioplasty or stenting. This will be immediately apparent, and is probably best treated by local thrombolysis. Surgical exploration, with thrombectomy and correction of the initial lesion is an option.

Congenital renal vascular anomalies

These are common, but rarely important. They are usually arterial, and comprise aberrant polar arteries. These are only important when encountered during operations on the kidney, or when identified on arteriograms.

Further reading

Bredenberg CE, Sampson LN, Ray FS *et al.* Changing patterns in surgery for chronic renal artery occlusive diseases. *Journal of Vascular Surgery*, 1992; **15:** 1018–1824.

Hansen KJ, Starr SM, Sands RE *et al.* Contemporary surgical management of renovascular disease. *Journal of Vascular Surgery*, 1992; **16:** 319–331.

Mailloux LU, Napolitano B, Bellucci AG *et al.* Renal vascular disease causing end-stage renal disease: incidence, clinical correlates and outcomes: a 20-year clinical experience. *American Journal of Kidney Disease*, 1994; **24:** 622–629.

Textor SC. Revascularisation in atherosclerotic renal artery disease. *Kidney International*, 1998; **53:** 799–811.

Plouin PF, Chatellier G, Darne B, Raynauld A. Blood pressure outcome of angioplasty in atherosclerotic renal artery stenosis: a randomized trial. EMMA Study Group. *Hypertension*, 1998; **31:** 823–829.

Van den Ven PJG, Kaatee R, Beutler JJ *et al.* Arterial stenting and balloon angioplasty in ostial atherosclerotic renovascular disease: a randomized trial. *Lancet*, 1999; **353:** 282–286.

SALIVARY GLAND CALCULI

Christopher Lattimer, Nitin Gureja

Silaolithiases is the commonest salivary gland condition occurring in adults, with an incidence of 12 per 1000 of adult population. It is most common in 40–60-year-old males, and involves the submandibular gland (80%) then the parotid (19%). In approximately 3% of cases the disease is bilateral.

Pathogenesis

This is multifactorial. It is believed that the larger Wharton's duct, with its 'up hill' course and its narrow orifice opening in a 'sump'; along with its higher pH concentration of saliva predispose the gland to more calculi formation. Other predisposing factors include reduced salivary flow rates, dehydration and changes in salivary pH.

A typical calculus is composed of an inner organic nidus and an external layer of calcium phosphate with smaller quantities of carbonate, aluminium and magnesium.

Salivary gland calculi are associated with diabetes mellitus in ~ 25% of patients, hypertension in ~ 20%, and chronic liver disease in ~ 10% of patients.

Clinical features

Rarely are salivary gland calculi asymptomatic. They often present with symptoms of gustatory pain and swelling; caused by the increased salivary secretion during meals being obstructed by the calculus. The glandular swelling often decreases in size after the meal. Intraglandular calculi may not cause any obstructive symptoms. Occasionally it is possible to palpate a calculus in the duct, especially if it lies distally. Massage of the gland is likely to produce a turbid, foul-tasting secretion.

Acute suppurative sialadenitis may also be a presentation. Ascending bacterial sepsis results in the gland being swollen and tender; the patient often presenting with features of pyrexia and pain. Examination may reveal a palpable calculus in the duct along with oedema of the duct orifice. Turbid secretions can be massaged from the gland.

Investigations

Intra-oral occlusive radiographs are used to demonstrate the calculi. Approximately 90% of submandibular calculi are radiopaque, compared to 20–30% of parotid calculi.

Sialography will demonstrate intraductal calculi, as well as any evidence of strictures and sialectasis. It should not be undertaken in acute sialadenitis.

CT scanning is effective in demonstrating calculi along with any associated intraglandular disease.

Treatment

Treatment depends on the clinical state, as well as the site of the stone.

In acute sialadenitis secondary to calculus obstruction (commonest cause), management is centred on pain relief and treatment of the infection with broad-spectrum antibiotics. This is augmented with frequent antiseptic mouth-washes and use of sialagogues to encourage drainage of the gland.

When infection has proceeded to abscess formation, incision and drainage of the gland is necessary, with definitive treatment of the stone once the acute infection has settled.

Definitive treatment depends on the site of the stone.

In the submandibular gland, calculi located in the terminal part of Wharton's duct are removed directly through the floor of the mouth, with an incision being made directly over the stone, and marsupialization of the duct ends. Intraglandular stones as well as stones in the proximal half of Wharton's duct are treated by excision of the submandibular gland and excision of the proximal portion of the duct.

Parotid gland calculi within 1 cm of the orifice of Stensen's duct are removed through a duct meatomy with marsupialization of the duct ends. Calculi more proximal to this may be successfully removed by using a Fogarty's embolic catheter. If this is unsuccessful then excision of the relevant portion of the parotid gland and duct is required.

Lately extra-corporeal shock wave lithotripsy has been advocated for use of calculi in the proximal part of the parotid gland, with variable results. This procedure is still in its infancy.

Further reading

Bodner L. Salivary gland calculi: diagnostic imaging and surgical management. *Compendium*, 1993; **14**(5): 574–576.

Deahl ST, Ruprecht A, Gilbaugh G. Management of submandibular gland sialoliths. *Iowa Dental Journal*, 1991; **77**(2): 13, 38.

Williams MF. Sialolithiasis. *Otolaryngologic Clinics of North America*, 1999; **32**(5): 819–834.

Related topic of interest

SALIVARY GLAND TUMOURS

Christopher Lattimer, Nitin Gureja

The majority of salivary gland tumours occur in the parotid gland (~80%), and of these the majority (~80%) tend to be benign.

The second most frequent site is the submandibular gland (~10%), with ~60% being benign.

The majority of tumours occurring in the minor salivary gland especially those lining the palate tend to be malignant.

The only risk factor for salivary gland tumours seems to be previous exposure to radiation.

Types

Benign	Malignant
Pleomorphic adenoma	Mucoepidermoid (low-grade)
Warthin's tumour	Acinic cell carcinoma (low-grade)
Oncocytoma	Adenoid cystic carcinoma (cylindroma)
	Pleomorphic carcinoma lymphoma
	Metastatic (lung, breast, kidney)

Histogenesis

Reserve cells give rise to the acinar cells, replacement intercalated duct cells and myoepithelial cells; whilst the basal cells give rise to the columnar and squamous cells lining the excretory duct.

It is now generally accepted that salivary gland tumours arise from either of these two main cell types.

Pleomorphic adenoma, Warthin's tumour, oncocytoma, acinic cell carcinoma and adenoid cystic carcinoma all arise from reserve cells. Squamous cell carcinoma and muco-epidermoid carcinoma arise from basal cells.

Benign salivary gland tumours

Pleomorphic adenoma (mixed cell tumour)

It is the most common benign tumour, accounting for ~80% of all benign tumours. It is virtually the only benign tumour to occur in the submandibular, sublingual and minor salivary glands. They tend to occur in the fifth decade, with an equal sex distribution.

Pleomorphic adenomas are made up of epithelial and stromal elements, and comprise a pseudo-capsule arising from compression of the surrounding gland tissue. They tend to be highly cellular, with areas containing cysts, and irregularly shaped and also have a high propensity to occur, especially if contents are spilled during surgery.

Presentation is often as a painless lump and are often slow growing with periods of rapid growth. Features of pain or facial nerve palsy should arouse the suspicion of malignancy.

Fine-needle aspiration and cytology often confirms the presence of pleomorphic adenoma. MRI scan allows location, showing as a low signal mass on T_1-weighted images, and an increased signal on T_2 images.

Treatment often depends on the position of the pleomorphic adenoma; if confined to the superficial lobe then superficial parotidectomy is sufficient after identification and preservation of the branches of the facial nerve. However if the adenoma is in the deep lobe then total parotidectomy is undertaken, with preservation of the branches of the facial nerve.

Enucleation of the pleomorphic adenoma is not carried out due to the high recurrence rate ~40% at 25–30 years.

In situations where the adenoma is adherent to the nerve trunk then post-operative radiotherapy is offered to minimize the risk of recurrence.

Recurrence is differentiated from post-operative fibrosis by the use of intravenous gadolinum and MRI scanning; increased uptake by gadolinum signifying recurrence. This is treated by use of radiotherapy.

Pleomorphic adenoma occurring in the submandibular and other minor salivary gland tumours is by excision of the gland.

Warthin's tumour (adenolymphoma)

It is only seen in the parotid gland, and tends to occur in the fourth to seventh decade, with a 7:1 male preponderance. Ten per cent can be bilateral but are often not synchronous. They often present as painless, fluctuant swellings usually in the tail of the parotid gland.

Histologically the tumour is composed of lymphoid stroma containing cysts and lymphoid follicles.

Treatment is often excision of the tumour with a cuff of normal tissue.

Oncocytoma

They occur in patients over 55 years, with a female preponderance of 2:1. They are made up of oncocytes (cells containing an abundance of mitochondria), and are probably more hyperplastic then neoplastic. Treatment is by excision only.

Malignant salivary gland tumours

Malignant salivary gland tumours are rare, occurring more frequently in women then men, and more common in the fifth to seventh decade.

Only 20% of parotid, 40% of submandibular, 50% of the minor salivary gland and most of sublingual tumours are malignant.

The tumours can be classed as high grade (adenoid cystic, squamous cell) or low grade (acinic) depending on mitotic rate, nuclear pleomorphism.

Mucoepidermoid

This is the most frequent of the malignant salivary tumours.

Histologically the tumour is composed of epidermal and mucous cells which secrete mucus into the stroma and hence form cysts. Tumours are graded as high if more then 90% of their area is made up of tumour cells and less than 10% of cysts. High-grade tumours have less then 40% 10-year survival rate, and low-grade tumours have ~80% 10-year survival rate.

Incidence of lymph node metastasis is ~40%.

Adenoid cystic

These slow-growing tumours occur in the sixth decade and have an equal sex distribution. They originate from reserve cells of the intercalated ducts. The tumour has a propensity to spread along neural sheaths and hence a large number (~30%) present with facial nerve palsy. Vascular dissemination is more a feature than lymphatic spread, hence metastasis especially to the lung is more common then regional lymph node involvement.

Five-year survival is between 60–80%.

Acinic cell carcinoma

Acinic cell carcinomas have a variable biological behaviour. They tend to be slow growing and ~3% will be bilateral. They have a 5-year survival of ~90%.

Malignant pleomorphic adenoma

This term actually designates three different types of tumours, two of them being malignant from the outset, and the third arising from the epithelial component of a mixed cell tumour–expleomorphic adenoma. The latter are the most common in this sub-group, and have often been present for several years. They have a high tendency to metastasize, and are associated with a poor prognosis; 5-year survival of ~40%.

Diagnosis and investigation

Presentation of a salivary gland tumour is best initially studied by FNAC. Trucut and incisional biopsy are to be condemned due to the risk of seedling along the tract. To date no evidence exists for any such risk associated with FNAC. Success of FNAC depends on the experience of the histopathologist.

MRI scan with intravenous gadolinium is better then CT scan in delineating the tumour along with gland structure and presence of lymph nodes.

Treatment of malignant parotid gland tumours

The basis of treatment is excision of the tumour with surrounding healthy parotid tissue.

In small tumours confined to the superficial gland, superficial parotidectomy is sufficient, otherwise a total parotidectomy with facial nerve sparing is carried out. In cases of suspected facial nerve involvement, frozen section is undertaken to confirm, prior to nerve excision and subsequent grafting.

A radical neck dissection is undertaken if lymph node involvement is present. Tumour invasion into skin and bone requires a radical excision with use of flaps to cover the defects.

Adjuvant therapy

Radiotherapy, often in the form of hyperfractionation or neutron therapy is used for high-grade tumours as well as those where there is doubt about the adequacy of clearance.

SCREENING

Nick Lagattolla

This may be defined as the detection of a disease in its early stages before the development of symptoms. The disease screened for may be benign or malignant. Screening of small at-risk patient groups for specific disorders is widespread at many levels of health care, for example the screening for familial polyposis coli in first-degree relatives of sufferers. However, this topic is concerned with the mass screening of unselected large populations for surgically treatable conditions.

Wilson's criteria

These define the principles of screening. The disorder must be prevalent, and must have a premorbid state which is readily detectable and easily treated. The screening tests must be acceptable to the population to be screened, simple to perform and interpret, and they must be reliable, offering a low rate of false-positive and false-negative results (high sensitivity and specificity for the disorder in question). There must be evidence of beneficial effects from a proposed screening programme in both economic (cost-effective) and health terms (reduced morbidity or mortality) before it becomes established practice.

Established national screening programmes

Cervical cancer

This was the first national programme established. Based on cytological diagnosis of dyskaryosis of a specially stained fixed cervical smear, the premorbid condition of cervical intra-epithelial neoplasia is determined, and minimally invasive surgery or laser ablation is used to prevent frankly invasive carcinoma, which would require radical surgery for a reduced chance of a cure. The benefits are beyond dispute, the only caveat being potentially difficult and subjective interpretation of cervical smears, requiring on-going quality control measures to establish consistency, sensitivity and specificity of results.

Breast cancer

Data from Scandinavia suggested that the result from surgery in mammogram-detected breast cancer patients was better than in clinically detected patients. This led to trials of mammography in the detection of early breast cancer, which has many ideal characteristics for screening: pre-invasive lesions may be detected mammographically, reasonably unequivocal cytological results can be obtained from fine-needle aspirates of suspicious sites, and potentially curable and cosmetically acceptable surgery is performed for localized disease.

Following the recommendations of the Forrest Report of 1982, women between the ages of 50–64 are offered single-view bilateral mammography every two years. The results have determined that screening is beneficial, with a reduced long-term mortality from breast cancer, though certain questions still remain about certain issues. These include considerable psychological morbidity inherent in the screening process, the determination of the optimal modes and frequency of mammography, the age-range for screening, and the application of both tumour and lead-time biases in the interpretation of results (vide infra).

Other conditions where screening is under investigation

Colorectal carcinoma

This is an ideal condition for screening, in terms of prevalence of disease, with colonic polyps being a readily identifiable and curable precursor condition. Tests currently under investigation include the Haemoccult stool test for faecal occult blood, with or without flexible sigmoidoscopy.

Prostate cancer

Blood tests for prostate-specific antigen and prostatic acid phosphatase form the basis of screening for prostatic carcinoma. Screening comprises blood testing combined with digital examination, followed by ultrasound-guided transrectal biopsy of suspicious lesions. The earliest stage (stage 1) may then be treated by radical prostatectomy. There is a clear health benefit to screening, though the cost–benefit ratio is rather loaded toward the cost element. A nationwide programme in the UK has only recently received government support.

Ovarian carcinoma

The CA-125 antigen is frequently elevated in this condition, and mass screening of middle-aged women has been proposed.

Aortic aneurysm

The initial results of screening selected populations with atherosclerosis were excellent, and screening programmes have been initiated on the population at large in certain areas. Aortic aneurysm is an ideal condition to screen for, as it is a silent and potentially lethal condition, yet is easily detected by ultrasound and carries a vastly reduced risk of death if operated electively.

Bias and the interpretation of results

Inherent to the practice of screening lie hidden biases that must be understood in order to correctly interpret the perceived benefits of screening. Any screening programme could be considered beneficial if cost were not a consideration and if any lives were shown to be saved. The question of cost and value are beyond the scope of this chapter. The interpretation of whether lives have been saved should be undertaken with tumour bias and lead-time bias in mind.

A screening programme will inevitably pick up a larger number of less malignant or lethal conditions as these will have a longer lifetime than very aggressive conditions carrying a high mortality. In this way, in the screened, treated and surviving population, there will be a proportionately greater number of individuals with less aggressive tumours or conditions, than in the population that has died in the same time period. This is termed tumour bias.

Lead-time bias reflects the time between the screened detection of a tumour or condition, and the point at which it would normally become clinically detectable. This length of time may be some months or years, depending on the natural history of the condition. Should the condition be incurable at the time of detection, death would ensue at the same point in time, whether detected clinically or by screening. However, there would be a considerably longer perceived survival time in a screened individual.

Further reading

Blanks RG, Moss SM, McGahan CE *et al.* Effect of NHS breast screening programme on mortality from breast cancer in England and Wales, 1990–8: comparison of observed with predicted mortality. *British Medical Journal*, 2000; **321**: 665–669.

Scholefield JH. Screening (ABC of colorectal cancer). *British Medical Journal*, 2000; **321**: 1004–1006.

Mini-symposium on screening. *Current Practice in Surgery*, 1993; **5**(1): 1–21.

SENTINEL NODE BIOPSY

Christopher Lattimer, Prakash Sinha

Definition

The sentinel node is the first lymph node on a direct drainage pathway from the primary tumour site. A tumour may drain to more than one sentinel lymph node.

Introduction

The sentinel node concept has radically changed our understanding of how cancers spread by lymphatics, and questions the practice of radical en bloc dissection of malignant tumours. Sentinel nodes have been identified at sites which do not correspond to the orderly drainage patterns demonstrated in anatomical books. For example, testicular tumours and breast tumours have had supraclavicular sentinel nodes, back melanomas have had pre-aortic sentinel nodes, occipital melanomas have had axillary sentinel nodes, rectal cancers have had inguinal sentinel nodes and medial breast cancers have had contralateral axillary sentinel nodes identified. Sentinel node surgery has been introduced as the ultimate staging modality of early cancers and to prevent the morbidity associated with radical lymphatic surgery.

History

In 1915, LR Braithwaite described the drainage pathway of a pigmented appendix (presumably a malignant melanoma) to the ileo-caecal, duodenal and greater curve gastric nodes. Ramon Cabanas in 1976 showed the existence of a specific draining lymph node, 'sentinel' lymph node, which could be identified after lymphangiography through the dorsal lymphatics of the penis. He confirmed that the first node visualized, the sentinel node, was the first site of metastases and reported that it was often the only affected lymph node. In 1992 Donald Morton and colleagues developed cutaneous lymphoscintigraphy as a method of identifying nodal areas at risk of metastases in patients with malignant melanoma. They showed preferential drainage to one or two nodes in a particular lymph node group. This concept was applied to breast cancer and it was expected that if malignant cells spread to a regional lymph node then they should follow the same route as lymph draining from the primary carcinoma. If the draining or sentinel node from a breast cancer or malignant melanoma can be identified and is free of metastasis then theoretically the other axillary nodes should also be free of disease.

Identification

Three techniques are used to identify sentinel nodes:

1. Lymphoscintigraphy. Dynamic and static acquisition scanning with a gamma camera after injection of a radioactive tracer.
2. The intra-operative use of a gamma probe after injection of a radioactive tracer.
3. Injection of blue dye. Blue lymphatics are followed into blue sentinel lymph nodes.

Technical considerations

- Site of injection: Intradermal lymphatic drainage is different to subcutaneous lymphatic drainage. Controversy exists as to whether there should be single or multiple injections, intratumoural, peritumoural, subcutaneous or intradermal injections. Most breast tissue (70%) drains into axillary nodes whereas nearly all the (99%) dermal lymphatics drain this way [b].
- Molecular weight of labelled colloid. Small particles travel fast but have shorter residency times. They may pass through sentinel nodes and travel to secondary or tertiary echelon nodes. Nano colloid and sulphur colloid are commonly labelled.
- Tumour massage after injection may improve sentinel node identification.
- A combination of patent blue dye and radioactive tracer techniques result in high rates of identification [c].
- False-positive sentinel nodes may occur if the primary lymphatic pathways are obstructed by tumour.
- Minute sentinel nodes may be missed with the blue dye technique. A tiny node may look like a diathermy mark.
- Sentinel node may be missed if they are close to the tracer injection site.
- The detection of background counts from the node excision site compared with a 10-fold or greater increase in counts from the excised node confirms sentinel node removal [c].
- The sentinel node technique requires close cooperation between surgeon, nuclear physician and pathologist.

Histology

It would be ideal to have the histology immediately so that if positive, the surgeon can proceed to a lymph node dissection. Unfortunately frozen section reports false-negative rates between 20 to 30% and is not reliable. Conventional paraffin waxed H&E staining takes days to report making second surgery necessary in positive patients. Immunohistochemical staining with antibodies (S-100, HMV 45 and Melan-A) and extensive multilevel sectioning are often essential in identifying micro-metastasis. There have been encouraging results with imprint cytology of bisected lymph nodes.

Breast cancer

Axillary lymph nodes status in patients with breast cancer is the single most important prognostic factor from which important clinical decisions are based [a]. In the absence of non-invasive techniques, staging of the axilla is performed either by a sampling technique (removal of at least 4 nodes), partial axillary dissection (level 1 or 2) or axillary clearance (level 3 – to remove all nodes) both to stage and treat the axilla. With the development of screening, increasing numbers of women are seen who are node negative. In these patients extensive axillary surgery is difficult to justify because 7 out of 10 women gain no significant benefit and suffer considerable morbidity (seroma, lymphoedema, cutaneous nerve impairment, shoulder pain and rarely lymphosarcoma) from the axillary surgery. Sentinel node biopsy offers a technique that assesses axillary lymph node status while minimizing morbidity.

In management of breast cancer sentinel node biopsy is a promising technique, but before it can be introduced into routine practice the technique of node identification and immediate histological evaluation needs to be optimized and it needs to be compared with other surgical options for axillary node staging. The false-negative rate is reported to be 3–5% in experienced hands[b]. If the procedure is optimized in experienced hands in invasive breast cancer it can be considered as an equal staging procedure as axillary dissection with reduced morbidity. The clinical relevance of micrometastasis found by immunohistochemistry is unknown. At the present time if the sentinel node is positive treatment of the axilla is advised.

Malignant melanoma

Nodal involvement is a vital prognostic factor in patients with invasive malignant melanoma. Although most of the patients present with clinically negative nodal basins, many of them actually harbour occult regional lymph node metastases. As a result, the optimal scope of surgical management has remained a controversial issue. Because only 20% of patients with a primary melanoma of intermediate thickness are expected to have metastases in their regional nodes, 80% of those undergoing elective lymph node dissection are risking complications without benefit. Therefore elective lymph node dissection has never been widely practised in the United Kingdom, where observation and therapeutic lymph node dissection for patients who develop metastasis have been preferred.

In malignant melanoma tumour thickness and ulceration are important prognostic discriminators in patients with negative sentinel nodes. In contrast, for patients with a positive SLN, neither tumour thickness nor any other factor provide additional prognostic information.

Other cancers

The role of sentinel node biopsies is also being evaluated in management of head and neck cancer, other skin cancers and gastrointestinal cancer.

In summary sentinel node biopsy concept in management of both malignant melanoma and breast cancer has proved to be valid; however before it can be introduced into routine practice results from randomized controlled trials should be awaited.

Further reading

Mohammed RS, Keshtgar PJ. Sentinel lymph node biopsy in breast carcinoma. In: Johnson CD, Taylor I (Eds) *Recent Advances in Surgery*, 2000; **23:** 109–123.

Pijpers R, Borgstein PJ, Meijer S, Hoekstra OS, Van Hattum LH, Teule GJJ. Sentinel node biopsy in melanoma patients: dynamic lymphoscintigraphy followed by intra-operative gamma probe and vital dye guidance. *World Journal of Surgery*, 1997; **21:** 788–793.

Rodier JF, Routiot T, Mignotte H *et al.* Lymphatic mapping and sentinel node biopsy of operable breast cancer. *World Journal of Surgery*, 2000; **24**(10): 1220–1225; discussion 1225–1226.

Veronesi U, Paganelli G, Galimberti V *et al.* Sentinel-node biopsy to avoid axillary dissection in breast cancer with clinically negative lymph-nodes. *Lancet*, 1997; **349** no. 9069: 1864–1867.

Related topics of interest

Breast cancer (p. 57); Malignant melanoma (p. 213).

SKIN COVER

Christopher Lattimer, Omar Faiz

The skin provides a competent barrier to infection and fluid loss. Extensive skin loss from burns, ulcers, pressure sores, trauma or radical cancer surgery can be replaced by a variety of methods when primary closure cannot be achieved. In all cases of tissue transfer patient factors that favour wound healing and promote adequate tissue bed vascularity, such as good nutritional status and cessation of smoking, should be optimized to maximize the chance of graft success.

Skin grafts

Skin grafts involve the transfer of skin from one part of the body (donor site) to another area (recipient site) where it must establish a new blood supply. Skin grafts can be either split-skin or full-thickness grafts.

Split-skin grafts

1. Principle. Split-skin grafts can be harvested to varying levels of dermal depth. In each case, the entire epidermis is taken with a variable portion of the dermis. Unlike the epidermis, the dermis is not capable of regeneration. The quality of the established graft therefore depends upon the initial dermal thickness. Thicker grafts require a greater blood supply and consequently take less easily than thinner grafts, however the eventual cosmetic outcome of the former is usually superior. In addition to the importance of graft thickness, recipient site factors such as adequacy of the bed vascularity, sterility and haemostasis, are essential components to eventual graft success.

2. Harvesting. The donor site chosen to resurface skin defects should aim to match the colour, texture and hair-bearing properties with those of the recipient sites. Commonly used donor sites include inconspicuous areas such as the buttocks and inner thighs. The lateral thigh is preferred in the elderly as the dermis is thick in this region, and access to dressings is facilitated. Extensive burn injuries can mandate the use of all available donor areas, including the scalp and the sole of the foot. Grafts are harvested with either a hand-held (Humby) knife or an electric or gas-powered dermatome. Thin grafts ensure rapid donor site re-epithelialization (7–10 days) and allow the same site to be used repeatedly. Intermediate and thick split-skin grafts may take 2–3 weeks for healing to occur. Re-epithelialization occurs most rapidly in a moist sterile environment. The latter is achieved by placement of a gas-permeable membrane (OpSite) over the donor site for 5–10 days.

3. Technique. The chosen donor site should be sterilized with chlorhexidine or savlon (iodine preparations interfere with lubrication) and smeared liberally with paraffin. Wooden boards flatten the desired skin surface whilst the operator of a hand-held knife harvests the graft. The harvesting technique involves short frequent slicing lateral movements rather than direct forward progression. The skin graft must then be fashioined and applied to the recipient bed. Good contact between the graft and recipient site is essential for capillary bud formation. The graft is then secured in place with either sutures or staples. Non-adherent gauze is applied directly over the graft surface, followed by generous layers of gauze and cotton wool. Crepe bandage is then used to effect pressure, and consequently minimize blood and seroma collection. The dressing should only be removed after 5–7 days unless collection or infection is suspected mandating earlier inspection.

Meshing

Meshing is a technique used to expand split-skin grafts. A graft can be expanded from 1.5 to 8 times its original size utilizing this technique. Such widely expanded autografts are ideal for covering extensive areas. In addition, the multiple perforations produced by passing a graft through the meshing machine permit the escape of blood and serum from the recipient bed and hence increase the likelihood of graft success. One major disadvantage however is the final latticed appearance produced by the healed graft perforations. This occurs as the graft interstices heal by epithelialization alone whereas the actual mesh component contains a thickness of dermis. If split skin grafts are placed directly on to a wound surface, the cosmetic defect remains fixed at the original size. A technique commonly employed is to permit wound contraction of full-thickness defects prior to skin grafting thereby significantly reducing ultimate graft size.

Full-thickness grafts

These grafts include both the epidermis and full dermis. They result in superior aesthetic appearance when compared to split-skin grafts and are consequently used to cover facial and genital defects. One disadvantage however, is that as no epithelial elements remain at the donor site, spontaneous re-epithelialization does not occur and primary closure is required.

Flaps

A flap is a term applied to tissue which is used for wound closure or reconstruction which retains, at least in part, its original blood supply. There are many different varieties of tissue flaps, which are commonly classified according to either blood supply (below), or tissue layer involvement (muscle, musculocutaneous, fasciocutaneous).

1. ***Random pattern flaps.*** This flap comprises undermined skin and subcutaneous tissue. In this type no specific regard is paid to blood supply. These flaps receive an arterial supply from vessels in the subdermal plexus. To avoid necrosis flap length should not exceed base width. An example of this type is that of the skin flaps fashioned during simple mastectomy.

2. ***Axial pattern flap.*** This is a modification of the previous variety which facilitates greater flap lengths by utilizing a known and dependable blood supply. The flap is fashioned such that the arterial supply courses the long axis of the flap. Examples of this type include rotation forehead flaps which are based on the supraorbital and supratrochlear arteries and the groin flap which is reliant on the superficial circumflex iliac artery.

3. *Axial island flap.* This flap allows for greater mobility than the axial pattern flap. It is detached cutaneously from its origin and maintained on an isolated artery and vein. An example of this type includes the latissimus dorsi flap breast reconstruction based on its supply by the thoracodorsal vessels.

4. *Free flap.* The advent of microvascular surgery has permitted the transfer of free flaps to remote regions by immediate arteriovenous anastomosis to named recipient artery and veins. An example of this type includes the radial forearm flap used for jaw reconstruction.

Tissue expansion

Tissue expansion is an effective method of increasing the available quantity of full-thickness skin. Sialastic balloons are placed beneath the dermis and inflated weekly with saline through a subcutaneous access port. When sufficient skin has been developed, the implant is removed and primary closure can then be achieved. Tissue expansion has also been utilized in breast reconstruction to good effect [b]. Early over-expansion of the reconstructed breast increases skin quantity such that, on deflation, the pendulous hang of the breast is reproduced. Complications associated with tissue expansion include: mechanical failure of the implant, port problems (such as rotation), and tissue necrosis due to rapid over-expansion.

Recent advances

Advances made in cell biology and tissues engineering over the last 15 years are revolutionizing the approach to skin cover. Keratinocyte culture techniques were the first major breakthrough. These techniques permit the in vitro manufacture of large confluent sheets of epidermis from just 1 cm of split skin in 2–3 weeks [b]. These grafts are now in use clinically for cover in patients where there is a paucity of donor skin. One major disadvantage however is that, without an underlying dermal layer, the graft is fragile and graft survival is consequently poor. Recent work has seen the development of bilayered grafts, whereby a polymeric scaffold is used to stabilize the epidermal surface [b]. Bilayered grafts could provide a solution to the problem of skin cover in the extensively burnt patient. Another important development in this field is the demonstration that peptide growth factors such as EGF, PDGF and TGF can, in animal models and limited human trials, enhance wound healing [b].

Further reading

Cairns BA, de Serres S, Peterson HD *et al.* The biotechnological quest for optimal wound closure. *Archives in Surgery*, 1993; **128**(11): 1246–1252.

Chang LD, Buncke G, Slezak *et al.* Cigarette smoking, plastic surgery, and microsurgery. *Journal of Reconstructive Microsurgery*, 1996; **12**(7): 467–474.

Hardesty RA. Plastic surgery. *Journal of the American College of Surgery*, 1998; **186**(2): 212–218.

Rudkin GH, Miller TA. Growth factors in surgery. *Plastic and Reconstructive Surgery*, 1996; **97**(2): 469–476.

Related topics of interest

THE SKIN AND SUBCUTANEOUS TISSUES

Christopher Lattimer, Omar Faiz

The skin is the largest organ of the body. It harbours a multitude of pathological processes that involve every clinical speciality.

Benign skin conditions

Papilloma

Otherwise known as skin tags, these pedunculated lesions are caused by benign overgrowth of all layers of the skin. Papillomas comprise a rugose epithelial covering (sometimes pigmented) with a central core of connective tissue, vessels and lymphatics.

Seborrhoeic keratoses

Also unflatteringly termed 'senile warts', these lesions arise due to an excessive overgrowth of the basal layer of the epidermis. This lesion can be picked or rubbed off to reveal pink skin below. As their colloquial name implies, seborrhoeic keratoses occur increasingly with advancing age.

Haemangioma

This general term encompasses multiple congenital lesions including: strawberry naevi, port-wine stains, spider naevi, vin rose patches and Campbell de Morgan spots. All of the above lesions arise secondary to aberrant skin capillary formation.

Keratoacanthoma

Also termed molluscum sebaceum this is a benign overgrowth of hair follicle cells. It arises as a skin swelling which develops an irregular keratinous central core. The appearance can be difficult to distinguish from that of a squamous cell carcinoma. The condition is however totally benign and, although the natural history is that of eventual spontaneous regression (albeit with scar formation), most keratoacanthomas are excised for cosmetic reasons as well as the exclusion of malignancy.

Dermatofibroma

Also termed a histiocytoma, this lesion is a benign tumour of dermal fibroblasts. These lesions are slow growing and occur most frequently on the limbs of young and middle-aged adults. There is commonly a history of previous mild trauma or insect bite suggestive that these are reactive lesions. They are firm in consistency and often have an erythematous sheen. When treatment is requested for cosmesis or there is diagnostic uncertainty simple excision is performed.

Pyogenic granuloma

This lesion arises as an excessive growth of granulation tissue from the site of a previous minor injury or insect bite. Often the initial injury is not recalled. The reason for this abnormality of tissue repair is not known but local infection is usually an associated factor. The lesion grows rapidly often discharging seropurulent fluid or bleeding when traumatized. Treatment is by excision.

Cylindroma

Also known as a *turban tumour* this lesion is relatively benign but gradually forms an extensive swelling over the scalp. Histologically these lesions are composed of cylinders of clear cells. These lesions can ulcerate and when this happens misdiagnosis for basal cell carcinomas commonly occurs.

Benign subcutaneous conditions

Lipoma

Lipomas arise as slow-growing benign tumours of fat cells and can occur anywhere in the body where there are fatty reserves. The subcutaneous tissues of the forearms and thighs are commonly affected. Lipomas *never* become malignant and should not be confused with liposarcomas which arise de novo preferentially in retroperitoneal fat. Lipomas are soft, lobulated, semi-fluctuant lesions which can grow to an enormous size. It is not uncommon for a patient to have more than one lipoma, however a minority of patients present with multiple tender subcutaneous lipomas – a condition known as Dercum's disease (adiposis dolorosa). The latter lesions can be difficult to distinguish from neurofibromas.

Fat necrosis

When traumatized fat necroses it manifests itself as an irregular, indurated lump. The breast is a common site for fat necrosis secondary to minor traumatic injury. Misdiagnosis with carcinoma is common.

Sebaceous cyst

This common skin tumour is commonly described as a retention cyst caused by obstruction of the mouth of the sebaceous gland by sebum. The latter explanation of the aetiology is now acknowledged to be an inaccurate oversimplification. More specifically, these cysts are derived from either the infundibular portion of the hair follicles (epidermal cysts), or from the hair follicle epithelium (trichilemmal cysts). Sebaceous cysts arise most commonly over the scalp, face and scrotum. They are typically fluctuant and cannot be separated from the overlying skin. There is usually a punctum on the skin overlying the cyst. The complications of sebaceous cysts include: infection; ulceration (also known as Cock's peculiar tumour when classically found on the scalp and often mistaken for a malignancy) and sebaceous horn formation. Treatment comprises cyst excision. Cyst recurrence is common if the entire capsule is not removed. Infected cysts require incision and drainage followed by elective excision.

Dermoid cyst

Implantation dermoids usually arise following penetrating injury resulting in the implantation of epithelial cells into the deeper subcutaneous tissues. These cysts arise commonly on the pulp of the fingers as subcutaneous swellings that are not attached either to the overlying skin or deeper tissues. *Sequestration dermoids* are subcutaneous swellings which occur commonly around the outer orbit, the root of the nose and in the midline. They result from aberrant inclusion of epithelial nests beneath the surface along a line of skin fusion. Suspected sequestration dermoids should be evaluated by CT prior to excision to exclude intracranial extension.

Ganglion

Ganglia occur most commonly around the wrist. Their aetiology is thought to be due to myxomatous degeneration of a joint capsule or tendon sheath. Ganglia are tense cystic swellings that contain clear gelatinous fluid. Treatment is by excision which is only usually curative if the entire ganglion wall is removed.

Nerve tumours

Neurilemmomas (schwannomas) arise from neurilemmal cells on peripheral nerves. These tumours can arise from a peripheral nerve anywhere in the body. They are soft and lobulated in appearance and classically give rise to tingling in the distribution of the affected nerve. *Neurofibromas* arise from the connective tissue of a nerve sheath. They arise on both peripheral and cranial nerves and can occur as solitary or multiple lesions. *Generalized neurofibromatosis* (Von Recklinghausen's disease) is an autosomal dominant condition characterized by café-au-lait spots, multiple neurofibromas and scoliosis. Sarcomatous change only occurs in a minority of patients with neurofibromatosis. Treatment is by excision for symptomatic, large lesions or lesions that have undergone malignant change.

Basal cell carcinoma (BCC)

Basal cell carcinomas (BCCs), or *rodent* ulcers, are the commonest type of skin cancers. They usually occur among the elderly in sun-exposed areas of the face and scalp. BCCs commonly present as a pearly nodular protuberance, often with a central depression and characteristic rolled edge. They can also be cystic, pigmented or be of the superficial spreading type (which classically give the 'field-fire' appearance). The inner canthus of the eye and the nasolabial fold are frequent locations for these lesions. The histological appearances are of basiloid cell clusters with peripheral palisading. The constituent cells of a BCC proliferate extremely rapidly but their rate of cell death is also high which falsely gives the impression of indolence. They are locally destructive tumours but metastases are extremely rare. Treatment involves local excision or radiotherapy. The cure rate for primary lesions is greater than 95%[a].

Squamous cell carcinoma (SCC)

These lesions also develop in areas exposed to solar irradiation. They are commoner in the immunosuppressed, within areas of actinic keratosis and in sites of Bowen's disease (carcinoma-in-situ), however most still arise de novo. Squamous cell malignant change in an area of ulceration (e.g. venous ulcer) is termed a *Marjolin's ulcer*. SCCs present classically as keratotic nodules with central ulceration and everted edges. The histological appearances are of protruding tongues of dysplastic squamous cells into the deep dermis or the subcutaneous fat. They are locally destructive, spread along peripheral nerves and involve regional nodes in 5–10% of cases. Therapy involves wide excision with block dissection of the draining nodal basin if it is involved. Recently, sentinel node biopsy has been employed to detect regional nodal involvement[c]. An adequate tumour excision margin is essential to prevent recurrence. SCCs are also highly radiosensitive and this can be used as an alternative form of therapy. Multiple early lesions can be coated with topical 5-fluorouracil to good effect[b].

Further reading

Fenton OM, Fenton L, Britto JA. The skin, skin tumours and plastic surgery. In: Burnand KG, Young AE (Eds). *The New Aird's Companion in Surgical Studies.* Edinburgh: Churchill Livingstone, 1998; 165–222.

Green A, Whiteman D, Frost I, Battistuta D. Sun exposure, skin cancers and related skin conditions. *Journal of Epidemiology*, 1999; **9**(6 Suppl): S7–13.

Wennberg AM. Basal cell carcinoma – new aspects of diagnosis and treatment. *Acta Dermatology and Venereology Suppl*, 2000; **209**(4): 5–25.

Related topic of interest

Malignant melanoma (p. 213).

SMALL BOWEL TUMOURS

Deya Marzouk

Small bowel hamartomas and benign tumours

Peutz–Jegher's syndrome

This is an autosomal dominant condition characterized by mucocutaneous pigmentation (circumoral, circumanal, palms and soles) and multiple hamartomatous polyps throughout the stomach, duodenum, small intestine and colon. The vast majority of these occur in the small bowel and can vary from a few millimetres in diameter to several centimetres. They are also prone to adenomatous polyps, which may undergo malignant change, particularly in the duodenum.

These polyps can cause colicky abdominal pains, act as lead points for intussusception and may present with small bowel obstruction. Treatment is by laparotomy, reduction of intussusception, with open polypectomy of the larger polyps, followed by operative endoscopic removal of most of the other polyps. Long-term follow-up with upper GI endoscopy and colonoscopy is needed to control gastric, duodenal and colonic polyps.

Benign tumours

Leiomyomas and lipomas are normally asymptomatic and are found incidentally during laparotomy for other causes. Occasionally these tumours are bulky and cause symptoms due to small bowel obstruction or initiate intussusception. Leiomyomas may be seen on small bowel contrast studies as ovoid intraluminal defects with intact mucosa. Treatment is by local resection and anastomosis. When in doubt about the nature of the tumour, it is best to treat it as a malignant lesion (commoner).

Tubular and villous adenomas occur especially in the duodenum and are often asymptomatic. Villous adenomas have malignant potential and occur in patients with familial polyposis and Gardner's syndrome, especially around the ampulla of Vater. These should be removed endoscopically. Haemangiomas also occur and may be multiple in Osler-Weber-Rendu syndrome. They may cause recurrent acute or occult GI bleeding.

Small bowel malignant tumours

Malignant tumours affecting small bowel may be metastatic in origin, a direct invasion from nearby malignancy, e.g. colonic cancer, or a primary small intestinal tumour. Primary small bowel malignancies are rare, accounting for only 1% of all GI malignancies. They include adenocarcinomas, leiomyosarcomas, lymphomas and carcinoid tumours. These tumours occur slightly more frequently in males and peak in incidence in the sixth and seventh decades of life. Predisposing factors include familial polyposis, Gardner's syndrome, Peutz–Jeghers syndrome and Crohn's disease. Immunosuppressed patients e.g. AIDS and those with IgA defeciency, also are at increased risk.

Metastatic malignancies

Metastases are more common than primary malignant tumours in the small bowel. Common primaries include colonic, ovarian, bronchial cancer and melanoma. They are usually part of widespread metastatic disease. The majority of these tumours (which can be multiple) remain localized, causing partial small bowel obstruction. Some may cause GI bleeding or perforate. Melanotic deposits may also spread to involve the small bowel mesentery and regional lymph nodes.

If the patient is expected to survive a few months or more, he or she may be treated by either resection or bypass.

Small bowel adenocarcinoma

Small bowel adenocarcinomas are more frequent in the duodenum and ileum. They may cause abdominal pain, weight loss, intestinal obstruction and occult or overt GI bleeding. Duodenal adenocarcinomas may present with gastric outlet obstruction or obstructive jaundice (usually intermittent). They may invade adjacent tissues. These lesions are diagnosed on endoscopy and small bowel contrast studies.

Treatment is by wide segmental resection with regional lymphadenectomy. Duodenal adenocarcinomas need a Whipple's pancreaticoduodenectomy. Bypass is needed in unresectable tumours. There is little role for radiotherapy and chemotherapy. Five-year survival is 20–30% after small bowel resection. Duodenal adenocarcinomas have 5-year survival rate of up to 40%.

Leiomyosarcoma

Small bowel sarcomas are more frequent in jejunum and ileum and account for 10% of small bowel malignancies. Leiomyosarcomas account for 75% of these lesions. Fibrosarcoma, angiosarcoma and liposarcoma also occur. They may invade nearby organs. Small bowel Kaposi's sarcomas may develop in AIDS patients.

They may present with colicky abdominal pain, upper or lower GI bleeding, anaemia, abdominal masses or intestinal obstruction. Small bowel enemas, CT scans and superior mesenteric angiography may be useful in establishing the diagnosis.

Treatment is by small bowel resection en bloc with involved adjacent organs. Wide mesenteric lymphadenectomy is unnecessary in these lesions, as they do not normally spread to regional nodes. Palliative resection is still the best treatment for bleeding or obstructing advanced lesions, otherwise bypass is the only option.

Lymphomas

1. Pathology and classification. Lymphomas affecting the GI tract may be primary (4–9%) or part of widespread lymphoma. Most are non-Hodgkin's lymphomas and occur most frequently in the ileum. Gut non-Hodgkin's lymphomas are generally classified into B-cell and T-cell lymphomas. B-cell lymphomas of the gut can be low grade or high grade. MALT (mucosa-associated lymphatic tissue) lymphomas represent about 27% of intestinal B cell lymphomas and they have a relatively good prognosis with 50% of patients surviving 10 years[b]. Enteropathy associated T-cell lymphoma (EATL) may occur as a complication of long-standing coeliac disease. It is an aggressive tumour that often ulcerates, bleeds and may perforate. It also tends to be resistant to treatment and have poor prognosis[c].

2. Clinical features. Lymphomas cause abdominal pain, weight loss, partial or complete intestinal obstruction and may perforate in up to 25% of patients. They also ulcerate and cause GI bleeding.

3. Treatment. Small intestinal lymphomas present with bulky disease in most patients. Thus surgical resection of the primary lesion and regional mesenteric lymph nodes is often needed for both diagnosis and treatment (even for low-grade lymphomas). Frozen section examination of the resection margins is advisable since these tumours tend to spread extensively submucosally.

Resection only may be sufficient for low-grade lymphomas, but most need post-operative chemotherapy usually using **CHOP** (**C**yclophosphamide, Doxorubicin (**H**ydroxydoxorubicin), Vincristine (**O**ncovin) and **P**rednisolone) chemotherapy. Prognosis is strongly influenced by grade and immunophenotype. The overall 5-year survival is about 20–23%.

4. Mediterranean lymphoma. Immunoproliferative small intestinal disease (IPSID), also known as Mediterranean lymphoma is a special form of MALT lymphoma, which is characterized by synthesis of alpha heavy-chain immunoglobulins and is seen in the Mediterranean basin and the Middle East. It affects young adults and presents with abdominal cramps, diarrhoea, steatorrhea and weight loss. This type usually affects the entire small bowel with predominance in jejunum and duodenum. The clinical course is characterized with exacerbation and remissions. Death occurs from malnutrition or progression to high-grade lymphoma. Proliferation of low-grade MALT lymphomas and IPSID may be driven by T-cells responding to specific *Helicobacter pylori*-derived antigens. Some low-grade IPSID and low-grade MALT lymphomas in stomach may respond to anti-*H. pylori* eradication therapy [c]. The usual treatment, however, remains combination chemotherapy.

Carcinoid tumours

Carcinoid tumours arise from neuroendocrine (Kulchitsky) cells which are identified histologically by silver stains (argentaffin cells). Of all GI carcinoids, 85% occur in the appendix, 13% in small bowel and 2% in the rectum. Most appendicular carcinoids are small and benign in behaviour and are found incidentally or at autopsy. In contrast most carcinoids in small intestine are malignant and eventually become symptomatic or metastasize.

Carcinoid tumours are slow-growing tumours. They may be endocrinologically inert or may produce a variety of vasoactive substances and thus give rise to carcinoid syndrome.

1. Carcinoid of the appendix. Appendiceal carcinoids less than 1 cm rarely metastasize and are adequately treated by appendectomy alone unless the appendix base is involved, which requires resection of part of the caecum as well. Appendiceal carcinoids 2 cm or more in size metastasize to lymph nodes and require a right hemicolectomy. Tumours less than 2 cm, but with apparent enlarged regional lymph nodes or invasion of the mesoappendix should also be treated by a right hemicolectomy.

2. Carcinoid of the small bowel. Carcinoids of the small bowel are typically yellow, golden or brown-grey intramural or submucosal nodules. They typically excite intense fibrotic reaction in the mesentery, which becomes shortened, thickened and fixed angulating the bowel. Obstructive symptoms develop because of narrowed bowel lumen as well as angulation. Mesenteric fibrosis rarely results in intestinal ischaemia.

Symptoms may be related to the primary, metastatic nodal or hepatic disease or the development of carcinoid syndrome. Most tumours only become symptomatic late in their course, when many already have metastatic disease.

Carcinoids of the small bowel metastasize even when 1 cm or less in size. They usually present with small bowel obstruction and are multiple in up to 30% of the patients. Careful inspection of the whole intestine during surgery is thus essential. Diagnosis on small bowel contrast studies may be possible, but more often CT scan suggests the diagnosis by demonstrating a mesenteric mass with stranding (nodal spread in the mesentery associated with stranding secondary to the fibrotic reaction) as well as liver secondaries. Urinary 5-HIAA (hydroxyindoleacetic acid) may be elevated especially in patients with carcinoid syndrome or bulky and metastatic disease. Localization by CT scan or nuclear medicine scans such as ^{131}I MIBG (metaiodobenzylguanidine) or ^{111}In-octreotide scans may be useful in mapping the extent of the disease.

Localized carcinoids are treated by small bowel resection and anastomosis with mesenteric lymphadenectomy or a right hemicolectomy depending on their site in the small intestine. Because of their slow growth resection is usually worthwhile even in the presence of hepatic secondaries.

Recurrent carcinoid tumours pose a significant surgical challenge since they excite intense fibrosis in the area of recurrence with multiple matted loops of small bowel and intense fibrosis and shortening of mesentery. Decision to offer surgery depends on patients' symptoms, response to symptomatic treatment, extent of metastatic disease and expected survival. In the absence of obstructive symptoms and presence of metastatic disease, treatment is symptomatic.

Prognosis is better than adenocarcinoma of the small bowel (slow-growing tumours). The 5-year survival rates for localized disease, patients with resectable liver secondaries and those with unresectable disease approach 90%, 66% and 33%, respectively.

Carcinoid syndrome

Metastatic or bulky carcinoids may secrete a variety of vasoactive substances, including serotonin, bradykinin, histamine, substance P, hydroxytryptophan and prostaglandins. These cause the symptoms associated with carcinoid syndrome.

1. Clinical features and diagnosis. This syndrome is characterized by episodic flushing, abdominal cramps and watery diarrhoea. Flushing is often dramatic affecting the face, arms and upper trunk. Less frequently sweating, wheezing, dyspnoea, abdominal pain, hypotension, right-sided heart failure (due to tricuspid regurgitation) or pulmonary stenosis (caused by endocardial fibrosis) may occur. Certain foods, alcohol, induction of anaesthesia or surgery may precipitate these symptoms. Occasionally these episodes are intense and may be life threatening (carcinoid crisis) and present with intense flushing, tachycardia, hypertension or hypotension, bronchospasm and diarrhoea. Carcinoid syndrome is diagnosed by urinary 5-HIAA, CT scans and octreotide or MIBG scintigraphy.

2. *Treatment.* Treatment depends on extent of disease and intensity of symptoms. Liver resection, debulking of liver metastases or hepatic artery ligation should be considered. More commonly, the disease is not amenable to surgery and either hepatic artery embolization or symptomatic treatment is offered instead. Loperamide may be useful for diarrhoea, octreotide 50 mg s.c. once or twice per day may control the diarrhoea and flushing. Alternatively octreotide long-acting repeatable (LAR) may be used 20 mg i.m. every 28 days with apparent similar efficacy [c]. Combin-ation chemotherapy (doxorubicin, 5-fluorouracil and streptozocin) is also sometimes used, but is not very effective with only 20–30% response rates.

Further reading

Cusack JC, Tyler DS. Small bowel malignancies and carcinoid tumours. In: Berger DH, Feig BW, Fuhrman GM, eds. *The M.D. Anderson Surgical Oncology Handbook.* Boston, Little, Brown & Company, 1995; 142–159.

Fischbach W, Tacke W, Greiner A, Konrad H, Muller-Hermelink. Regression of immunoproliferative small intestinal disease after eradication of *Helicobacter pylori. Lancet,* 1997; **349:** 31–32.

Godwin JD II. Carcinoid tumours: an analysis of 2837 cases. *Cancer,* 1975; **36:** 560–569.

Kvols LK, Moertel CG, O'Connell MJ, Schutt NJ, Rubin J, Hahn RG. Treatment of malignant carcinoid syndrome: evaluation of a long-acting somatostatin analogue. *New England Journal of Medicine,* 1986; **315:** 663–666.

Sarr MG. Small intestinal neoplasms. In: Greenfield LJ, Mulholland MW, Oldham KT, Zelenock GB, Eds. *Surgery. Scientific Principles and Practice.* 1st edition. Philadelphia: JB Lipipincott Company, 1993; 753–762.

SOFT TISSUE SWELLINGS
Nick Lagattolla

Musculoskeletal

1. Ganglion. This is a cystic swelling arising from the synovial lining of a joint or a tendon sheath. They occur commonly around the wrist, on digits, and on the dorsum of the foot and can be excised under local infiltration if small, or under Bier's block if larger.

2. Bursae. These may develop into cystic swellings which may become acutely or chronically inflamed or infected (bursitis). They are frequently found around the knee (housemaid's knee if prepatellar, and parson's knee if infrapatellar) or over the olecranon. If they are symptomatic, they may be excised. Abscesses must be drained.

3. Baker's cyst. A cystic swelling in the medial part of the popliteal fossa in children and young adults is likely to be a semimembranous bursa. This is often termed Baker's cyst, though this is erroneous, and the term should be reserved for inflammatory swellings in the popliteal fossa. These arise as a complication of arthritis of the knee from posterior rupture of inflamed synovium, or from a communicating existent popliteal bursa.

4. Synovial swellings. The synovium may be inflamed as a result of systemic disease, such as rheumatoid or sarcoidosis. Benign 'brown tumours' may occur, and rarely malignant synovioma may result.

Benign soft tissue tumours

1. Lipomas. These are very common benign tumours of adipose tissue. They are classified according to their anatomical layer. They may be subcutaneous, extrafascial, subfascial, intramuscular, subperiosteal, extraperitoneal, subserosal, submucosal, or retroperitoneal. Malignant change to liposarcoma is a rare occurrence.

Lipomas are frequently lobulated by fibrous septa. They are soft and may feel fluctulant. The edge of a subcutaneous lipoma, the most common variety, can be displaced laterally under the examining finger. This 'slipping' sign is said to be typical.

Lipomas can easily be excised under local anaesthesia. Larger lipomas on the trunk are almost always related to deep fascia. They are often much larger than initially thought. These are best dealt with under a general anaesthetic. Multiple spontaneously painful subcutaneous lipomas is Dercum's syndrome, or adiposis dolorosa.

2. Neurofibromas, neurilemmomas and schwannomas. These are neural tumours arising from supporting cells of the sensory component of peripheral nerves. The three types are differentiated on histological appearance. They present as lumps, usually on a limb, which may cause altered sensation distally. Clinically, they are fixed in the plane parallel to the axis of the nerve, and are mobile perpendicular to this. When palpated, tingling may be felt along the distribution of the nerve.

3. Neurofibromatosis. This is Von Recklinghausen's disease, comprising multiple (up to many hundreds) of small, soft, sessile, cutaneous neurofibromas, freckling of the axillary skin, and oval café-au-lait patches. It may be associated with central nervous system gliomas, cranial nerve neuromas, and phaeochromocytomas. Neurofibromatosis is a congenital disorder of the neuroectoderm, one of a group called phakomatoses (others are Von-Hippel Lindau and Sturge–Weber syndromes, ataxia telangiectasia, and tuberous sclerosis). Larger neurofibromas with a broad base and a fissured surface may occur on the trunk or a limb girdle. These are plexiform neurofibromas and should be observed carefully for increase in size or the development of hard areas which may signify sarcomatous change.

4. Neuroma. This may arise following trauma to a nerve. Peripheral nerves regenerate if damaged, however the regeneration may become disordered, and a tangled mass of neuronal tissue can evolve. These are most often seen in amputation stumps, or at the edges of surgical wounds. They may be a source of constant pain and can be successfully treated by injection of local anaesthetic. Permanent relief may follow phenolic ablation if local anaesthetic infiltration is successful.

5. Desmoid tumours and the fibromatoses. These are rare and sporadic but may be seen as part of the familial polyposis coli syndrome. They are localized collections of well-vascularized fibrous tissue which are not malignant, but which often recur after excision. They commonly occur in the abdominal wall where they are said to arise from aponeurotic tissue. They may occur in the neck. Desmoid tumours may respond to radiotherapy if they recur following wide excision.

Desmoid tumours may occur as part of a diffuse fibrotic condition known as fibromatosis. This includes other fibrotic conditions such as Dupuytren's contracture of the palmar and plantar fascia, retroperitoneal and mediastinal fibrosis, Peyronie's disease of the penis, Reidel's thyroiditis and keloid scarring.

6. Leiomyomas. These can occasionally present as slow-growing subcutaneous lumps.

Malignant soft tissue tumours: sarcomas

1. Clinical features. The majority of sarcomas encountered arise from bone, cartilage or periosteum, however soft tissues may also give rise to malignancies. The incidence of soft tissue sarcomas rises with age, and peaks in the seventh decade. They present as painless masses that increase in size. They feel firm or rubbery, and their edge is indistinct. They may be warm to the touch, and there may be an overlying bruit. They spread by local invasion through tissue planes and via the bloodstream to the lungs.

2. Investigation and treatment. MRI is the investigation of choice, although CT is adequate. The sarcoma appears as an encapsulated solid mass. The diagnosis may be obtained by core biopsy in 90% of cases. Definitive surgical resection entails wide resection beyond the sarcoma pseudocapsule, which frequently contains tumour. In a limb, this usually takes the form of a 'compartmentectomy'. Adjuvant treatment in the form of radiotherapy to the tumour bed results in reduced recurrence rates. Chemotherapy may also be used, though it is often reserved for unresectable or recurrent tumours.

3. **Classification.** Sarcomas may be classified according to the tissue of origin. Varieties include fibrosarcoma, malignant fibrous histiocytoma, liposarcoma, rhabdomyosarcoma, Kaposi's sarcoma, lymphangiosarcoma, synovial sarcoma, malignant schwannoma, and malignant mesenchymoma. The more common varieties are discussed.

- *Malignant fibrous histiocytoma.* This arises from fibroblasts. It is the most commonly diagnosed sarcoma, arising from many tissues, including bone. Dermatofibrosarcoma protruberans is best considered a less malignant, but locally invasive form of MFH, will recur if it is not widely excised, but histologically typically having a high mitotic rate. It occurs on the trunk as a progressively enlarging smooth, bulbous, lobulated mass, often with ulceration of the overlying skin.
- *Liposarcoma.* These are rare malignant tumours arising from adipose tissue and mostly occurring in the region of the limb girdles and in the retroperitoneum. There is some debate as to whether larger lipomas can become malignant, but if a patient is thought to have a large lipoma, and clinically there are hard areas within it, this must be excised.
- *Kaposi's sarcoma.* Also known as cutaneous haemorrhagic angiosarcomas, these tend to occur in particular races, especially the Eastern Europeans, Jews and sub-Saharan Africans. They are purple or red-coloured cutaneous papules and tend to be multiple. They are common in AIDS when they are often very small and may occur on any mucosal surface as well as the skin. Gastrointestinal Kaposi's sarcomas may bleed.
- *Rhabdomyosarcoma.* These arise from skeletal muscle, and embryonal and mature histological types are described. The commonest sarcomas of childhood, they are found in the head and neck, genitourinary tract and, in older children, in the trunk and limbs.

Further reading

Pittam MR, Thomas JM. Sarcomas of soft tissue and bone. In: Burnand KG, Young AE (eds) *The New Aird's Companion in Surgical Studies*. Edinburgh: Churchill Livingstone, 1992; 179.

Related topics of interest

The skin and subcutaneous tissues (p. 303); Vascular malformations and tumours (p. 353).

THE SPLEEN

Nick Lagattolla

This is a highly vascular lymphatic organ occupying the lieno-renal ligament in the dorsal meso-gastrium. It lies under the cover of the left ninth to eleventh ribs in the midaxillary line. It has a very fragile capsule. Accessory splenic tissue, or splenunculi, may be found in the ventral mesogastrium or in the greater omentum, occurring in approximately 10% of individuals.

The spleen has immunological, haemopoietic, phagocytic and erythrocyte storage functions. The major immunological function is one of phagocytosis of a variety of immunologically identified particles, both foreign and intrinsic. It also removes effete red blood cells from the circulation, whilst acting as a store of immature red cells. It is a source of erythropoiesis, and platelet and monocyte production, though not for lymphopoiesis. It is however a store of both B- and T-lymphocytes.

Idiopathic thrombocytopenic purpura

This may occur as an isolated condition, or part of a systemic disorder. The spleen is typically not enlarged. Conservative treatment includes transfusion, steroids, or infused gammaglobulins. Splenectomy may be curative, particularly if the condition is not severe, the patient is young, and there has been a reasonable response to steroids. Should platelets need to be transfused perioperatively (remembering that the counts are very likely to be low through hypersplenism), then they should be transfused only once the splenic pedicle has been clamped or ligated. Otherwise the perfused spleen will happily demolish the newly infused platelets.

Haemolytic anaemias

Splenectomy is the treatment option of choice in hereditary spherocytosis. This is performed after the age of six to reduce the risk of post-splenectomy infection (vide infra). A careful search for splenunculi is mandatory, as functional residual splenic tissue will negate the effects of surgery. Hereditary elliptocytosis may also be treated by splenectomy in severe cases. The beta thalassaemias, particularly the major type, result in splenomegaly and potentially very severe anaemia. Repeated transfusion can cause severe iron overload, and splenectomy may be of value in reducing the requirement for transfusion.

Hypersplenism

Splenic overactivity may result in thrombocytopenia and anaemia with detectable circulating immature haemopoietic cells. This usually occurs as part of a diffuse haematological disorder, such as lymphoma and some leukaemias. A variety of conditions giving rise to an enlarged spleen may also result in hypersplenism. Hypersplenism does not necessarily implicate a massive spleen, though splenomegaly is typical. However, not all enlarged spleens are overactive. Conservative treatment depends on the underlying cause of the hypersplenism. Once conservative measures fail and transfusion requirements become too great, the treatment is splenectomy.

Massive splenomegaly

Certain conditions predispose to massive enlargement of the spleen. These include myelofibrosis, malaria, schistosomiasis, visceral leishmaniasis, beta thalassaemia major, and chronic myeloid leukaemia. Massive spleens do not necessarily result in hypersplenism, and in fact, splenic function is often normal; however, symptoms of abdominal discomfort can arise from the sheer volume of spleen present, or pain may ensue from segmental splenic infarction. The risk of splenic rupture is increased in splenomegaly. Splenectomy may be indicated in symptomatic massive splenomegaly and if hypersplenism is present. This operation is hazardous due to the inevitability of multiple peritoneal adhesions to the splenic capsule and adherence to the diaphragm. This is therefore surgery for the specialist interest surgeon.

Trauma

Blunt trauma to the left lower chest with or without overlying rib fractures frequently traumatizes the spleen. Patterns of injury range from subcapsular haematoma, simple or multiple lacerations, stellate fracture and frank rupture. Any of these injuries may be associated with haemoperitoneum, and massive blood loss may ensue.

A pathologically enlarged spleen for whatever reason, from lymphoma to infectious mononucleosis, is more prone to traumatic injury. Pathological spleens have been reported to rupture spontaneously.

Management of splenic injury

If the patient with a splenic injury is haemodynamically unstable, a laparotomy and splenectomy must be undertaken as a potentially life-saving procedure. Signs of diffuse peritonism suggest a haemoperitoneum has developed, and even if the patient is haemodynamically stable, bleeding is likely to continue, and a laparotomy is indicated. However, if a patient is stable, with absent or localized signs, and imaging indicates a localized injury, such as a subcapsular or contained perisplenic haematoma, conservative management may be instigated. This revolves around careful monitoring, repeated non-invasive imaging, serial haemoglobin estimation, and the availability of cross-matched blood should haemorrhage supervene.

Splenic conservation

Splenectomy may not be required in all cases of splenic injury. The immunological benefits to splenic preservation are clear, particularly in the very young. At laparotomy, should the spleen contain a localized injury, such as a capsular tear or simple laceration, simple suturing with or without haemostatic plugging has been recommended. Wrapping the spleen in a vicryl mesh or a commercially available haemostatic sheet has been advocated for more diffuse splenic injuries. Partial splenectomy has been undertaken in injuries to either splenic pole, though in practice this is a difficult procedure to undertake in emergency conditions.

Emergency splenectomy

This involves firstly the mobilization of the spleen by incision of the tethering peritoneum posterior to the spleen, the so-called lieno-renal ligament. This is frequently undertaken blindly by long scissor dissection. Occasionally as spleen may be mobile with a long lieno-renal ligament. The spleen is then easily pulled forward into the abdominal incision. The gastrosplenic ligament is incised exposing the structures at the splenic hilum, which can then be gently dissected out. The splenic vein and artery are separate, and should be clamped and tied independently. Care should be taken not to injure the tail of the pancreas which lies in the lieno-renal ligament. The remaining short gastric vessels are carefully clipped and tied, and the spleen should then be free.

Splenic tumours, cysts and abscess

Splenic cysts probably result from organized haematomas, though simple cysts undoubtedly also occur. Hydatid cysts are common in endemic areas. Splenic abcesses may occur. Primary focal splenic tumours are very rare, are usually benign, and include dermoids. The definitive treatment for any undiagnosed splenic lesion is splenectomy.

Secondary tumours include involvement in generalized lymphomas and disseminated carcinomas, usually intraperitoneal in origin. Unless lymphoma is recognized as the cause, these are best treated by splenectomy. Lymphoma may be diagnosed only once an enlarged or frankly neoplastic spleen has been removed, though solitary splenic lymphoma is unusual.

Overwhelming post-splenectomy infection

The absence of a spleen reduces phagocytosis and antigenic presentation and removes an entire B-lymphocyte source, predisposing to certain bacterial infections. The infections may be severe, hence the term 'overwhelming post-splenectomy infection' or OPSI. This term was first utilized in 1969 by Diamond, and it serves admirably to emphasize the potential severity of the condition, and to remind one of the predisposition following splenectomy. The incidence may be as high as 5%, the risk is greater in childhood, and the mortality is high, ranging from 25–75%.

The infecting organisms are predominantly encapsulated bacteria, typically *Streptococcus pneumoniae*, but also *Haemophilus influenzae*, *Neisseria meningitidis* and *Escherichia coli*. A wide variety of organisms have been implicated in OPSI, however. The risk of OPSI varies with the reasons for splenectomy, with underlying lymphoreticular diseases and haemolytic anaemias carrying the greatest risk, and trauma the least. The vaccinations and prophylactic antibiotics prescribed post-splenectomy are geared to reducing the risk of OPSI.

Post-splenectomy instructions

It is very important to council a patient who has recently undergone a splenectomy. The incidence of serious systemic infection is higher then in the normal population, and patients must be vaccinated against certain bacteria including meningococcus (Groups A and C), pneumococcus (23 valent pneumococcal polysaccharide vaccine) and *Haemophilus influenzae* Type b (Hib vaccine). An alert card should be presented to the patient indicating that a splenectomy has been carried out, which might be of particular use in an emergency. Oral penicillin is presbied at a reduced (prophylactic) dose and this is recommended for life. The patient is informed to be particularly aware of any focal or systemic infection, and to present to the GP at the first sign.

Splenosis

In cases where the spleen has ruptured, spillage of splenic tissue may result in seeding of splenic cells within the peritoneal cavity. These may form microscopic nests of splenic tissue and retain their function. Splenic physiology may thus not necessarily be lost in those who have had a splenectomy.

Further reading

Reviews

Bickerstaff KI, Morris PJ. Splenectomy for massive splenomegaly. *British Journal of Surgery*, 1987; **74:** 346–349.

Cooper MJ, Williamson RCN. Splenectomy: indications, hazards and alternatives. *British Journal of Surgery*, 1984; **71:** 173–180.

Cullingford GL, Watkins DN, Watts ADJ, Mallon DF. Severe late post-splenectomy infection. *British Medical Journal*, 1991; **78:** 716–721.

Ghosh S, Symes JM, Walsh TH. Splenic repair for trauma. *British Journal of Surgery*, 1988; **75:** 1139–1140.

McMullin M, Johnston G. Long term management of patients after splenectomy. *British Medical Journal*, 1993; **307:** 1372–1373.

Observational study

The splenic injury group. Splenic injury: a prospective multicentre study on non-operative and operative treatment. *British Journal of Surgery*, 1987; **74:** 310–313.

Related topic of interest

Abdominal trauma (p. 1).

TESTICULAR TUMOURS

Christopher Lattimer, Adrian Simoes

Testicular cancer is relatively rare, accounting for about 1% of all cancers, but is the commonest malignancy in males in the age group of 15 to 35 years. It is one of the most curable solid neoplasms with figures above 90% 5-year survival even with metastatic disease[b].

Classification

Primary

    Germ cell tumour (GCT) (90–95%)
        Seminoma
        Embryonal carcinoma
        Teratoma
        Yolk sac tumour
        Choriocarcinoma

    Non-germ cell tumour (NGCT)
        Leydig cell tumour
        Sertoli cell tumour
        Gonadoblastoma
        Miscellaneous

Secondary

    Lymphoma
    Leukaemic infiltration of the testis
    Metastatic

Risk factors

Cryptorchidism is known to be associated with an increased risk of tumorigenesis. Previously it was estimated that the risk was 48 times that of men with normally descended testis but recently this figure was found to be much lower, i.e. 3 to 14 times[b]. Five to ten per cent of patients with history of cryptorchidism develop malignancy in the contralateral, normally descended testis. The relative risk for malignancy is highest for the intra-abdominal testis (1 in 20) in comparison to inguinal testis (1 in 80) and orchipexy does not alter its malignant potential[b]. Testicular neoplasms are more common in the right testis than in the left in keeping with the slightly greater incidence of right-sided cryptorchidism. Approximately 2 to 3% of testicular tumours are bilateral and 50% occur in those with history of cryptorchidism. Approximately 5% of men with testicular cancer have carcinoma-in-situ (CIS) of the opposite testicle and this is thought to progress to invasive GCT.

Presentation

Men usually present in the third (teratoma) or the fourth (seminoma) decade with a testicular nodule or painless swelling. In 10% of the patients, acute pain is the presenting symptom. Another 10% present with manifestations due to metastases including supraclavicular lymph node mass, chest symptoms, bulky retroperitoneal disease, skeletal metastases, central and peripheral nervous system lesions and lower limb swelling due to venous obstruction or thrombosis or lymphoedema. Gynaecomastia is seen in 5% of patients and precocious puberty is the presentation in Leydig cell tumour.

Investigations

Ultrasonography may pick up impalpable lesions. Tumour markers help in the diagnosis, staging and future monitoring of the disease and include alpha-fetoprotein (AFP), beta-human chorionic gonadotrophin (β-HCG), lactic acid dehydrogenase (LDH), placental alkaline phosphatase (PLAP) and gamma-glutamyl transpeptidase (GGT). Chest X-ray and CT scanning of the thorax, abdomen and pelvis are required for staging.

Staging

The growth rate among germ cell tumours is very high with doubling times of 10 to 30 days. Immediate orchidectomy through a groin incision to clamp the cord at the internal ring is performed unless the patient is unwell with metastatic disease in which case chemotherapy takes preference. A testicular prosthesis should be offered to all patients. Biopsy should be considered in patients with a remaining small testis, low sperm count and ultrasound abnormality of the remaining testis, and in young patients (< 30 years) and those with a history of maldescent. Once the disease has been staged and the histology graded, treatment plans are formulated.

pT0	no evidence of primary tumour
pT1	tumour limited to testis and epididymis without blood or lymphatic vascular invasion
pT2	tumour limited to testis and epididymis with vascular invasion or tumour extending through tunica albuginea to involve tunica vaginalis
pT3	tumour invasion of spermatic cord
pT4	tumour invasion of scrotum

RMH Staging (Royal Marsden Hospital)

I	No evidence of disease outside the testis
IM	As above but with persistently raised tumour markers
II	Infradiaphragmatic nodal involvement
III	Supra and infradiaphragmatic node involvement
IV	Extralymphatic metastases

Management

Stage I seminoma needs a high orchidectomy. The inguinal approach allows early control of the vascular and lymphatic supply as well as en bloc removal of the testis with its tunics. Secondly, a scrotal incision risks implanting cancer in the scrotal tissue and may allow lymphatic spread to occur to the inguinal nodes which are otherwise never involved. There is a 15% probability of recurrence in 3 years and hence close surveillance is necessary. Prophylactic irradiation of the para-aortic nodes is recommended as the early diagnosis of relapse is difficult in the absence of a reliable tumour marker. Initial results with adjuvant chemotherapy (single agent carboplatin) are encouraging. Radiation therapy to para-aortic and ipsilateral pelvic lymph nodes (dog leg) is recommended for the treatment of stage II disease along with high orchidectomy. Chemotherapy is usually instituted if patients have bulky lymphadenopathy. Patients with stage III and IV seminoma are treated with high orchidectomy and a platinum-based multi-drug chemotherapy regimen.

Patients with stage I teratoma of the testis with no high-risk features should be managed by surveillance following inguinal orchidectomy. Adjuvant chemotherapy should be offered to patients with high risk. All other stages require multi-drug chemotherapy. Cisplatin, etopside and bleomycin are commonly used. Nerve sparing retroperitoneal lymph node dissection (RPLND) is commonly performed in the USA but considered to be overtreatment in the UK.

Fertility issues

A significant proportion of men with testicular tumours will have low sperm counts. Both chemotherapy and radiotherapy may result in infertility as well as biopsy of the contralateral testis to exclude CIS. Consequently, sperm storage should be offered to men.

Further reading

Duchesne GM, Horwich A, Dearnaley DP, Nicholls J, Jay G, Peckham MJ, Hendry WF. Orchidectomy alone for stage I seminoma of the testis. *Cancer*, 1990; **65:** 1115–1118.

Loehrer PJ Sr, Williams SD, Einhorn LH. Status of chemotherapy for testis cancer. *Urologic Clinics of North America*, 1987; **14:** 713–720.

Oliver RT, Lore S, Ong J. Alternatives to radiotherapy in the management of seminoma. *British Journal of Urology*, 1990; **65:** 61–67.

Related topics of interest

Penile conditions and scrotal swellings (p. 251); Undescended testis (p. 335).

THYROGLOSSAL TRACT ANOMALIES

Nick Wilson

The thyroid gland develops from the thyroglossal duct (median bud of the pharynx) during the fourth embryonic week and passes ventrally from the foramen caecum at the back of the tongue to the pharynx, just below the position of the developing hyoid cartilage. This line of descent is called the thyroglossal tract. The thyroglossal duct thus formed usually degenerates, but its incomplete regression results in the following congenital abnormalities which are rarely evident at birth.

Thyroglossal cyst

- May occur with patent or closed thyroglossal duct.
- May occur at any age, but 40% present in the age group 0–10 years.
- Incidence: male = female.
- Midline usually, but may deviate slightly.
- Commonest midline cervical tumour in infants.
- Does not usually transilluminate.
- Usually situated just above or below the hyoid bone.
- Moves up on protrusion of tongue.

It is lined by squamous or ciliated pseudostratified epithelium and may contain thyroid or lymphoid tissue which may be dysplastic in the wall. The diagnosis is made on clinical grounds but many surgeons request an ultrasound or radioisotope scan preoperatively to exclude ectopic thyroid tissue[c].

Thyroglossal sinus

This is not congenital but results from infection in or inadequate excision of a thyroglossal cyst.

- Midline orifice with tract leading cranially.
- Crescentic fold of skin (concavity faces down) at skin orifice.
- Mucopurulent discharge.
- Recurrent infection.
- Lined by columnar epithelium.

Sistrunk's operation

This is the operation of choice for thyroglossal cyst and sinus. A transverse incision is made over the cyst (transverse elliptical incision around the mouth of a sinus) and the tract followed up between the strap muscles to the hyoid bone. The tract, duct, cyst or sinus is then excised with the central portion of the hyoid bone (or recurrence is likely). For suprahyoid cysts or sinuses, the tract should be followed to the base of the tongue.

Lingual and aberrant thyroid

A lingual thyroid gland represents failure of descent of part or all of the embryonic thyroid gland from the foramen caecum. In most cases it represents the only thyroid tissue present. It may remain symptomless or develop any of the recognized thyroid abnormalities. Clinical problems occur most commonly in young women when physiological hypertrophy at the time of pregnancy or the development of an adenoma occur. Symptoms and signs include:

- Dysphagia.
- Speech impairment.
- Respiratory obstruction.
- Haemorrhage.
- Smooth, vascular dark red projection at the back of the tongue.

Symptomless glands should be left alone. If treatment is required, an iodine or technetium isotope scan should be performed to determine the presence of any other thyroid tissue. Glands may be reduced in size by antithyroid drugs, thyroxine, or radioiodine. Excision is required if malignant change occurs.

Aberrant thyroid tissue may occur in any site along the thyroglossal tract and this may be the only thyroid tissue present. If a non-cystic mass is found during Sistrunk's operation, the procedure should be abandoned and an isotope scan performed subsequently to determine the site of all thyroid tissue.

The term 'lateral aberrant thyroid gland' is a misnomer, the thyroid tissue found in these lateral sites being cervical node metastases from a papillary thyroid carcinoma.

Further reading

Brewis C, Mahadevan M, Bailye CM, Drake DP. Investigation and treatment of thyroglossal cysts in children. *Journal of the Royal Society of Medicine*, 2000; **93:** 18–21.

Young AE. The neck. In: Burnand KG, Young AE (eds) *The New Aird's Companion in Surgical Studies* (2nd Edn). London: Churchill Livingstone, 1998; 447–457.

Young AE. The thyroid gland. In: Burnand KG, Young AE (eds) *The New Aird's Companion in Surgical Studies* (2nd Edn). London: Churchill Livingstone, 1998; 459–483.

Related topics of interest

Goitre (p. 150); Hyperthyroidism – treatment (p. 173); Thyroid neoplasms (p. 324).

THYROID NEOPLASMS

Nick Wilson

Thyroid neoplasms present as a solitary nodule, in common with many benign processes that affect the gland, 5% of Western populations having a palpable thyroid nodule. The incidence of thyroid malignancy is low but may be rising (1.5% of all malignancies – 4/100 000 per year).

Benign

1. Follicular adenoma.
- The majority of benign neoplasms.
- Differentiation from malignant follicular tumours is difficult.
- Scintiscanning may show a 'solitary cold nodule'.
- Cytological distinction from follicular carcinoma impossible.
- Treatment is by total hemithyroidectomy with frozen section to exclude malignancy.

2. Teratoma.
- Rare.
- Arise from all three primitive germ layers.
- Benign in children.

Malignant – differentiated (account for 80% of neoplasms)

1. Papillary.
- 70% of all thyroid cancers.
- Peak incidence 20–40 years.
- Female to male ratio 3 : 1.

Tumours tend to be multifocal and unencapsulated, but there is a spectrum from occult intrathyroid tumours (< 1.5 cm diameter) to locally invasive and metastatic tumours. They invade lymphatics and spread to cervical lymph nodes early. Distant metastases rarely occur. The misnamed 'lateral aberrant thyroid' is invariably a cervical metastasis from a papillary tumour. Tumours may occur with a mixed papillary and follicular pattern and should be treated as papillary tumours, even if the predominant element is follicular. Diagnosis is by FNAC.

Total lobectomy is satisfactory if the tumour is confined to a single lobe. More extensive tumour necessitates total thyroidectomy, allowing subsequent diagnosis and treatment of metastases by radioiodine. Lymph node involvement should be treated by modified cervical block dissection or by 'cherry-picking' (removing nodes individually), particularly for node recurrence. Radioiodine should be given if the tumour extends beyond the thyroid capsule. Thyroxine suppresses residual tumour and is necessary after lobectomy and total thyroidectomy. External radiotherapy is of value where there is residual metastatic disease after radioiodine or where there is no iodine uptake, or if there is a large, unresectable tumour. The prognosis for patients with intrathyroid tumours is similar to that of the normal population. The 10-year survival for patients with extrathyroid disease is 55%.

2. Follicular.
- 15% of thyroid malignancies.
- Older age group than papillary tumours (mean age 45 years).
- Female : male ratio is 3 : 1.
- Commoner in endemic goitrous regions.

These tumours are usually solitary, encapsulated, and metastasize by haematogenous spread to lung and bone. Local lymph nodes are involved late. Malignancy is diagnosed by capsular invasion and vascular spread and cannot be assessed by FNAC.

If the diagnosis is uncertain preoperatively, total lobectomy should be performed, proceeding to completion total thyroidectomy if frozen section reveals malignancy. Where the frozen section is uncertain, completion total thyroidectomy is performed at a second procedure if frank invasion is demonstrated by paraffin sections, enabling radioiodine to be given. Modified block dissection should be performed only if nodes are involved. Lifelong thyroxine suppression/replacement is given. Thyroglobulin is a marker for both recurrent papillary and follicular tumours.

3. Medullary.
- Arises from the parafollicular cells (C-cells) which synthesize calcitonin.
- 5–10% of thyroid neoplasms.
- Wide age range.
- Most are sporadic, but 10% are familial, occurring both with and without the other features of multiple endocrine neoplasia (MEN) types IIa or b.
- Lymph node metastases are present in 25%.

The tumours secrete calcitonin and carcinoembryonic antigen and a range of other peptide hormones causing diarrhoea in some patients. If a medullary tumour is suspected, other abnormalities of the MEN II syndromes should be sought. The diagnosis is made by FNAC.

Total thyroidectomy should be performed with ipsilateral modified block dissection regardless or node status or bilateral if the disease appears multicentric. Calcitonin levels should be measured to monitor recurrence for which radioiodine, radiotherapy and chemotherapy are reserved. All relatives should have their calcitonin levels measured. The 5-year survival is 90% or 50% in node-negative and node-positive disease respectively.

4. Lymphoma.
- Rare.
- Primary or secondary.
- Usually diffuse B-cell. Must be distinguished from small cell anaplastic carcinoma.
- Occur in old age, affecting women more often than men.
- Usually a history of a rapidly growing goitre.

Pre-existing Hashimoto's disease is found in 30% (few cases of Hashimoto's thyroiditis progress to lymphoma). Primary lymphoma is treated by total thyroidectomy with postoperative radiotherapy. Patients with extrathyroid disease are best treated with radiotherapy. Secondary or recurrent disease is treated by chemotherapy. In primary disease, the 5-year survival is 85% falling to 40% for metastatic disease.

5. Squamous.
- Very rare.
- Must be distinguished from squamous metaplasia of papillary tumours.
- Arise in embryonal remnants.
- Very aggressive.
- Treatment usually ineffective.

6. Sarcoma.
- Very rare.
- Poor prognosis.

7. Teratoma.
- In adults these are highly malignant.
- Few patients survive 1 year.

8. Metastatic.
- Rare.
- Malignant melanoma, breast.

Malignant – anaplastic
- Peak incidence 60–70 years.
- Women are affected slightly more often than men.
- Commoner in endemic goitrous regions.
- Invariably a long history of goitre.

These extremely aggressive tumours usually arise from a differentiated carcinoma, or occasionally a benign adenoma. There is usually a hard, fixed mass involving the trachea and adjacent structures. There may be stridor or hoarseness from recurrent nerve invasion.

Distinction from lymphoma is important and a biopsy rather than FNAC is usually required. Treatment by total thyroidectomy is seldom feasible, local debulking and tracheal decompression being the only option. The response to radiotherapy is usually poor. Chemotherapy (doxorubicin) may be useful in younger patients. Few patients survive 1 year.

The solitary nodule
- Clinical diagnosis unreliable.
- Malignancy suggested by male, young patient, cervical lymphadenopathy, hoarseness, pain or dysphagia.
- In children, the incidence of malignancy in a solitary nodule approaches 50%.
- Multinodularity and/or thyrotoxicosis make malignancy unlikely but still possible.

Ultrasound scanning should be performed to confirm the solitary nature of the nodule (50% are dominant nodules in a multinodular goitre), to detemine whether it is cystic, or solid. If needle aspiration resolves the cyst completely, no further treatment is necassary. If the nodule is incompletely removed or recurs, excision is necessary. If repeated FNAC indicates benign disease only, thyroidectomy is not required unless symptoms determine otherwise. If FNAC indicates a follicular nodule, total lobectomy should be performed with frozen section. Other tumours are dealt with as described above.

Further reading

Young AE. The thyroid gland. In: Burnand KG, Young AE (eds) *The New Aird's Companion in Surgical Studies* (2nd Edn). London: Churchill Livingstone, 1998; 459–483.

Related topics of interest

Goitre (p. 150); Hyperthyroidism – treatment (p. 173); Thyroglossal tract anomalies (p. 322).

TRAUMA MANAGEMENT

Nick Wilson

Trauma is the cause of 545000 hospital discharges and 14500 deaths annually in the UK. Road traffic accidents account for 850000 hospital bed nights and in 1985 cost the British economy £2.8 million.

Death from trauma has a trimodal distribution. The first peak occurs within seconds or minutes of injury and is caused by severe neurological, cardiac or vascular injuries. Few of these patients are salvageable. The second peak occurs within the first few hours ('the golden hour') following injury as a result of extra- or subdural haemorrhage, haemopneumothorax, splenic or hepatic injury or severe haemorrhage. Many of these deaths are preventable and it is hoped that the widespread adoption of the Advanced Trauma Life Support (ATLS) approach will improve the management and survival of such patients. The third peak occurs weeks or months following injury and is caused by sepsis or multisystem organ failure.

Experience in the USA has indicated that a network of designated trauma centres, staffed by senior trauma specialists and the use of helicopters for transporting severely injured patients significantly improve the outcomes for trauma patients, but similar findings have not been reproduced in the UK.

Triage and trauma scoring systems

Triage is the sorting of patients based on the need for treatment. Ideally, the number of patients and the severity of their injuries do not exceed available facilities. Injury severity should be assessed and an estimate of survival probability made so that management can be instituted with the appropriate degree of urgency and in the appropriate place. In general, the most severely injured patients are treated first. Where the number of patients and/or the severity of their injuries exceed available facilities, those patients with the greatest chance of survival requiring the least expenditure of time, equipment and personnel should be treated first.

Injury severity score (ISS)

In this system, injuries in six anatomical regions are scored on a 1–5 scale at death or discharge. The sum of the squares of the three highest values is taken (maximum score is 75). The ISS is an accurate predictor of mortality, time to death or discharge and the degree of residual disability.

Trauma score (TS)

This score is based on five variables: respiratory rate, respiratory effort, systolic blood pressure, capillary refill, Glasgow coma score. Patients with a score of 12 or less should be transferred to a trauma centre. Survival is closely relate to the TS for blunt and penetrating injuries.

Revised trauma score (RTS)

The Glasgow coma scale, systolic blood pressure and respiratory rate are recorded. Each measurement is assigned a coded value which is weighted according to regression analysis derived from the Major Trauma Outcome Study (26 000 patients). The RTS provides a more accurate assessment for triage than the TS.

Paediatric trauma score (PTS)

A score between −1 and +2 is assigned according to the weight of the child, airway quality, systolic blood pressure, conscious level, type of fractures, and extent of cutaneous injury. A PTS of 8 or less indicates potentially high mortality and morbidity and the need for management in a trauma centre.

TRISS method

The RTS and ISS are plotted against each other for a given patient on a graph. A standard regression line on the graph indicates the division between patients expected to survive and perish. Unexpected deaths and successes can thus be identified for audit purposes.

Principles of management

A standard format for the management of severely injured patients is essential to ensure that all injuries are detected and treated correctly. The ATLS system is used here.

Primary survey

The primary survey is undertaken to identify life-threatening conditions. Management of these injuries should be simultaneous.

A. Airway maintenance with cervical spine control. Assume cervical spine fracture and stabilize in patient with multisystem trauma.
B. Breathing and ventilation. A bag-valve device should be used via a mask or endotracheal tube to deliver oxygen at an FIO_2 greater than 0.85. Tension or open pneumothorax and flail chest must be recognized and treated.
C. Circulation. The state of conciousness, skin colour and pulse are valuable in rapidly assessing haemodynamic status. External bleeding should be controlled with direct pressure.
D. Disability – neurological status. A rapid neurological evaluation to determine the level of conciousness: A – alert; V – vocal stimuli; P – painful stimuli; U – unresponsive. Good oxygenation should be achieved for the assessment.
E. Exposure. The patient must be fully undressed and examined thoroughly.

Resuscitation

Oxygenation, control of haemorrhage and volume replacement are the priorities. Oxygen therapy to achieve an FIO_2 greater than 0.85. Cricothroidotomy may be required if the airway is obstructed. Two large-bore intravenous catheters (16 gauge or larger) are sited and blood withdrawn for crossmatch, full blood count, urea and electrolytes. Two litres of crystalloid fluid should be infused initially and, if necessary, type-specific or low titre type-O blood may be used whilst cross-matched whole blood is prepared.

A urinary catheter and nasogastric tube should be inserted providing there are no indications of urethral rupture or cribriform plate fracture.

Regular monitoring of ventilation, pulse, blood pressure, arterial blood gases, electrocardiograph, and urine output should be undertaken.

Secondary survey

The head, eyes, face and neck should be further examined for any undetected injuries. Any faciomaxillary trauma indicates the possibility of a cervical spine injury and the neck should be immobilized until such an injury has been excluded.

The chest should be re-examined for pneumothorax, flail segment, haemothorax, and cardiac tamponade. An erect chest radiograph must be obtained.

Frequent re-evaluation of the abdomen should be undertaken in the face of blunt trauma to exclude a visceral or vascular injury that may not be initially apparent. Rectal examination should be undertaken to detect blood in the bowel lumen, any rectal defect, anal sphincter laxity, a pelvic fracture or a high riding prostate.

Extremities, the chest wall and pelvis should be examined for fractures and the presence of peripheral pulses noted. Appropriate radiographs should be taken at this stage.

A comprehensive evaluation of motor and sensory systems, a reassessment of the level of conciousness and pupils and scoring on the Glasgow scale are performed.

Continuous re-evaluation of the patient is vital to detect emerging signs of injury.

Definitive care

Injuries detected should be treated and where local expertise is unavailable, discussion with or transfer to a specialist unit should take place.

Further reading

ATLS Core Book. American College of Surgeons, Chicago, 1993.
Report of the Working Party on the Management of Patients with Major Injuries. Royal College of Surgeons of England, London, 1988.
Rowlands BJ, Barros D'Sa AAB. Principles in the management of major trauma. In: Burnand KG, Young AE (eds) *The New Aird's Companion in Surgical Studies* (2nd Edn). London: Churchill Livingstone, 1998; 127–151.

Related topics of interest

Abdominal trauma (p. 1); Chest trauma (p. 81); Head injury (p. 158); Vascular trauma (p. 357).

ULCERATIVE COLITIS

Nick Lagattolla

This is an inflammatory condition of the colon of unknown cause that affects any age group, though the peak incidence occurs in the third and fourth decades. Females are affected more than males. Ulcerative colitis always involves the rectum and may involve a variable extent of proximal colon. The rectosigmoid is the only site of inflammation in 60% of cases, colitis up to the splenic flexure occurs in a further 25%, and there is total colitis in the remaining 15%. The colon is always affected in continuity, such that skip lesions characteristic of Crohn's disease are never seen.

Presentation

Ulcerative colitis presents with diarrhoea with the passage of blood and mucus per rectum. Abdominal pain may occur, and the patient often feels generally unwell. The abdomen may be tender over the affected colon. There may be systemic signs characteristic of chronic inflam-matory bowel disease. The patient may have oedema from hypo-albuminaemia and pallor from anaemia.

Ulcerative colitis can take one of a number of clinical courses. Acute colitis may occur once and not recur, but more often there are relapses, often with a back-ground, persistent, low-grade colonic inflammation. Rarely, it is fulminant, with toxic dilatation of the colon necessitating emergency colectomy.

Investigation

- Full clinical examination and sigmoidoscopy will demonstrate typical changes including mucosal erythema, contact bleeding, granularity of the mucosa and luminal pus.
- Biopsy will confirm the diagnosis of colitis.
- FBC may show leucocytosis or anaemia.
- Disease activity may be monitored by ESR and C-reactive protein levels, both typically
  rising in acute episodes.
- Stool culture may exclude infective colitis.
- Colonoscopy or barium enema will assess the extent of the disease once the acute episode has settled.

Pathology

Macroscopically there is erythema of the mucosa and ulceration with adjacent areas of regenerating mucosa which appear polypoid (pseudopolyps). Histologically there is predom-inantly mucosal acute and chronic inflammation with some specific features, including Paneth cell metaplasia and goblet cell depletion. Granulomata and transmural inflammation are not seen (this is important in differentiating ulcerative from Crohn's colitis). In severe ulcerative colitis, fissuring ulcers may be seen with inflammatory changes present deep to the mucosa, leading to diagnostic confusion with Crohn's disease. It may be impossible to determine the nature of colitis histologically, and the description indeterminate colitis may be used.

Dysplasia and malignancy

Ulcerative colitis predisposes to colorectal carcinoma. This does not arise as a consequence of the polyp–cancer sequence, but directly from dysplasia occurr-ing in the colonic epithelium. Areas of dysplasia are usually not apparent macroscopically, and the diagnosis can only be established in multiple biopsies taken from different sites.

The risk of malignancy rises in proportion to the extent of the disease, the duration of colitis, and the degree of epithelial dysplasia. There is no risk of carcinoma until the dur-ation of disease passes 10 years, and thereafter there is a steady rise in risk. Those with total colitis are at greater risk. The carcinomas are often poorly differentiated, plaque-like or stricturing, and more likely to be multifocal and locally advanced at presentation than spor-adic carcinomas.

Toxic megacolon

This is severe, intractable, progressive acute colitis. Tachycardia, pyrexia, abdominal distension and tenderness result. The colon is seen to distend increasingly on sequential plain abdominal X-rays, which must be performed daily. A transverse diameter of 6 cm or greater is indicative of a toxic megacolon. Perforation and faecal peritonitis will ensue unless emergency colectomy is undertaken. It may complicate colitis of any cause, although it is most commonly associated with ulcerative colitis.

Treatment

1. *Medical*

- *Anticolitics.* 5-Aminosalicylic acid (5-ASA) forms the basis of oral anticolitic drugs. The drug is formulated in different ways. 5-ASA bonded to the sulphonamide sulfapyridine is Salazopyrin, which has excellent anticolitic properties, but may cause infertility in males. The molecule is cleaved in the colon to release the active 5-ASA. Olsalazine is two 5-ASA molecules joined by a diazo bond. The molecule is cleaved by colonic flora and thus acts locally. Mesalazine is enteric-coated 5-ASA. This may be of greater benefit in those with terminal ileal chronic inflammatory disease as the active molecule is liberated in the distal small bowel. These drugs should be continued to prevent relapses at lower doses.
- *Steroid preparations (hydrocortisone foam or prednisolone enemas).* These may be instilled per rectum to treat acute episodes with good effect but must not be used on a long-term basis. Should 5-ASA and local steroid instillations not control symptoms, then oral or intravenous prednisolone should be started in high doses. This will improve severe colitis in most patients.
- *Antidiarrhoeal drugs.* These may be prescribed to reduce bowel frequency, but they will not modify the course of the disease. Total alimentary rest and parenteral feeding via a tunnelled feeding line are indicated in severe colitis.

2. Surgical

The indications for surgery are:

- Toxic megacolon.
- Failure of medical treatment to control symptoms.
- Presence of mucosal dysplasia.
- Development of carcinoma.

The operation in all these situations is essentially the same, amounting to at least a subtotal colectomy to the level of the rectum. The rectum and proximal ileal end are dealt with differently according to the circumstances.

1. *Proctocolectomy and permanent ileostomy (panproctocolectomy).* Dysplasia or carcinoma necessitates removal of all colonic mucosa (deemed to be unstable and premalignant). A proctocolectomy with formation of a permanent right iliac fossa spouted ileostomy (Brooke ileostomy) is required. The anus and adjacent rectum should be excised, and the perineal wound is closed as with an abdomino-perineal excision of the rectum. This is also the definitive operation for those who have failed medical treatment.

2. *Sub-total colectomy mucous fistula, and permanent ileostomy.* This is usually undertaken for toxic megacolon. The rectum is brought out as a mucous fistula, and a spouted end ileostomy is fashioned in the right iliac fossa. This allows the option of a later elective ileorectal anastomosis, ileorectal pouch, or proctectomy if symptoms persist from the retained rectum. Persistent rectal disease can usually be controlled with instillation of anticolitics or steroid.

3. *Restorative proctocolectomy.* Younger patients need to be considered for restorative proctocolectomy. This is a three-stage procedure that avoids a permanent ileostomy by the formation of a pelvic ileal reservoir acting as a neorectum. The first stage is a subtotal colectomy and end ileostomy. The second stage involves the creation of the ileal reservoir. The residual rectum is denuded of its mucosa (mucosectomy) and the pouch is placed within the rectal muscle tube and anastomosed to the upper end of the anal canal. The pouch is defunctioned by a split (loop) ileostomy. The third stage is ileostomy reversal after confirmation of an intact reservoir and pouch-anal healing by contrast radiology. Restorative proctocolectomy should only be performed if the patient is keen and well motivated and accepts the possibility of complications or failure of the procedure. Success also depends on satisfactory anal tone, the length of the anal canal and a preserved anorectal angle, and patients should undergo anorectal physiological tests pre-operatively. Complications include continued inflammation ('pouchitis'), pelvic sepsis from anastomotic dehiscence, dehydration and electrolyte imbalance, and adhesion obstruction. Ten per cent of cases will continue to have mucus leakage, and the operation fails outright in approximately 5%. Over 75% of those operated will have satisfactory bowel evacuations up to six times a day with good control.

Other surgical options include sub-total colectomy with ileorectal anastomosis which has few indications since the development of restorative proctocolectomy and the ileorectal pouch. Patients have difficulty controlling their motions, and many require conversion to an end ileostomy. There is a risk of carcinoma developing in the rectal stump which must be screened at regular intervals.

The Koch continent ileostomy is an end ileostomy leading into an ileal reservoir, the two linked via an invaginated spout of ileum acting as a valve to maintain continence. The reservoir is emptied at intervals using a catheter.

Water, sodium and potassium depletion may easily arise from continued loss of small bowel fluid. This fluid and electrolyte imbalance can occur imperceptibly, and complications must be pre-empted by careful monitoring of ileostomy output volume. Ileostomies may retract, prolapse, and develop parastomal hernias. The most common and troublesome complication is excoriation of the peristomal skin due to enzymatic digestion from contact with ileal effluent. This is minimized by the spouting of the ileostomy to direct the effluent into the stoma bag.

Further reading

Golligher J. Ulcerative colitis. In: *Surgery of the Anus, Rectum and Colon*, 5th edn. London: Baillière Tindall, 1984.

Ghosh S, Shand A, Ferguson A. Ulcerative colitis, *British Medical Journal*, 2000; **320:** 1119–1123.

Saga PM, Taylor BA. Pelvic ileal reservoirs: the options. *British Journal of Surgery*, 1994; **81:** 325–332.

Schofield PF. Inflammatory disease of the large bowel. *Surgery*, 1990; **85:** 2020–2026.

Tjandra JJ, Fazio VW. The ileal pouch – indications for its use and results in clinical practice. *Current Practice in Surgery*, 1993; **5:** 22–28.

Related topics of interest

Colorectal carcinoma (p. 91); Crohn's disease (p. 103); Lower gastrointestinal haemorrhage (p. 207).

UNDESCENDED TESTES

Christopher Lattimer, Omar Faiz

Evidence suggests that the incidence of infertility in undescended testes is reduced by early placement of the testicle in its natural location within the scrotum[(b)]. Orchidopexy is usually performed between 1 and 3 years of age in an attempt to promote normal subsequent development.

Definitions

Confusion arises in the classification of this condition. An *undescended* testis is any testis that fails to descend into the scrotum, and it includes those which adhere to the normal path but fail to descend fully (incomplete or arrested descent) as well as those found in locations remote from the normal path (ectopic). Approximately 3% of male infants have an undescended testicle at birth whereas this figure drops to 1% by the age of one year [(b)]. *Ectopic* testes account for 10% of extrascrotal testes. They usually lie in one of four positions: superficial inguinal (7.1%), base of penis, perineal or femoral (crural). An *incompletely descended* testis can be intra-abdominal (3.4%), intracanalicular (71.5%), emergent or high scrotal. *(The above percentages relate to percentages of total patients with undescended testes.)*

Development

The testes originate from the posterior abdominal wall mesoderm, the urogenital (Wolffian) ridge, and migrate into the scrotum via the inguinal canal. They are directed along this path by the gubernaculum. The accepted theory is that failure to follow the correct fibromuscular gubernacular strand leads to an ectopic testis whereas maldevelopment of the gubernaculum produces an incompletely descended testis.

Incidence

Genuinely undescended testes (*cryptorchism*) occur in 1% of males, however 4–5% of males undergo orchidopexy. This dichotomy suggests diagnostic confusion between undescended and retractile testes resulting in a proportion of the latter group undergoing unnecessary operations.

Complications

The complications of undescended testis include: associated inguinal hernia (50%), trauma, infertility (40% if unilateral, 70% bilateral), failure of development of secondary sexual characteristics (if bilateral and testes very immature) and malignant change (35 fold)[(b)]. The predisposition to malignancy (germ cell tumours) and infertility is considered a secondary effect to abnormal testicular location; however, some testes are dysplastic from the start. Returning a testis to the scrotum has not conclusively been shown to prevent malignant change, but the testis is made more accessible to screening (palpation and/or ultrasound) thereby improving earlier detection of testicular lesions. Despite the increased risk of malignant change it is important to note that only one boy out of 120 with undescended testes will actually develop malignancy throughout his lifespan[(b)].

Diagnosis

The diagnosis of cryptorchism is made by the exclusion of a retractile testis. Incomplete descent should be suspected when the scrotum is underdeveloped. In contrast, normal scrotal development and the presence of scrotal rugae suggest a retractile testis. The examination should take place in a warm room on a relaxed child by a competent clinician. The bony landmarks are first identified and then with the flat of one hand the testis is milked into the scrotal neck whilst the other catches it and records the lowest limit to which it can be drawn. All retractile testes can be placed deep into the scrotum in this way.

Treatment

By 1 year all testes should be palpable within the scrotum. If not, orchidopexy is recommended prior to three years of age as, beyond this age, secondary testicular degeneration is believed to be irreversible[b]. An inguinal incision identifies the testis. The gubernaculum is divided well below the low-lying vas and the inguinal canal is opened. The cord is mobilized to the level of the deep ring by: division of peritoneal adhesions; ligation of a concurrent inguinal hernia; and trimming of any restricting cremasteric fibres. A Dartos pouch is fashioned through a transverse scrotal incision and the mobilized testis then button-holed through the Dartos to lie within the pouch (ensuring that the testicular sinus remains in the lateral position). The testis is then anchored with a suture through the tunica albuginea to prevent torsion and displacement. Testicular atrophy is a recognized surgical complication and occurs in 5%. It can sometimes be avoided by meticulous dissection and preventing fixation under tension, however the incompletely descended testicle can be associated with an unpredictable blood supply. In most cases the above procedure will enable the testis to be brought to lie within the scrotum. In a minority of patients however, other procedures will be required to lengthen the cord. These include the:

1. *High retroperitoneal approach.*   This approach is routinely performed for the high testis. It maintains the integrity of the superficial inguinal ring and allows a more proximal dissection to be carried out. Staged operations are required for the very high testis.

2. *Fowler-Stephens.*   This procedure involves proximal ligation of the testicular artery to increase cord length. This procedure relies on the assumption that the artery to the vas and other collaterals will be sufficient to supply the testis. The latter supply should be tested by temporary clamping of the testicular artery.

3. *Silber-Kelly.*   This procedure involves testicular artery and vein division with direct microvascular anastomosis to the internal epigastric vessels.

Orchidectomy is only required in a minority of cases. It may be considered when a normal contralateral testis is present in the patient with a hypoplastic testicle, and/or the patient who has successfully passed puberty. In the latter groups, the undescended testis serves no function and poses only an unnecessary risk of malignant change.

When orchidectomy is required a testicular prosthesis, matched to the size of the contralateral testicle, can be used to preserve cosmesis.

The impalpable testis

The principal causes of impalpable testes are: congenital absence; intra-abdominal testis; and dysplastic testis. Neither ultrasonography, CT or MRI have demonstrated consistent efficacy for the localization of an impalpable testis[b], however testicular venography reliably demonstrates the absence of a normal venous plexus in the congenitally absent testis group (4% of impalpable testes)[b]. Laparoscopy has proven the most sensitive investigation for true intra-abdominal testes[b]. Surgical exploration can reveal a blind-ending vas or a streak gonad.

Hormone therapy

Human chorionic gonadotrophin (hCG) or luteinizing hormone-releasing hormone (LHRH) have been used experimentally to encourage testicular descent[c]. Unfortunately, the efficacy of hormonal manipulation for true undescended testes is unclear as randomized controlled trials have yielded conflicting results[a]. This ambiguity may be explained, in part, by the inadvertent inclusion of patients with retractile testes in the undescended testes study group.

Further reading

Davenport M. ABC of general paediatric surgery. Inguinal hernia, hydrocele, and the undescended testis. *British Medical Journal*, 1996; **312**(7030): 564–567.

Gill B, Kogan S. Cryptorchidism. Current concepts. *Paediatric Clinics of North America*, 1997; **44**(5): 1211–1227.

Leissner J, Filipas D, Wolf HK, Fisch M. The undescended testis: considerations and impact on fertility. *BJU International*, 1999; **83**(8): 885–892.

Related topics of interest

Common paediatric conditions (p. 96); Inguinal hernia (p. 179); Testicular tumours (p. 319).

UPPER GASTROINTESTINAL HAEMORRHAGE

Christopher Lattimer, Simon Gibbs

Although improved acid suppression over the last 20 years has led to an overall fall in the incidence of upper GI haemorrhage in the UK, it still remains a major cause of morbidity and mortality. Approximately 70–80% of upper gastrointestinal bleeds will stop spontaneously. A further 10–15% will stop with endoscopic intervention. Surgery remains a necessity in 5–10% depending on local endoscopic expertise. The aim of all therapies is to stop continuing haemorrhage and decrease the risk of a rebleed.

Peptic ulceration is the leading cause of haemorrhage. The percentage of variceal bleeders increases in inner city areas. Upper gastrointestinal haemorrhage frequently occurs in hospital patients being treated for unrelated conditions. Of these, 25% bleed from acute erosive gastritis and 50% from peptic ulcers.

Cause	UK incidence (%)
Duodenal ulcer (DU)	30
Gastric ulcer (GU)	25
Acute erosive gastritis	10
Oesophageal varices	10
Mallory-Weiss tear	10
Oesophagitis, duodenitis, tumour, other	15

Haematemesis of fresh blood often indicates a significant bleed. Melaena usually indicates an upper gastrointestinal cause, as the blood has been digested by the small bowel. Bloody stools occur as the only feature of bleeding in 10% of patients.

Resuscitation

Resuscitation proceeds with diagnosis in a designated resuscitation area if possible. Inspired oxygen is administered and pulse oximetry and non-invasive blood pressure measurement are commenced. Large-bore intravenous access is established. The features of alcoholic liver disease should be sought (spider naevi, palmar erythema, ascites, hepatosplenomegaly, jaundice) although over 20% of patients with known varices bleed from a peptic ulcer. Patients are often elderly and tolerate blood loss poorly. Blood is taken for urgent FBC, U&E, LFT, cross-match and clotting studies, and if liver disease is suspected vitamin K and fresh frozen plasma are administered. Thrombocytopenia should be corrected with platelet transfusion after urgent advice from a haematologist. The preferred volume replacement fluid is blood, and in severe cases with profound hypotension O negative blood can be given without cross-match. However when possible, cross-matched blood should be given. Crystalloids and colloids disturb fluid balance in patients prone to ascites, but can be started whilst cross-matched blood is awaited, particularly if hypotension is minimal. Nasogastric aspiration of stomach contents allows gastric contraction and reduces the chances of aspiration. The absence of blood in the aspirate does not exclude an upper gastrointestinal cause. Head down and semi-prone positioning protects against an aspiration pneumonia which is the commonest cause of death in these patients. A central venous line and a urinary catheter allow better assessment of circulatory filling pressure.

Endoscopy

Emergency endoscopy may be both therapeutic and diagnostic. Performed early it identifies the cause of bleeding in 90% of cases. Naso-gastric evacuation of retained blood with lavage may greatly aid visibility. The diagnostic yield decreases with time following the initial bleed. Emergency endoscopy should therefore be performed promptly. Rapid exsanguination calls for an immediate endoscopy and in most cases the bleeding lesion is obvious. Endoscopic therapy can then be initiated if appropriate (injection sclerotherapy, argon beam coagulation, diathermy, laser, heater probe), or the patient taken directly to surgery, with the surgeon now able to plan the appropriate operative approach. It will also allow diagnosis of conditions for which conservative management is more appropriate (Mallory-Weiss tear, erosive gastritis) and those in which surgery is usually inappropriate (varices). The best form of endoscopic therapy is not known and many trials exist comparing one against another, often with varying results. The modalities available at each centre also vary widely. In most UK centres injection sclerotherapy remains the most commonly used therapy.

Pharmacology

There is no evidence that pharmacological intervention can alter the clinical course once bleeding starts. Antacids, H_2 antagonists, and proton pump inhibitors are ineffective in arresting haemorrhage from a spurting vessel or a ruptured varix. Vasopressin and somatostatin have been shown to lower portal pressure in patients with varices and are thus used in conjunction with other haemostatic maneouvres. Haemoglobin is an effective natural buffer which can neutralize gastric pH without the need for additional anti-acid therapy. The time-honoured conservative treatment for upper gastrointestinal bleeding was bed-rest and the antacid effect of a full diet.

Peptic ulcer

Peptic ulcer disease is decreasing but the number of operations for bleeding ulcers remains unchanged. Widespread H_2 receptor antagonist use appears to have had little success in decreasing the incidence of bleeding peptic ulcers. Rebleeding can be predicted by the endoscopic findings and several clinical factors. A visible vessel indicates an early rebleeding rate of over 50%.

Endoscopic	Clinical
Visible vessel	Shock (systolic < 90 mmHg)
Clot in ulcer base	Haemoglobin < 8 g/dl
Black or red spots	Haematemesis
Left gastric artery location	Age over 60 years
Gastroduodenal artery location	

Endoscopic therapy can effectively reduce the incidence of rebleeding and allow an elective operation, with its reduced mortality, to take place. It is not yet known whether endoscopic therapy will be a true substitute for operation. A visible vessel (which is really a protruding clot overlying a rent in a non-protruding vessel) is seen in 45% of cases of ulcer haemorrhage but is present in 85% of deaths due to this condition. Surgery for bleeding DU usually involves a duodenotomy and underrunning of the bleeding vessel. The ulcer, if possible, is excluded from the gastrointestinal tract by suturing the mucosa over the ulcer. Bleeding GU can be treated in a similar fashion by gastrotomy and under-running although partial gastrectomy may be necessary if the ulcer is very large or looks malignant. Most patients are elderly however and thus the less one does to give haemostasis is often for the better. Truncal vagotomy is rarely employed now although may be useful in combination with under-running in patients with bleeding DU who have already been on or who are not compliant with PPI therapy.

Oesophageal varices

Ninety per cent of variceal bleeding occurs within 2 cm of the gastro-oesophageal junction. Most varices bleed acutely in the small hours of the morning as portal pressure is at a peak in its diurnal variation. Evidence of a recent bleed is seen by finding a transparent fibrinous clot on the surface of a varix. Long-term survival is dependent on the severity of the liver disease (Child's classification). The therapeutic armamentarium is considered below.

1.   Intravariceal sclerotherapy/banding.   Sclerotherapy is the method of choice for acute bleeding control. Ethanolamine oleate is injected directly into the varix. Banding is now most often used to control varices electively at a later date.

2.   Vasopressin/somatostatin.   These both lower portal pressure and are used as intravenous therapies in the acute situation.

3.   Sengstaken-Blakemore/Minnesota tube.   Balloon tamponade of the varices by a gastric balloon, filled with 200 ml of saline, pressed firmly up against the diaphragm is only a temporary manoeuvre prior to definitive sclerotherapy. The oesophageal balloon, if required, is attached to a mercury manometer and inflated to not more than mean arterial pressure. It should be deflated every 2 hours to prevent iatrogenic ulceration.

4.   Portasystemic shunts.   Mesocaval or splenorenal shunts decrease portal pressure. The more proximal the shunt, the more effective it is, but this is paralleled by a progressive increase in hepatic encephalopathy. Shunts are considered after two failed sessions of sclerotherapy.

5.   Transjugular intrahepatic portasystemic anastomosis (TIPS).   Portasystemic shunts may be performed intrahepatically under radiological control to lower portal venous pressure.

6.   Major surgery.   Oesophageal transection and reanastomosis with a stapler through a small gastrotomy is combined with a devascularization procedure. Its indications are rare as the operation carries a much higher mortality than shunting.

Acute erosive gastritis

This is caused by stress conditions like burns (Curling's ulcer), head injury (Cushing's ulcer), major trauma, sepsis, MOF or by the ingestion of injurious substances like alcohol or NSAIDs. Haemorrhage from the latter group can be arrested with a platelet transfusion in occasional cases. Endoscopic appearances are of multiple brown-coloured areas the size and shape of tea leaves. Pharmacological suppression of acid secretion is the mainstay of therapy. Sucralfate has been used in this situation but there is little convincing evidence that it is useful. A gastrectomy is rarely indicated.

Mallory-Weiss tear

These are found at the gastro-oesophageal junction on the lesser curve in 80% of cases. The cause is usually violent vomiting after the consumption of a large meal with alcohol. In 90% of cases the bleeding stops spontaneously. Endoscopic electro-coagulation is indicated or operative underrunning in resistant cases.

Aorto-enteric fistula

Almost all occur in the first two centimetres of jejunum. They should be considered in all patients with an aortic graft. There is usually a history of a minor painless haematemesis (herald bleed). Treatment involves graft removal with either extra-anatomical bypass or in-situ replacement with a rifampicin-bonded graft. Adequate graft coverage with the aneurysm sac, periaortic fat and omentum at the time of the aortic surgery will help to reduce this complication.

Gastrointestinal stromal tumours (GIST)

Leiomyomas or leiomyosarcomas are the commonest tumours to cause major upper gastrointestinal bleeds. They are recognized at endoscopy as a yellowish polyp with an ulcer crater on the surface. Treatment by local excision is curative. Gastric carcinomas, in contrast, ooze slowly causing anaemia.

Dieulafoy malformation

This rare hamartomatous lesion presents with a large painless haematemesis. Endoscopy is often negative. The lesion can be in any portion of the upper GI tract but is commonest in the stomach. The lesion consists of a large blood vessel in the submucosa which bleeds easily and intermittently. If recognized, argon beam coagulation can be curative, otherwise diagnosis is often only found at surgery.

Further reading

Palmer KR, Choudari CP. Endoscopic intervention in bleeding peptic ulcer. *Gut*, 1995; **37**: 161–164.

Rockall TA *et al*. Incidence of and mortality from acute upper GI haemorrhage in the United Kingdom. *British Medical Journal*, 1995; **311**: 222–226.

Steele RJC. The treatment of non-variceal upper gastrointestinal bleeding. In: Griffin SM, Raines SA (eds) *Upper Gastrointestinal Surgery – A Companion to Specialist Surgical Practice*. W.B. Saunders, London, 1999; 361–390.

Related topics of interest

Blood transfusion (p. 53); Gastric cancer (p. 135); Gastro-intestinal polyps (p. 142); Peptic ulceration (p. 255).

URINARY CALCULI

Adrian Simoes

The last century has seen a rising incidence of renal calculi and a falling incidence of bladder calculi. Urinary calculi are polycrystalline aggregates composed of varying amounts of crystalloids and organic matrix. It has been suggested the lifetime risk of stone formation is 10–15% in men and 5–10% in women. Urinary calculi are commonly composed of:

- Calcium oxalate;
- Calcium phosphate;
- Magnesium ammonium phosphate;
- Uric acid;
- Cystine;
- Xanthine;
- Matrix.

Aetiology

Many factors are involved in the formation of urinary stones and can be broadly categorized under three main headings.

1. Urinary inhibitors and promoters.   Urinary crystals are a common occurrence as urine is normally supersaturated. It has therefore been postulated that various constituents present in urine may act as inhibitors or promoters of crystal nucleation and growth to form stones. Citrate, magnesium, pyrophosphates, nephrocalcin and uropontin are considered to be inhibitors and Tamm-Horsfall protein and glycosaminoglycans act as inhibitors as well as promoters.

2. Anatomical features.   Urinary stasis due to anatomical anomalies can result and encourage stone formation. Hence in various conditions such as pelvi-ureteric junction obstruction, infundibular narrowing of a calix or collecting tubular dilatation in medullary sponge kidney, stone formation in the region of stasis is common.

3. Metabolic defects.   Various metabolic errors leading to cystinuria and primary hyperoxaluria (both being autosomal recessive disorders) and renal tubular acidosis are associated with stone formation.

Presentation

Renal stones may be asymptomatic and incidentally noted on an abdominal radiograph or ultrasound. Often there is a continuous or intermittent dull ache in the loin with microscopic or frank haematuria. Occasionally the patient may present with urinary tract infection, pyocalycx, pyonephrosis and perinephric abscess. Obstruction of a calyx by an impacted stone causes pain and a hydrocalyx. The differential diagnosis should exclude muscloskeletal pain and gall bladder pathology.

Ureteric stones classically present with ureteric colic, which is unilateral, severe, arises in the loin and radiates to the groin, testis or the tip of the penis. A writhing fetal posture with vomiting is typical and so also is haematuria. The differential diagnosis of ureteric colic includes a leaking abdominal aortic aneurysm, prolapsed intervertebral disc, Munchausen's syndrome and analgesia abuse.

Investigation

Urine dipstix and culture. Plain abdominal radiograph and tomograms will identify radio-opacities. An IVU will indicate whether the radio-opacity is a stone or not, its site, size and the shape and the degree of obstruction. In addition it will also delineate any abnormality of the urinary tract. In the case of hypersensitivity to intravenous contrast, an unenhanced spiral CT will be equally informative. Ultrasound is a non-invasive modality identifying stones and back pressure effects. The use of Doppler scanning allows the resistive index of the kidney to be calculated to indicate obstruction. In certain patients renal isotope scanning needs to be done to evaluate renal function. Rarely retrograde pyelography and ureteroscopy are needed to confirm the presence of a ureteric stone. In addition, especially in recurrent, multiple and bilateral calculi a metabolic screening test on blood and urine needs to be performed.

Management

The management of urinary calculi depends on the size, site, shape, number and chemical composition of the stone. Patient factors include degree of symptoms, coexisting anatomical abnormalities, metabolic defects and renal reserve. Infection of an obstructed kidney is a surgical emergency and needs to be managed aggressively with antibiotics and drainage either by ureteric stenting or percutaneous nephrostomy.

Definitive stone treatment may be carried out by a variety of procedures.

1. ESWL (extracorporeal shock wave lithotripsy). This involves the production of shock waves extracorporeally which are focused on the stone using either radiological or ultrasonographic localization. The shock waves are created by lithotriptors and the principle behind them is electrohydraulic, electromagnetic or piezoelectric. Steinstrasse (German for 'street of stone') may result following ESWL due to the accumulation of multiple stone fragments within the ureter. Percutaneous nephrolithotomy involves making a percutaneous tract into the renal pelvis by a Seldinger technique under radiological guidance and subsequent extraction of the stone either intact or following fragmentation. Ureteroscopy and stone extraction, if required, are achieved by using intraureteral lithotripsy which includes ultrasonic, electrohydraulic, laser and ballistic techniques.

Open procedures are necessary for less than 5% of stone disease and include both open and laparoscopic ureterolithotomy.

2. Pyelolithotomy and extended pyelolithotomy (Gil-Vernet technique). Stones in the renal pelvis and at times those in a major calyx may be extracted by incising open the renal pelvis and extending the incision on to the renal sinus for added exposure to the stone (extended pyelolithotomy).

3. Anatrophic nephrotomy. Renal stones are extracted by cutting open the kidney longitudinally. The site of incision on the kidney is planned after demarcating the junction of the renal tissue supplied by the anterior and posterior branch of the renal artery. The renal artery is clamped to provide a bloodless field. The warm and cold (core temperature of 20°C) ischaemic times are 30 minutes and 3 hours respectively.

4. *Paravascular radial nephrotomy.* Once again renal ischaemia is required and the incisions on the kidney are radial and achieve good access to calices. The healing also is considered to be better with a fine scar but multiple nephrotomies may be necessary to approach multiple calices.

5. *Partial nephrectomy and nephrectomy.* These procedures are rare and are undertaken when there is significant damage to a part or the whole of renal tissue in relation to the calculus and is associated with non-function or poor function. Prior to resorting to these procedures adequate efforts need to be made to salvage renal tissue to make sure that following this procedure the renal function is not significantly compromised.

Bladder stones

Aetiology

Common in children in India, Thailand, Egypt and Turkey and is attributed to malnutrition and episodes of severe dehydration. In the West they are seen in adults suffering from bladder outflow obstruction, bladder diverticulum, neurogenic bladders, chronic infection, foreign bodies or renal stones retained in the bladder.

Presentation

The calculus may be found incidentally in investigating men with lower urinary tract symptoms. Dull or sharp suprapubic pain with intermittent, painful voiding associated with terminal haematuria is common. In addition to this pain the flow of urine may be interrupted and relief may be achieved on assuming a recumbent position. Recurrent urinary tract infection may be the presenting picture. Children sometimes present with priapism and nocturnal enuresis.

Diagnosis

Historically they were diagnosed during bladder instrumentation with a metal 'sound'. Now an abdominal radiograph, ultrasound and intravenous urogram will reveal the stone. Occasionally a cystoscopy is necessary to arrive at the diagnosis.

Management

Treatment involves correction of the underlying pathology and cystoscopic extraction of the calculus after its fragmentation using mechanical crushers or various other energy sources. Rarely open cystolithotomy is necessary for large stones.

Further reading

Pak CY. Etiology and treatment of urolithiasis. *American Journal of Kidney Disease*, 1991; **18:** 624–637.

Prien EL. Crystallographic analysis of urinary calculi. A 23 year survey study. *Journal of Urology*, 1963; **89:** 917–924.

Springmann KE, Drach GW, Gottung B, Randolph AD. Effect of human urine on aggregation of calcium oxalate crystals. *Journal of Urology*, 1986; **135:** 69–71.

Related topic of interest

Bladder outflow obstruction (p. 49).

VARICOSE VEINS

Nick Wilson

Varicose veins are defined by the World Health Organization as saccular dilatations of veins that are often tortuous. This excludes dilatations of small intradermal subcutaneous veins and tortuous dilated veins that are secondary to thrombophlebitis or arteriovenous fistula.

Epidemiology

1. Race and sex. Approximately 2% of Western populations have primary varicose veins, the problem being much less common in Eastern populations particularly Africans and Indians. Women are affected 3–4 times more frequently than men.

2. Age. The prevalence of varicose veins increases with age with a peak frequency between 50 and 60 years of age.

3. Pregnancy. Pregnancy predisposes (incidence 8–20%), second and subsequent pregnancies compounding the risk. Rising levels of progesterone during pregnancy encourage smooth muscle relaxation and venous distension, possibly resulting in the development of varicose veins. Compression of the iliac veins by the gravid uterus may also be important.

4. Heredity. Heredity is an important factor with many patients having at least one parent affected. The mode of inheritance is, however, unclear and is probably polygenetic. Varicose veins are a human condition, being unreported in any animal species, including bipeds.

5. Other factors. Although it has frequently been suggested that extremes of height and weight predispose there is little evidence to support this. Occupations involving prolonged periods of standing probably predispose.

6. Secondary varicose veins. Secondary varicose veins are caused by post-thrombotic damage, pelvic tumours, acquired arteriovenous fistulae and congenital venous anomalies including the Klippel Trenaunay syndrome, Parkes–Weber syndrome and congenital valvular agenesis.

Aetiology

The principal aetiological theories advanced are valvular deficiency, defective vein wall structure and arteriovenous fistulae, the last of which can now largely be discounted. Saphenofemoral valvular incompetence as cited by Trendelenburg is probably a secondary effect, being the result of ascending reflux caused by a primary vein wall structural defect. Histological features of the vein wall and the histochemical features of reduced collagen and increased muscle and hexosamine content of varicose veins suggest that a structural abnormality of the vein wall is the primary defect[c].

Clinical features

1. **The distribution of varicose veins.** The long saphenous venous system is most commonly affected, but the stem vein itself is frequently spared, the tributaries showing the most pronounced varicosis. The short saphenous vein is less commonly affected and the anatomical course of this vein is frequently less obvious, particularly if the varicosities are recurrent. The varicose process starts in the distal veins and ascends proximally.

2. **Symptoms.** The commonest symptoms caused by varicose veins are unsightliness and aching. Mild ankle oedema is also common. More severe leg pain is usually caused by other conditions such as peripheral vascular disease or osteoarthritis.

3. **Complications.** These include haemorrhage, superficial thrombophlebitis and the calf pump failure syndrome (pigmentation, eczema, lipodermatosclerosis, ulceration). Any history of deep vein thrombosis, pulmonary embolism, or associated events must be elicited and any previous treament for varicose veins should be recorded.

4. **Examination.** Firstly, a thorough inspection of the legs for the site of all major varicosities, the presence of a saphena varix, ankle oedema, signs of calf pump failure, angiomata, arterial insufficiency, joint disease, and previous trauma or surgery to the leg is made. It is important to distinguish long saphenous, short saphenous and communicating vein incompetence. The cough impulse test indicates the presence of valvular incompetence in the vein under examination and the percussion test is useful for demonstrating the origin of a varicose vein. The tourniquet test is extremely useful in determining the system of origin of varicose veins, although it appears insensitive when compared with duplex scanning.

5. **Investigations.** Where there is continuing doubt about the presence of superficial venous reflux a hand-held Doppler probe is of considerable benefit. Duplex ultrasound is used for demonstrating reflux, for identifying the saphenopopliteal junction, for mapping the anatomy and for imaging the deep veins. Where there is the possibility of previous deep vein thrombosis, imaging with ascending phlebography or duplex ultrasound is mandatory to demonstrate post-thrombotic damage and to exclude deep vein obstruction. Where this is present, it must be assumed that any varicose veins must be secondary to the obstruction and should not be removed. Where the short saphenous vein is varicose it is important to identify the site of the saphenopopliteal junction as this is very variable. Varicography can be used as an alternative to duplex ultrasound for demonstrating anatomy and provides an easily interpretable permanent record that can be referred to in the operating theatre.

Treatment

1. **Indications.** These include the relief symptoms, the relief and prevention of complications and correction of unacceptable cosmetic appearance. Approximately 30% of patients attending a varicose vein clinic will not require treatment. It is generally assumed that untreated varicose veins will continue to enlarge and involve other adjacent veins in the varicose process.

2. **Results.**   Results of treatment are very variable and the chances of recurrence at 5 years are 8–50%. Patients should be warned appropriately before being offered treatment. Greater use of preoperative imaging techniques, attention to anatomical variants and improved surgical techniques will hopefully improve the long-term results.

3. **Principles.**   The principles of treatment include the reduction of transmural venous pressure gradient, disconnection of superficial veins from the deep veins at sites of reflux (saphenofemoral, saphenopopliteal, communicating vein ligation) and abolition of visible varices (obliteration or excision).

4. **Compression hosiery.**   Patients who are unsuitable for surgery and pregnant women can be treated using class I or II graduated compression stockings. Below knee stockings are usually adequate and should be worn at all times other than in bed. Patients should be supplied with two pairs which should be replaced every 6 months. Stockings are inconvenient to wear and, although often relieve discomfort, most patients find them unacceptable.

5. **Injection sclerotherapy.**   This has been used to treat all forms of varicose veins but in the United Kingdom is employed mainly for the obliteration of tributary vein varicosities with saphenofemoral or saphenopopliteal incompetence being treated surgically. Contraindications include oral contraception, pregnancy, a history of severe allergy, foot veins (because of the risk of intra-arterial injection). The technique depends on the induction of a chemical inflammation in the vein endothelium following injection of a sclerosant agent. The detergent sodium tetradecyl sulphate (STD) remains the most popular agent in use although newer agents including Aethoxysclerol and Scerovein are also used. It is vital that the sclerosant is only injected into the vein lumen. Extraluminal sclerosant induces a brisk tissue reaction resulting in the formation of indolent ulcers that are painful, slow to heal and frequently leave residual pigmentation. Other complications include vasovagal attacks, allergic reactions, deep venous thrombosis and intra-arterial injection. Following injection compression bandages are applied for a variable period (3–6 weeks) although the role and importance of this in producing variceal obliteration is unclear. Patients should be warned about the risks of extravasation, the need to be bandaged (they may wish to avoid this during hot weather or holiday periods) and the tenderness and swelling of the vein that accompanies the inflammatory process. It may take 6–12 weeks for the swelling to resolve.

6. **Surgery.**   Surgery is preferable if there is clear saphenofemoral or saphenopopliteal incompetence, if the varices are large and if there is communicating vein incompetence. Most surgical procedures in common use are best performed under general anaesthesia, although local and regional techniques have been used. Many healthy patients can be treated as day cases, but patients requiring extensive bilateral surgery with recurrent or communicating vein disease may require longer admission. Saphenofemoral ligation is performed where the saphenofemoral junction is incompetent and there are long saphenous system varicosities. Before ligation, the femoral vein must be clearly identified and all tributaries should be ligated and divided. Stripping of the long saphenous vein is advisable as the recurrence rate

is lower than achieved by saphenofemoral ligation alone. The vein should be stripped to just below the knee, but no further to avoid damage to the saphenous nerve. This procedure is usually performed with local avulsions of the most prominent varicosities performed through small incisions placed in the direction of Langer's lines. Saphenopopliteal ligation is performed with the patient prone and with the aid of a saphenogram or duplex scan to demonstrate the position of the junction. This vein is also usually stripped.

Communicating vein interruption is best performed using subfascial endoscopic perforating vein surgery (SEPS), although in the UK, this is usually reserved for patients with skin changes or ulceration[c]. Having demonstrated the presence of incompetent communicating veins by duplex ultrasound and/or by phlebography an endoscope is passed subfascially through a small incision on the medial side of the calf just below the knee. The perforating veins are clipped under direct vision. This technique avoids the wound healing problems associated with standard open subfascial perforating vein surgery (Cockett's operation, Linton's operation).

Considerable care and skill is required for the optimum treatment of many patients with varicose veins, particularly those with short saphenous or recurrent varicose veins. Frequently this is left to the most junior members of the surgical team.

Further reading

Browse NL, Burnand KG, Irvine AT, Wilson NM. *Diseases of the Veins* (2nd edn.) Edward Arnold, London, 1999.
Gloviczi P. Subfascial endoscopic perforator vein surgery: indications and results. *Vascular Medicine*, 1999; **4:** 173–180.

Related topics of interest

Calf pump failure and venous ulceration (p. 66); Deep vein thrombosis (p. 113); Lymphoedema and the management of the swollen leg (p. 210); Vascular imaging and investigation (p. 350); Vascular malformations and tumours (p. 353).

VASCULAR IMAGING AND INVESTIGATION

Nick Lagattolla

Arterial

Inspection may reveal pulsatile aneurysms. The extremities may be pallid and cool to the touch, particularly on elevation, in chronic arterial insufficiency, with cyanosis of the foot on dependency (Buerger's sign). The presence of fixed mottling of the skin, arterial ulceration, pregangrenous dusky discoloration or frank gangrene amounts to critical ischaemia, and the limb will be lost unless urgent revascularization is undertaken. A pulse will not be palpated distal to an arterial occlusion or a tight stenosis, which can be differentiated from an occlusion by the presence of a bruit. A clear distribution of the patent, stenotic and occluded segments of the arteries of a limb may thus be obtained clinically.

*1. **Doppler ultrasound and pressures.*** The patency of an artery or graft is confirmed with an audible Doppler signal. Low amplitude prolonged signals indicate reduced flow, suggesting filling from collaterals in the presence of a proximal arterial occlusion, or reduced flow distal to a stenosis. A high amplitude abrupt signal suggests non-compliant calcified arteries. A proximal sphygmomanometer cuff gradually inflated until the Doppler signal disappears reveals the pressure in the artery. The brachial systolic pressure is also assessed. The ratio of the best pedal measurement on either foot to the brachial pressure is the ankle–brachial pressure index (ABPI). Generally, normal arterial ABPI ranges from 0.9 to greater than 1.0, and critically ischaemic limbs have an ABPI of less than 0.5.

ABPI is important in the assessment of effects of surgery or angioplasty. It is useful to confirm vascular disease not evident in the quiescent patient by measuring ABPI under resting and exercise conditions.

*2. **Duplex scanning.*** The combination of B-mode and Doppler ultrasound is duplex scanning. It is used in the assessment of carotid stenoses, arterial graft surveillance, and in the localization of peripheral arterial disease. In the carotid artery, the ultrasound detects plaques, and their content may be deduced from the appearance. The Doppler principle allows the velocity and flow to be calculated. This is used to calculate the percentage stenosis of an artery.

*3. **Radiology.*** CT and ultrasound scans are invaluable in the assessment of aneurysms, gauging their diameter accurately, and indicating the presence of mural thrombus. Magnetic resonance angiography (MRA) can image the arterial tree in a totally non-invasive fashion.

*4. **Contrast angiography.*** Views of both legs plus the aorta can be obtained by direct needle puncture of the aorta (translumbar aortography) or by a transfemoral catheter advanced proximally. Direct arterial puncture carries complications, including dissection of the artery, distal embolization of thrombus or atheromatous debris, arterial thrombosis, and haemorrhage, which may be life-threatening if it occurs in the retroperitoneum.

5. *Digital subtraction arteriography (DSA).* DSA provides better resolution films than conventional contrast angiography. DSA can be achieved through the intravenous (i.v. DSA) or intra-arterial (i.a. DSA) route. In i.v. DSA, the aorta and its branches are well visualized, as are the femoral and popliteal arteries. The crural arteries cannot be visualized beyond their origin with clarity. An i.a. DSA will show vessels down to the foot with great clarity. Thus, for patients with aorto-iliac or carotid artery disease, i.v. DSA is usually sufficient, but those with critical ischaemia, who have distal arterial disease by implication, will need an i.a. DSA. Care should be taken in patients with renal failure, as large boluses of intravascular contrast are nephrotoxic, and i.v. DSA should be avoided.

Venous

Visible varicosities will be seen in the back of the calf in short and the thigh and anterior and medial lower leg in long saphenous incompetence. These must be confirmed by tourniquet tests. Gentle palpation in the popliteal fossa with the patient standing with the knee slightly flexed will demonstrate an enlarged and incompetent short saphenous vein.

Incompetent communicating veins may be seen on the medial aspect of the leg. These may be primarily incompetent, or a manifestation of deep venous insufficiency. Other stigmata of deep venous insufficiency are swelling, dermatoliposclerosis (induration and pigmentation of the skin), eczema, and venous ulceration. Some may develop pale scarring of the skin with punctate or reticular red vascular tufts (atrophie blanche).

1. *Duplex scanning.* This has become the optimal non-invasive method of assessment of the venous system of the lower limb. Sources of superficial venous incompetence and the presence of incompetent perforating veins are confirmed. The deep veins are assessed with regard to patency and the presence of venous reflux. This may be due to primary valvular incompetence, but it is usually due to post-thrombotic damage to the venous valves.

2. *Venous function tests.* The filling and emptying of the veins of a limb change the limb volume. This can be measured by venous plethysmography. These tests include foot volumetry by water displacement, and strain-gauge plethysmography, air-, photo- or impedance-plethysmography, depending on the physical method of determining venous filling of a limb. Light reflection rheography works along the same principles as photoplethysmography, using infrared light to penetrate the dermis of the skin of the leg, recording the amount reflected back, which is in proportion to the filling of the dermal vessels. Dermal capillary flow can be measured by laser Doppler fluximetry.

3. *Varicography.* The injection of varicosities enables visualization of the source of varicose vein filling. This is particularly useful in recurrent varicose veins when the source is difficult to determine clinically.

4. *Ascending phlebography.* This is the optimal method of assessing the anatomy of the deep venous system, particularly in the detection of postphlebitic deep vein damage. It is useful in detecting incompetent perforating veins, but not all may be detected.

5. Descending phlebography. Deep venous reflux may be assessed by descending phlebography. Reflux is classed according to Kistner's grading 0–IV. Grade I is reflux into the superficial femoral vein and is deemed normal, and grade IV is gross reflux down to the calf veins.

Lymphatic

Lymphoedema results in swelling of the lower limb, which can range from as little as mild swelling of the dorsum of the foot to gross swelling of the entire limb. There is usually squaring of the toes. In advanced cases, the skin develops filiform and nodular excrescences. Classically, chronic lymphoedema is said not to pit with pressure, though this is not true in all cases. Lymphoedema due to lymphatic obstruction at the level of the groin nodes with patent lymphatics distally may produce swelling of the thigh and leg with sparing of the foot. This is important to detect clinically and to confirm by special investigations, as this may be amenable to surgical bypass using an entero-mesenteric bridge.

1. Isotope lymphography. This provides rapid confirmation of a clinical diagnosis of lymphoedema. A reduced isotope uptake in the lymph vessels and nodes of the groin confirm lymphoedema, and additionally an obstructive pattern may be discerned. A higher uptake than the normal range may be indicative of a venous cause for swelling.

2. Contrast lymphography. This is performed under general anaesthesia. Dorsal pedal lymphatics are dissected and cannulated using an operating microscope, and lipid-soluble contrast is slowly infused. It is time-consuming and expensive, and cannot be used to confirm all cases of suspected lymphoedema. It should be used only when there is clinical and isotopic evidence of proximal lymphatic obstruction.

Further reading

Beard JD, Scott DJA. Investigation of chronic lower limb ischaemia. *Hospital Update*, 1991; **June:** 496–506.
Donelly R, Himwood D, London NJM. Non-invasive methods of arterial and venous assessment. *British Medical Journal*, 2000; **320:** 698–701.
Nicolaides AN. Assessment of leg ischaemia. *British Medical Journal*, 1991; **303:** 1323–1326.

Related topics of interest

Aneurysms (p. 24); Critical leg ischaemia (p. 100); Deep vein thrombosis (p. 113); Intermittent claudication (p. 187); Lymphoedema and the management of the swollen limb (p. 210); Varicose veins (p. 346).

VASCULAR MALFORMATIONS AND TUMOURS

Nick Lagattolla

Malformations

These may have arterial, venous or lymphatic elements, or they may be mixed. The majority are congenital, in which case they are hamartomatous in origin and not neoplastic. Acquired vascular malformations are usually traumatic in origin.

Congenital arteriovenous fistulae

These are rare, and can arise in any part of the body but are more frequent on the head and neck and in the upper limb. They vary in size, and may be very unsightly and distressing. An appreciable increase in size may occur at the time of puberty. The swelling caused by the malformation is usually warm, soft and pulsatile, with a palpable thrill and a bruit. Occlusion of the fistula by compression may result in a bradycardia from the transiently reduced venous return (Branham's sign). There is often an erythematous hue of the overlying skin. Tissues distal to an arterio-venous fistula may become ischaemic as a result of the 'steal' of oxygenated blood, and ulceration or haemorrhage may occur. The diagnosis can be confirmed by arteriography, which might enable therapeutic embolization of the feeding vessels. This is a risky undertaking which may lead to further ischaemia of the distal tissues, or inadvertent embolization into vital structures. Simple ligation of the feeding vessels is rarely successful in controlling the malformation. Excision of an arteriovenous malformation is hazardous as blood loss may be enormous. Quilting sutures may be successful in reducing the size of a malformation.

Parkes–Weber syndrome

This comprises multiple deep arteriovenous fistulae resulting in a generally swollen and often lengthened limb, which is warm to the touch, and mildly red in colour. Bruits and thrills are rare because the fistulae are small. The diagnosis is confirmed by angiography. Symptoms may be controlled by repeated angiography and embolization, which reduces the shunting of arterial blood to the venous system and thus prevents or delays the onset of high-output cardiac failure, which is a serious complication.

Venous angioma

These malformations vary widely in appearance, and may occur virtually anywhere. If superficial, they may present as a bulky, blue-coloured, compressible mass. Deeper angiomas may be painful, and manifest only by diffuse swelling with a hint of blue discoloration. Frequently, the abnormality extends further than can be appreciated by external examination. CT scan after injection of contrast or magnetic resonance venography will demonstrate the true extent, and involvement of muscle groups and joints may be identified. Excision can result in symptomatic or cosmetic improvement, although lesions are rarely completely excised.

Klippel–Trenaunay syndrome

This condition is essentially a triad of venous, bone and lymphatic congenital anomalies. The lower limb is most commonly affected, followed by the arm then the pelvis. The overriding abnormality is usually venous, although the extent of venous, bone and lymphatic involvement varies widely. The affected limb is swollen, and often longer, with an extensive cutaneous venous haemangioma following a metameric distribution. There are usually grossly dilated and incompetent superficial varicosities. Support hosiery remains the most effective and simple treatment. Deep venous abnormalities may be present, and this must be excluded by phlebography should surgery be planned for symptomatic superficial varicosities.

Cystic hygroma

This is a bulky swelling lymphatic present in the root of the neck at birth. It is soft and cystic on examination, and transilluminates. The management is conservative as resolution often occurs by the age of four. Aspiration and injection with sclerosants may be required for recalcitrant lesions.

Lymphangioma circumscripta

This is a cutaneous lesion comprising multiple, small, cutaneous vesicles in very close approximation to each other. They are usually colourless but are occasionally blood-filled. They contain lymph, and may be a manifestation of an underlying chronic lymphatic abnormality. They may cause troublesome seepage of fluid, and may act as a source of infection. Excision of a patch of vesicles is unlikely to prevent recurrence, though symptoms may be temporarily relieved.

Haemolymphangioma

This is a diffuse congenital abnormality of the lymph-atics, usually affecting a limb, and most commonly the leg. The abnormality is present in the subcutaneous tissues, but may also involve deeper structures. The limb is swollen, indurated and discoloured, and some degree of disability usually results. Because of the diffuse nature of the abnormality, excision is not feasible although reduction of limb volume may be of help.

Tumours

Glomus tumour

These are benign vascular tumours that typically occur on extremities. They arise from the dermal glomus apparatus, a vascular organ that has a role in temperature regulation. The majority affect upper limb, and 50% occur on the finger, one-third of which are sub-ungual. They present as exquisitely painful and tender lesions. Pain may result from very minor disturbances, particularly changes in temperature and on pressure. They are often purple or red in colour, though they may appear colourless if sub-ungual. Although they are often very small, often only millimetres in diameter, they may be localized on examination by their intense point tenderness. Treatment is by excision.

Carotid body tumour

These are also known as chemodectomas. They are rare tumours arising from the chemoreceptor cells of the carotid body. Exceptionally, they may arise from chemoreceptor tissue at other sites. They are highly vascular. Ten per cent are bilateral. They affect males and females equally and at all ages, although the peak incidence is at 50. They present as a painless, often long-standing mass below the angle of the jaw, which will be compressible with gentle sustained pressure, and refills when pressure is released (the 'sign of emptying' of a vascular mass). The diagnosis is confirmed by intravenous digital subtraction angiogram (DSA), which shows characteristic splaying of the carotid bifurcation, or by CT scan. Macroscopically they appear as featureless oval masses, leading to the description 'potato tumour' although on cut section they are red or brown.

The treatment is by excision by an experienced vascular surgeon, as the internal carotid artery may need to be shunted or even resected and grafted, though the latter is unusual. Their behaviour is unpredictable, with the majority not recurring following excision, though a proportion will have frank evidence of malignancy with local invasion. If left unresected, 10–20% will develop metastases. Radiotherapy may be of use in the elderly or unfit patient, or in the treatment of local recurrence.

Glomus jugulare tumour

These are similar to chemodectomas but arise in the jugular bulb in association with the ninth, tenth and eleventh cranial nerves. They are slow growing but locally invasive. Presentation is with pulsatile tinnitus, or as a lump anterior to the mastoid process. Surgical excision is a major undertaking that risks facial and other cranial nerve palsies, and radiotherapy is an alternative option.

Haemangio-pericytoma

These are purple nodular subcutaneous tumours which usually occur on extremities, most often on fingers or toes. They are histologically benign, but are prone to local recurrence. They may be treated by repeated resection or amputation of the affected digit. They may become frankly sarcomatous.

Kaposi's sarcoma

This is a malignant tumour arising from vascular tissue that is histologically a haemangiosarcoma. It sporadically arises in middle-aged Mediterranean and African populations and in Eastern European Jews. Men are mostly affected. It is frequently found on the leg and trunk and is commonly multiple. It appears as a red or bluish usually painless papule. The incidence of this has risen greatly with the increase in HIV infection, which predisposes to the appearance of Kaposi's sarcoma in the skin and throughout the intestinal tract. It responds initially to cytotoxic chemotherapy and radiotherapy, but spreads readily to the liver and lungs, carrying a dismal prognosis.

Angiosarcoma

Sarcomatous change is a very rare complication in a long-standing angioma. Rapid enlargement and induration of the lesion will occur. Primary angiosarcoma also occurs in the liver in children and young adults.

Leiomyosarcoma

Leiomyosarcoma may arise from the vena cava, and more rarely from the iliac or femoral veins. The sarcoma invades locally and may present with pain. There may be symptoms from venous obstruction. These tumours should be treated by excision and interposition grafting as necessary. Further local control may be achieved by radiotherapy. However local recurrence is usual, and the prognosis is poor.

Lymphangiosarcoma

This is a rare primary malignancy arising from lymphatic vessels. It may occur in long-standing lymphoedematous limbs, in which case it is known as Stuart–Treeves syndrome. Rapid growth is characteristic, and the prognosis is poor.

Further reading

Allison DJ, Kennedy A. Peripheral arteriovenous malformations. *British Medical Journal*, 1991; **303:** 1191–1194.

Halliday AW, Mansfield AO. Congenital arteriovenous malformations. *British Journal of Surgery*, 1993; **80:** 2–3.

Related topics of interest

The skin and subcutaneous tissues (p. 303); Soft tissue swellings (p. 312); Vascular imaging and investigation (p. 350).

VASCULAR TRAUMA

Nick Wilson

Mechanism of injury

Urban, terrorist and military violence involving blunt and penetrating arterial and venous injuries is increasingly common. Road traffic accidents may also result in penetrating injuries, but commonly cause fractures and dislocations that damage adjacent vessels. Low-velocity penetrating injuries (pistols, knives) produce localized, direct injury to vessels. High-velocity injuries (high-velocity rifles) produce a shock wave effect resulting in widespread tissue destruction. Secondary missiles (bullet or bone fragments) can produce further damage. Iatrogenic injuries occur with the increasing use of invasive or minimally invasive procedures. Vessels may also be injured by chemical agents and by cold.

Types of vessel injury

- Contusion.
- Puncture.
- Laceration.
- Partial division.
- Transection.

Effects of vessel injury

- Haemorrhage. Primary, reactionary or secondary. Revealed or concealed.
- Occlusion. Thrombosis, dissection, external compression, spasm.
- False aneurysm.
- Traumatic arteriovenous fistula.

Clinical assessment

The history of injury is usually clear. External haemorrhage or expanding haematoma are usually evident. Weak or absent distal pulses are an important sign but distal ischaemia is uncommon in isolated arterial injuries and pulses are present in 20% of patients with arterial wounds. Duplex ultrasound and/or arteriography may be helpful but should not delay the control of severe haemorrhage.

Indications for surgical exploration

- Weak or absent distal pulse.
- Persistent arterial bleeding.
- Large expanding haematoma.
- Ischaemia.
- Bruit.

Treatment

1.   Principles of repair.   Major vascular injuries in a haemodynamically unstable patient require immediate operation. Direct pressure should be used to control bleeding initially whilst intravenous access is gained for the infusion of electrolyte solutions until blood is available. Vertical incisions enable easy extension if necessary and reduce the likelihood of injury to adjacent neurovascular structures. Control proximal and distal to the site of injury will allow control where a large haematoma obscures the site of injury. In major vessel transection a heparin-bonded shunt may be used to re-establish arterial and/or venous continuity whilst adjacent fractures are stabilized, or more life-threatening injuries are repaired. Careful embolectomy proximal and distal to the site of injury should be performed before the repair is completed. Ultrasound or arteriography should be used to confirm distal patency if there is any doubt. Systemic anticoagulants are best avoided in patients with multiple injuries. Synthetic grafts should be avoided in contaminated wounds. Small and medium sized veins can safely be ligated but axial outflow veins should be repaired and continuity established to prevent subsequent thrombosis with swelling and aching, providing the patient is stable. Reperfusion injury may occur after revascularization of an ischaemic limb and fasciotomy should be employed liberally.

2. Techniques of repair
- Simple suture – for small holes.
- Lateral suture – for small tears.
- Patch repair – where direct closure would cause stenosis.
- End to end anastomosis – for complete transection or where excision of a short segment of damaged vessel is necessary.
- Interposition graft – where there is significant loss of vessel length. Use autogenous vein if possible.

Iatrogenic injury

1. Ligation. Unexpected arterial injury at operation may result in ligation of a major artery. Removal of the ligature (or repair of the artery where appropriate) should be undertaken rather than relying on collateral circulation.

2. Compression from plasters and splints. These problems should be prevented by adequate padding, splinting and monitoring of the limb.

3. Arterial puncture. Cardiac catheterization via femoral or brachial arteries results in sporadic arterial injuries which can be minimized by careful dissection, compression and suture where necessary. Distal ischaemia is usually caused by thrombosis or dissection and is treated by exploration, embolectomy/thrombectomy and repair of the damaged segment by patch or interposition graft.

4. False aneurysms. Arterial puncture for insertion of angioplasty catheters results in a relatively large hole in the artery which may result in a false aneurysm. Until recently these were repaired surgically, but increasingly they are managed by utrasound-guided thrombin injection which thromboses the false aneurysm sac.

5. Intra-arterial injection. Barbiturates, sodium tetradecyl sulphate and substances used by drug abusers inadvertently injected into an artery may cause thrombosis and distal ischaemia. A dextran infusion should be started immediately the injury is recognized. Systemic anticoagulants, sympathetic block, prostaglandin infusion and thrombolysis should also be considered.

Venous injury

Damage to major veins frequently accompanies arterial injury. Data from military and civil conflicts have demonstrated enhanced limb salvage and function where concomitant venous injuries are repaired rather than ligated[c]. Venous injury is usually caused by penetrating trauma, although hepatic vein injuries result from blunt shearing forces. Injuries to major thoracic, abdominal and pelvic veins carry a high mortality. Repair of venous limb injuries should only be undertaken in haemodynamically stable patients[c]. Anticoagulation or the construction of a temporary arteriovenous fistula may be necessary to maintain patency.

Frostbite

Frostbite affects the distal extremities not adequately protected from cold. The fingers and toes redden at about 15°C because of a relative oxygen surplus. Below 10°C the skin becomes painful and hypersensitive. At 2.5°C the skin becomes anaesthetic and ice crystals form. Tissue destruction occurs between −4 and −10°C. Slowing of blood flow leads to thrombosis and gangrene. Pain and swelling occur as the tissues rewarm and blisters form as plasma seeps out of the damaged microcirculation. The use of properly insulated garments together with movement and, if necessary, enforced exercise will usually prevent frostbite. Rapid whole body rewarming in a whirlpool at 37–40°C is the preferred treatment. Dextran, heparin or thrombolysis may be required to treat thrombosis. The place of hyperbaric oxygen is unclear. Local amputations should be performed when demarcation lines have become evident.

Immersion foot

Explorers and vagrants are prone to this condition which occurs in those wearing constrictive footwear in cold wet environments. The extremities become numb causing the sensation of walking on cotton wool. Feelings of cramp and constriction occur and the skin becomes inflamed, then pale, blue and finally black. The footwear should be removed and the feet gently rewarmed, but kept dry. The feet should be elevated until the swelling has resolved. Smoking should be prohibited and sympathectomy may be of benefit. Local amputation may be necessary, but should be delayed until demarcation of dead tissue has occurred.

Further reading

Browse NL, Burnand KG, Irvine AT, Wilson NM. *Diseases of the Veins* (2nd Edn). London: Arnold, 1999; 711–729.

Burnand KG, Taylor PT, Murie JA, Callum K. The arteries. In: Burnand KG, Young AE (eds) *The New Aird's Companion in Surgical Studies* (2nd Edn). London: Churchill Livingstone, 1998; 223–306.

Chant ADB, Barros D'Sa AAB. *Emergency Vascular Practice*. London, Arnold, 1997.

Related topics of interest

VASOMOTOR AND VASCULITIC CONDITIONS

Nick Wilson

The vasospastic conditions affect the small arteries of the extremities causing local ischaemia, ulceration and sometimes gangrene. They may be primary or secondary. The arteritic conditions are characterized by an inflammatory infiltrate of the arterial wall (lymphocytes, plasma cells and histiocytes) causing luminal narrowing or obliteration. Different patterns of ischaemia result depending on the size and distribution of vessels affected. The vasculitic conditions systemic lupus erythematosis, scleroderma and polyarteritis nodosa are not widely encountered in surgical practice and are not discussed.

Vasomotor conditions

Raynaud's disease

Attacks of bilateral digital ischaemia occur comprising a blanching phase (white) caused by arterial spasm, a cyanotic phase (blue) and a reactive hyperaemia phase (red). Cold or emotion are the precipitating causes and the condition is generally most severe during winter months. Young women (12–45 years) are most commonly affected (M : F = 1 : 9). The hands are usually involved, but feet are affected in 40% of cases. In severe cases, trophic changes including ulceration and gangrene may occur. The ischaemia is caused by spasm of the digital arteries, but the cause is unknown.

The diagnosis is made by exclusion of factors implicated in (secondary) Raynauds phenomenon. Patients should be advised to avoid getting their hands and feet cold and to avoid smoking and betablockers. Calcium antagonists (nifedepine), serotonin receptor antagonists (ketanserin), alpha-adrenoceptor blockers (prazosin), methyldopa, prostaglandin analogues and transdermal glyceryl trinitrate have been tried with varying success[c]. Prostglandin infusions and plasmapheresis are sometimes required. Surgical cervical sympathectomy is effective initially, but symptoms generally recur within 6 months[c]. Occasionally, local debridement or amputation is required. The Raynaud's association is able to supply patients with useful practical information.

Raynauds phenomenon

This term is used where the features of Raynauds disease are secondary to another condition.

- Connective tissue disorders: scleroderma, systemic lupus erythematosis (SLE), dermatomyositis, polyarteritis nodosa, rheumatoid arthritis.
- Arterial disease: atherosclerosis, arteritis, thoracic outlet symdrome.
- Physical: neurovascular compression, vibration-induced white finger, frostbite.

- Haematological abnormalities: cryoglobulinaemia, cold agglutinins, poly-cythaemia, thrombocythaemia.
- Drugs: beta blockers, sympathomimetics, nicotine, ergot, oral contrceptive, cytotoxics.

Acrocyanosis

There is a generalized cyanosis of the hands (and sometimes feet) which is exacerbated by exposure to cold. Women are principally affected. The vasospasm affects smaller arteries and arterioles than are affected in Raynaud's disease and the stagnant hypoxia that occurs in the capillary bed causes the marked cyanosis. Trophic changes do not occur. Avoidance of cold is the main treatment, drugs and sympathectomy giving only marginal relief.

Livedo reticularis

Men and women of all ages are affected. Cyanotic mottling of the skin occurs, especially of the leg and foot. Spasm of the arterioles and dilatation of the capillaries and venules causes local stagnation of blood resulting in a reticular pattern. There is a perivascular infiltrate of inflammatory cells. Ulceration may occur which is painful and indolent. Some variants of livedo are associated with SLE, anticardiolipin antibody, PAN and syphilis.

Erythrocyanosis (Pernio)

This condition typically affects obese young women. The legs develop dusky erythematous patches just above the ankles, although the skin over triceps may also be affected. The erythematous patches may become indurated and nodular ('chilblains'). Ulceration may occur. Histologically these lesions show fat necrosis and scanty giant cells. Treatment is by cold avoidance and weight loss.

Erythromelalgia

Erythema and a burning pain of the extremities occur in this condition which may be primary or associated with gout, SLE, rheumatoid arthritis, PAN, vascular disease, diabetes mellitus, neurological conditions and vasoactive drugs. Symptoms are exacerbated by warmth and limb dependency and relieved by cooling and rest. The cause is unknown, but a platelet-mediated arteriolar inflammation has been proposed following the marked response to aspirin obtained in some cases.

Hyperhidrosis

Excessive sweating of the hands and sometimes feet and axillae occur in this condition. Sweating may be so severe as to make letter writing and other manual and social pastimes virtually impossible. Sweating can be reduced by regular application of aluminium hexachloride. Thoracoscopic sympathectomy provides effective and long-lasting relief of palmar sweating, but compensatory hyperhidrosis of the trunk sometimes occurs[c]. Lumbar sympathectomy is similarly effective for plantar sweatimg. Axillary sweating can be treated by repeated intradermal injection of Botulinum toxin or excision of axillary skin[c].

Vasculitic conditions

Buerger's disease

This condition is also known as thromboangiitis obliterans and typically affects male smokers between 20 and 45 years. The distal, medium-sized arteries of the upper and lower limbs are obliterated by a transmural round cell infiltration and intimal proliferation which lead to luminal thrombosis. Depositions of collagen are often found around the vessels. Patients present with chronic low-grade digital infection, indolent ulceration or gangrene. The principal trunk arteries are usually intact, but the foot pulses are frequently missing. The condition must be differentiated from diabetic arterial disease, atherosclerosis, or embolic ischaemia. Arteriography shows a typical distal distribution of occlusive disease with collateral vessel formation and intact proximal arteries.

Patients must be strongly advised to stop smoking to avoid progressive ischaemia and amputation. Sympathectomy is effective at relieving rest pain and healing ulceration. Arterial bypass is usually impractical and patients who do not stop smoking frequently require distal amputations. Prostaglandin infusions sometimes provide short-term relief.

Temporal arteritis

This condition usually affects men and women over 60 years and frequently starts with a fever and myalgia. A frontal headache develops and the region of the affected temporal artery becomes tender. The superficial temporal artery may be thickened and palpable. The retinal artery and its branches may become involved and if left untreated, occlusion resulting in blindness may develop.

The diagnosis is usually confirmed by temporal artery biopsy which shows round cell infiltration and scattered giant cells. Treatment with high-dose steroids to prevent blindness should not be delayed.

Takayasu's disease

This arteritis of unknown aetiology typically affects the large vessels of the aortic arch (type 1), but may affect the thoracic and abdominal aorta (type 2). Involvement of the arch, thoracic and abdominal aorta can occur (type 3); any of these patterns may be associated with involvement of the pulmonary circulation (type 4). Women of childbearing age are typically affected. Patients often report a preceding infection and symptoms include transient ischaemic attack, stroke, and arm claudication. Immunosuppression with steroids, cyclophosphamide or methotrexate is helpful during the acute inflammatory phase. Surgical bypass to revascularize the ischaemic territory yields good results and the disease process often resolves itself over several years.

Further reading

Belch JJF. Temperature-associated vascular disorders: Raynaud's phenomenon and erythromelalgia. In: Tooke JE, Lowe GDO (eds) *A Textbook of Vascular Medicine*. London: Arnold; 1996; 329–352.

Fiessinger J-N. Buerger's disease or thromboangiitis obliterans. In: Tooke JE, Lowe GDO (eds) *A Textbook of Vascular Medicine*. London: Arnold; 1996; 275–286.

Related topics of interest

Critical leg ischaemia (p. 100); Vascular imaging and investigation (p. 350).

WOUNDS: HEALING, CLOSURE AND SUTURES

Nick Lagattolla

Normal healing

Wounds fill with blood, the coagulation cascade is activated and platelets degranulate, releasing transforming growth factor-β and platelet-derived growth factor from their α-granules. These are potent regulators of subsequent events. The fibrin clot loosely seals the wound edges, and acts as a matrix for the adhesion of migrating cells. Local vessels leak protein-rich fluid into the matrix.

Vessels contract under the influence of locally produced histamine. Platelet plugs are formed to occlude open vessels, and the coagulation cascade is initiated. Within hours of wounding neutrophils enter the wound matrix. They phagocytose contaminating bacteria and debris for the first few days until circulating monocytes enter the wound matrix.

Migrating monocytes enter the wound under chemotaxis by growth factors. These become activated macrophages which also phagocytose debris, produce more growth factors, and recycle the provisional wound matrix, releasing degradation products that are also chemotactic.

Stimulated by transforming growth factor-β, fibroblasts migrate into the provisional wound matrix producing the collagen and glycoproteins that form the definitive extracellular matrix. Endothelial buds sprout from capillaries forming capillary loops. Basic fibroblast growth factor is a major stimulant of this process of angiogenesis. The new vessels are visible macroscopically as red, friable granulation tissue which bleeds easily on contact, and this is a hallmark of a healthy wound.

The matrix undergoes organization into mature fibrous tissue. Specialized myofibroblasts contract the wound. Continuous collagen deposition and degradation by matrix proteinases allow connective tissue deposition in bundles. This strengthens the wound, though only reaching about 80% of the strength of unwounded skin. This fibroplasia results in a scar. The underlying fibrous scar tissue eventually loses its vascularity and changes in colour from red to white.

During the last two phases of wound healing, or as the principal event if there is only a superficial wound, epithelialization of the exposed new dermis occurs from the wound edges. This is under control of local growth factors, such as basic fibroblast growth factor-7 (known as keratinocyte growth factor) and epidermal growth factor. Keratinocytes migrate through and attach to a wound matrix, as well as dividing and encroaching from the wound edge.

Wound classifiation

Wounds can be classified according to their degree of or potential for being contaminated. This is of practical importance, as it will have a bearing on the treatment and closure of a wound.

1. Infected wound. A frankly infected wound bears the hallmarks of acute inflammation (tumour, calor, dolor, and rubor, the signs of Celsus) and there may be cellulitis in the surrounding tissues. There may be pus in the wound, necrotic tissue in the wound base, and if the infecting organisms include anaerobes, there may be an offensive odour. Surgical wounds are said to be infected or 'dirty' if the operative field contains pus or faecal contamination.

2. *Contaminated wound.* A wound that has been exposed to a source of bacteria is a contaminated wound. These clearly have the potential to become infected. Surgical wounds are contaminated if surgery is being undertaken on an infected viscus, or there is a breach in the sterility of the operation, such as spillage of faeces during a colonic resection. Traumatic wounds are usually considered contaminated, a good example being stab wounds.

3. *Clean wounds.* These are wounds that are sterile from start to finish, and are usually only encountered in surgical procedures on non-infected sites. An example is an elective cholecystectomy. Clean wounds made at operation can be classified as 'clean-contaminated' if a source of bacteria is operated upon during the course of the procedure, but potential for contamination is limited by meticulous surgical technique.

Wound closure

If wounds are closed by means of sutures, then healing is said to occur by primary intention.

1. *Primary intention*

1. *Primary closure.* If a wound is closed at the time of surgery, or following trauma, this is called primary closure. This must only be performed on wounds that are clean and healthy. Unhealthy tissue at a wound edge, whether it is devitalized following trauma, or old scar tissue from previous surgery, must be debrided. Sutures in the scalp or face should be removed after 4 days. Those in the leg or back may need to be left for 2 weeks, and those closing a laparotomy wound should be left for 10 days. Most other sutures can be removed after 1 week.

2. *Delayed primary closure.* Sometimes a wound is contaminated and yet controlled closure by sutures is desirable. The wound may be treated with antiseptic dressing and sutures placed after 3 or 4 days, by which time the wound should be free of potentially infecting organisms. This is delayed primary closure.

2. *Secondary intention.* If wounds are left alone to heal, healing is said to occur by granulation or secondary intention. Grossly contaminated or infected wounds are debrided and left to granulate. Wounds following the excision of pilonidal disease in the natal cleft or excision of axillary or groin skin for hidradenitis or hyperhidrosis may heal satisfactorily in this way. The process is that of normal wound healing, but this takes longer than in wounds that have been closed. Prominent scars may result.

Inhibition of wound healing

Various medical conditions may inhibit normal wound healing. Treatment with steroids, diabetes mellitus, uraemia, carcinomatosis, jaundice, vitamin deficiency particularly vitamin C, trace metal deficiency, for example zinc, have all been incriminated. If a wound fails to heal, it becomes chronic. Some chronic wounds have a clear aetiology; for example, the majority of chronic leg ulcers are arterial, venous (or mixed) or are secondary to rheumatoid or other connective tissue, autoimmune, or vasculitic disease. Treatment should be aimed at dealing with the underlying cause. Venous ulcers require compression, arterial ulcers may need vascular reconstruction, and steroids may be required if there is a vasculitis.

Scarring

1. *Hypertrophic scarring.* Scarring always results in full-thickness wounds. The degree of scarring may vary, however. Some scars become hypertrophic, resulting in unsightly and disorganized scars within 3 months of wounding. These are common, and the changes do not extend beyond the confines of the scar. The best form of treatment is avoidance, and this may be achieved by recognition of the potential for scarring. Burn wounds frequently become hypertrophic, and elasticated compression stockings worn following treatment reduce the likelihood of this.

2. *Keloid scarring.* This results in a mass of fibrous tissue at the site of a wound (though some appear to arise spontaneously), which continues to expand and apparently involve skin beyond the confines of the original wound. These are more common in African people, and in the young. Keloids often recur after excision. The development of keloid scarring may be inhibited by radiotherapy or intralesional triamcinolone injection. Removal of an established keloid scar may require reconstructive surgery.

Sutures: size and application

As suture diameter increases, the number decreases: 2/0 is a wider and more robust suture than 6/0. Sutures larger than 2/0 are 0, 1 and 2. The largest sutures in common general surgical practice are usually 0 and 1, and these are often used to close the abdominal wall after a laparotomy. The finest sutures are 10/0 and 12/0, used in microscopic repairs of small vessels and nerves, or in ophthalmic surgery.

Suturing the skin of the face requires 6/0 for ideal cosmesis, 5/0 may be used on the neck, 4/0 is ideal for use on digits, and 3/0 on the leg or arm. Suturing the skin of the trunk requires 3/0 or 2/0.

2/0 is an ideal size for sutures placed in subcutaneous tissues and fascial layers. For intestinal anastomoses, 2/0 or 3/0 is generally used. Aortic anastomoses require 2/0 or 3/0, with smaller sutures for distal anastomoses.

Needles for arterial suturing are taper-pointed and round in cross-section to avoid tearing the vessel wall. Tougher tissues such as skin are sutured with cutting-edged needles (triangular cross-section).

Composition and properties

- *Permanent.* Synthetic sutures that are non-resorbable are polyamine (nylon) and polypropylene (prolene). Nylon and prolene sutures combine strength with slenderness. Nylon stretches more than prolene, and thus prolene is the ideal suture for vascular anastomoses, and nylon is often the choice for closing the musculature of the abdominal wall. For skin closure, prolene is best for sub-cuticular running sutures, and nylon is ideal for interrupted sutures. Both need to be removed. Stainless steel sutures are occasionally used.

- *Resorbable.* Resorbable synthetic sutures are polyglycolic acid (dexon), polyglactin (vycril) and polydioxanone (PDS). Dexon and vycril are resorbed after about 3 weeks, PDS in 3 months. These are used internally, for example, all three can be used to anastomose bowel, and vycril and dexon are often used as ligatures. PDS lasts long enough to be used to close the abdominal wall, with the additional advantage of being resorbed.

- *Natural sutures.* Silk is non-resorbable, catgut is totally resorbable and linen, which is often termed simply thread, is very slowly and only partially resorbable. Catgut is composed of sheep intestinal collagen. Plain catgut lasts only a matter of days unless treated to produce chromic catgut, which lasts for approximately 10 days. All these are used as ligatures. Catgut sutures are frequently used internally, including intestinal anastomoses. Silk sutures were once commonly used on the skin, though synthetic monofilament sutures are superior.

- *Suture structure.* Sutures are monofilament or braided. Nylon, prolene and PDS are monofilaments. For extra strength, nylon is also available in a braided form (ethibond), and prolene and nylon are available as looped sutures. Mono-filament synthetic sutures slip easily through tissues, and are thus ideal for skin closure. However, natural sutures have better handling qualities, and are usually preferred as ligatures. Silk is braided, and allows bacteria to flourish in its inter-stices, and thus minor degrees of infection are common when used on the skin.

- *Wound clips.* Staples may be used to close wounds. These are quick to apply, and this is their main advantage over sutures. Care must be taken to ensure that the wound edges are everted during the application of the clips.

- *Steristrips and tissue adhesives.* Steristrips are adhesive strips that can often be used to close clean, well opposed wound edges. They are ideal for use on the face and neck, and in children. They are often applied in addition to subcuticular sutures, to close any gaps that might be present. Tissue adhesives may be used to close skin wounds. This is methyl methacrylate (essentially superglue) and should be used with care.

Further reading

Eden CG. A classification of suture material and needles. *Surgery*, 1991; **91**: 2179.
Eden CG. Properties of individual suture materials. *Surgery*, 1991; **95**: 2271.
Forrester JC. Wounds and their management. In: Cuschieri A, Giles GR, Moosa AR (eds) *Essential Surgical Practice*. London: Wright, 1988.
Kingsnorth AN, Slavin J. Peptide growth factors and wound healing. *British Journal of Surgery*, 1991; **78**: 1286–1290.

Related topics of interest

Burns (p. 62); Skin cover (p. 300); The skin and subcutaneous tissues (p. 303).

INDEX

Murphy's sign, 130

Nasogastric tubes, 265, 266
Necrotizing fasciitis, 183
Nelson's syndrome, 109
Nephroblastoma, 283
Neuroblastoma, 15
Neurofibromatosis, 312
Neuroma, 305
Neuropathic bladder, 51
Nissen fundoplication, 148, 225
Non-specific abdominal pain, 231, 232
Nutrition, 233–236

Obturator hernia, 177
Oesophageal dilation, 148, 244
Oesophageal dysmotility, 242–245
Oesophageal intubation, 240
Oesophageal manometry, 147, 242
Oesophageal varices, 262, 263, 338–340
Oesophagitis, 146, 147, 338
Ogilvie's syndrome, 198
On-table colonic lavage, 196
Orchidopexy, 97, 335, 336
Organ support, 183–186
Organ transplantation, 246–247
Osteitis fibrosa cystica, 171
Oxygen free radicals, 229

Paget's disease, 58
Pain relief, 270–273
Pancreas divisum, 8, 84
Pancreatic trauma, 2
Pancreatic abscess, 11
Pancreatic cancer, 248–250
Pancreatic pseudocyst, 10, 86
Pancreatitis
    acute, 8–12
    chronic, 84–86
Paralytic ileus, 268
Paraphimosis, 251
Parathormone, 170
Parathyroid adenoma, 170
Parathyroid carcinoma, 172
Parathyroid hyperplasia, 170
Parathyroid localization, 171
Para-umbilica hernia, 177
Parkes–Weber syndrome, 353
Parotid calculi, 288
Patient-controlled analgesia, 265, 271

Peptic ulceration, 226, 255–258
Percutaneous endoscopic gastrostomy (PEG), 234
Percutaneous nephrolithotomy, 343
Percutaneous transhepatic cholangiography (PTC), 205
Percutaneous transluminal angioplasty, 188
Perforated peptic ulcer, 256
Periductal mastitis, 46
Perineal hernia, 178
Peritoneal lavage, 1, 43
Peritonitis, 4, 42, 256
Peutz–Jeghers syndrome, 142, 144
Peyronie's disease, 252
Phaeochromocytoma, 14
Pharyngeal pouch, 243
Phimosis, 251
Phlebography, 351
Pilondial disease, 259–261
Pleomorphic adenoma, 289
Pneumothorax, 81, 82
Poly-cancer sequence, 143
Polyps, 142–145
Portasystemic shunting, 263
Post-cricoid web, 237
Postoperative complications, 266–269
Pre-emptive analgesia, 272
Pre-operative assessment, 274–276
Pressure sores, 185
Priapism, 252
Pringle's manoeuvre, 2
Proctocolectomy, 333
Prostanoids, 102
Pseudo-obstruction, 198–200
Pugh's classification of portal hypertension, 262
Pulmonary collapse, 266
Pulmonary embolism, 3, 115, 267
Pyloric stenosis, 96, 129, 257
Pyogenic granuloma, 303

Radiolabelled red cell scanning, 208
Radiation enteritis, 195
Ramstedt's operation, 96
Raynaud's phenomenon, 359
Rectal bleeding, 207
Rectal shelf of Blummer, 203
Rejection, 247
Renal artery stenosis, 284
Renal calculi, 342–344
Renal perfusion, 184
Restorative proctocolectomy, 333